ABEL SYMPOSIA

Edited by the Norwegian Mathematical Society

More information about this series at http://www.springer.com/series/7462

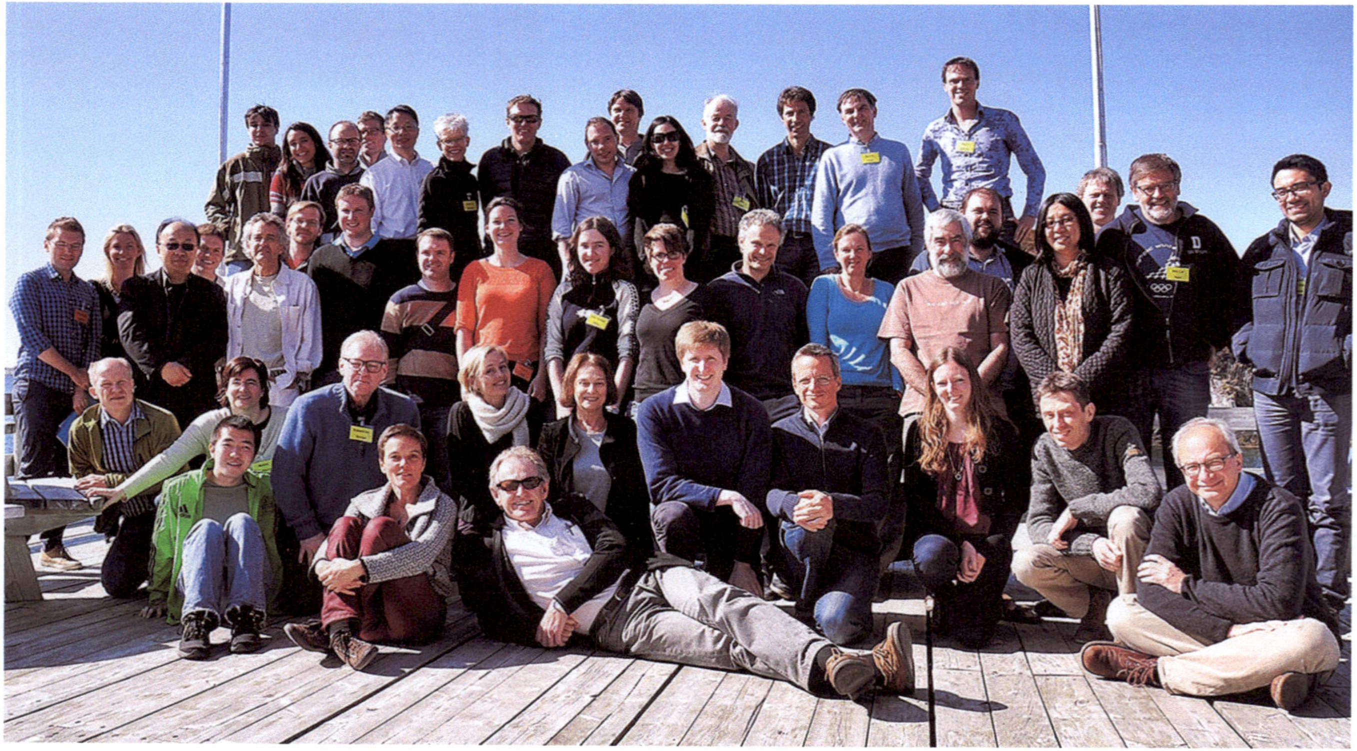

Participants at the 2014 Abel Symposium at Nyvågar.
Photo taken by Mette Langaas

Arnoldo Frigessi • Peter Bühlmann •
Ingrid K. Glad • Mette Langaas •
Sylvia Richardson • Marina Vannucci
Editors

Statistical Analysis for High-Dimensional Data

The Abel Symposium 2014

ABEL
PRISEN

Springer

Editors
Arnoldo Frigessi
Oslo Centre for Biostatistics and Epidemiology
University of Oslo
Oslo, Norway

Peter Bühlmann
Seminar for Statistics
ETH Zürich
Zürich, Switzerland

Ingrid K. Glad
Department of Mathematics
University of Oslo
Oslo, Norway

Mette Langaas
Department of Mathematical Sciences
Norwegian University of Science and Technology
Trondheim, Norway

Sylvia Richardson
MRC Biostatistics Unit
Cambridge Institute of Public Health
University of Cambridge
Cambridge, UK

Marina Vannucci
Department of Statistics
Rice University
Houston
Texas, USA

ISSN 2193-2808 ISSN 2197-8549 (electronic)
Abel Symposia
ISBN 978-3-319-27097-5 ISBN 978-3-319-27099-9 (eBook)
DOI 10.1007/978-3-319-27099-9

Library of Congress Control Number: 2016931284

Mathematics Subject Classification (2010): 62F15, 62H30, 62P10, 62F99, 62H99, 62J99

Springer Cham Heidelberg New York Dordrecht London

Printed on acid-free paper

Springer International Publishing AG Switzerland is part of Springer Science+Business Media (www.springer.com)

Foreword

The Norwegian government established the Abel Prize in mathematics in 2002, and the first prize was awarded in 2003. In addition to honoring the great Norwegian mathematician Niels Henrik Abel by awarding an international prize for outstanding scientific work in the field of mathematics, the prize shall contribute toward raising the status of mathematics in society and stimulate the interest for science among school children and students. In keeping with this objective, the Niels Henrik Abel Board has decided to finance annual Abel Symposia. The topic of the symposia may be selected broadly in the area of pure and applied mathematics. The symposia should be at the highest international level and serve to build bridges between the national and international research communities. The Norwegian Mathematical Society is responsible for the events. It has also been decided that the contributions from these symposia should be presented in a series of proceedings, and Springer Verlag has enthusiastically agreed to publish the series. The Niels Henrik Abel Board is confident that the series will be a valuable contribution to the mathematical literature.

Chair of the Niels Henrik Abel Board Helge Holden

Preface

The 11th Abel Symposium on "Statistical Analysis for High-Dimensional Data" was held at Nyvågar Rorbuhotell, near the village of Kabelvåg, in the Lofoten archipelago, Norway, from Monday, May 5, to Friday, May 9, 2014. This Abel Symposium Proceedings contains a selection of papers within this field.

There were 53 participants, and participation was by invitation only. The scientific committee for the symposium consisted of the editors of this Abel Symposium volume: Peter Bühlmann, Arnoldo Frigessi, Ingrid K. Glad, Mette Langaas, Sylvia Richardson, and Marina Vannucci.

The symposium had 23 invited talks:

Yoav Benjamini	Addressing statistical woes affecting replicability
Peter J. Bickel	Asymptotic analysis of unlabeled networks and an application
Leonardo Bottolo	Bayesian hierarchical mixture models
Tony Cai	Sparse PCA: optimal rates, adaptive estimation, and computational challenges
Mathias Drton	Ising model selection with Bayesian information criteria
Edward I. George	Spike-and-slab variable selection
Jelle J. Goeman	A global $\times$ global test for association between two high-dimensional data sets
Chris Hans	From a conditional Lindley's paradox to poly-hyper-g priors in Bayesian regression
Trevor Hastie	Sparse models and coordinate descent
Nicolai Meinshausen	Maximin effects for heterogeneous large-scale data
Xiao-Li Meng	The potential and perils of preprocessing: building new foundations
Sach Mukherjee	High-dimensional approaches for investigating disease heterogeneity

Peter Müller	A Bayesian feature allocation model for tumor heterogeneity
Susan A. Murphy	Micro-randomized trials and off-policy reinforcement learning
Judith Rousseau	Asymptotic properties of empirical Bayes procedures in parametric and nonparametric models
Richard Samworth	Independent component analysis via nonparametric maximum likelihood estimation
Terence P. Speed	Removing unwanted variation for prediction
Sara van de Geer	Confidence sets for the graphical lasso
Martin J. Wainwright	Randomized sketches of high-dimensional convex programs: practical schemes and sharp rates
Mike West	Dynamic sparsity modeling
Bin Yu	Relating developmental transcription factors (TFs) based on *Drosophila* embryonic gene expression images

The participants not giving invited talks had the possibility to give a short presentation of their work. Contributed talks were given by Magne T. Aldrin, Bettina Kulle Andreassen, Elja Arjas, Lamiae Azizi, Linn Cecilie Bergersen, Peter Bühlmann, Jan Christoph Ernest, Arnoldo Frigessi, Ingrid K. Glad, Clara-Cecilie Günther, Kari K. Halle, Kristoffer H. Hellton, Eric B. Laber, Mette Langaas, Tonje G. Lien, Ole Christian Lingjærde, Keli Liu, Edgar A. Muro Jimenez, Christian M. Page, Andrea I. Riebler, Sylvia Richardson, Daniel P. Simpson, Nicolas Städler, Øystein Sørensen, Marina Vannucci, Valeria Vitelli, Verena Zuber, and Erik W. van Zwet.

The full list of participants follows:

Aldrin, Magne T.	Norwegian Computing Center
Andreassen, Bettina Kulle	University of Oslo
Arjas, Elja	University of Oslo
Azizi, Lamiae	University of Cambridge
Benjamini, Yoav	Tel Aviv University
Bergersen, Linn Cecilie	University of Oslo
Bickel, Peter J.	University of California at Berkeley
Bottolo, Leonardo	Imperial College London
Bühlmann, Peter	ETH Zürich
Cai, Tony	University of Pennsylvania
Drton, Mathias	University of Washington
Ernest, Jan Christoph	ETH Zürich
Frigessi, Arnoldo	University of Oslo
George, Edward I.	University of Pennsylvania
Glad, Ingrid K.	University of Oslo

Goeman, Jelle J.	Leiden University
Günther, Clara-Cecilie	Norwegian Computing Center
Halle, Kari K.	Norwegian University of Science and Technology
Hans, Chris	Ohio State University
Hastie, Trevor	Stanford University
Hellton, Kristoffer H.	University of Oslo
Hjort, Nils Lid	University of Oslo
Laber, Eric B.	North Carolina State University
Langaas, Mette	Norwegian University of Science and Technology
Lien, Tonje G.	University of Oslo
Lingjærde, Ole Christian	University of Oslo
Liu, Keli	Harvard University
Low, Mark G.	University of Pennsylvania
Meinshausen, Nicolai	ETH Zürich
Meng, Xiao-Li	Harvard University
Mukherjee, Sach	Netherlands Cancer Institute
Müller, Peter	University of Texas, Austin
Muro Jimenez, Edgar A.	ETH Zürich
Murphy, Susan A.	University of Michigan
Page, Christian M.	University of Oslo
Richardson, Sylvia	University of Cambridge
Riebler, Andrea I.	Norwegian University of Science and Technology
Rousseau, Judith	Université Paris Dauphine
Rue, Håvard	Norwegian University of Science and Technology
Salomond, Jean-Bernard	Université Paris Dauphine
Samworth, Richard	University of Cambridge
Simpson, Daniel P.	Norwegian University of Science and Technology
Sørensen, Øystein	University of Oslo
Speed, Terence P.	Walter and Eliza Hall Institute of Medical Research
Städler, Nicolas	The Netherlands Cancer Institute
Thoresen, Magne	University of Oslo
van de Geer, Sara	ETH Zürich
van Zwet, Erik W.	Leiden University
Vannucci, Marina	Rice University
Vitelli, Valeria	University of Oslo
Wainwright, Martin J.	University of California, Berkeley
West, Mike	Duke University
Yu, Bin	University of California, Berkeley
Zuber, Verena	University of Oslo

We thank the Norwegian Mathematical Society for nominating our application and the Board for the Niels Henrik Abel Memorial Fund for deciding to support it.

We also thank the organizing committee, consisting of the participants Magne T. Aldrin, Bettina Kulle Andreassen, Arnoldo Frigessi, Ingrid K. Glad, Clara-Cecilie Günther, Kristoffer H. Hellton, Mette Langaas, Tonje G. Lien, Christian M. Page, Øystein Sørensen, and in addition Elisabeth H. Seland. Further; we would like to acknowledge the excellent service we received from the staff at the Nyvågar Rorbuhotell during our stay.

Special thanks goes to the contributors to this volume and to the participants and the speakers for their part toward the success of the symposium. Finally, we would like to thank Springer and Ruth Allewelt, for great patience and service during the preparation of this volume.

Oslo, Norway	Arnoldo Frigessi
Zürich, Switzerland	Peter Bühlmann
Oslo, Norway,	Ingrid K. Glad
Trondheim, Norway	Mette Langaas
Cambridge, UK	Sylvia Richardson
Houston, TX, USA	Marina Vannucci
October 2015	

Contents

Some Themes in High-Dimensional Statistics

Arnoldo Frigessi, Peter Bühlmann, Ingrid K. Glad, Sylvia Richardson, and Marina Vannucci

Abstract The symposium covered a broad spectrum of themes on High-Dimensional Statistics. We present here a short overview of some of the topics discussed at the symposium: high-dimensional inference in regression, high-dimensional causal inference, Bayesian variable selection for high-dimensional analysis, and integration of multiple high-dimensional data, but this categorization is not exhaustive. The contributions by some of the participants, appearing as chapters in the book, include both in-depth reviews and development of new statistical methodology, applications and theory.

A. Frigessi (✉)
Oslo Centre for Biostatistics and Epidemiology, University of Oslo, Oslo, Norway
e-mail: frigessi@medisin.uio.no

P. Bühlmann
Seminar for Statistics, ETH Zürich, Zürich, Switzerland
e-mail: buhlmann@stat.math.ethz.ch

I.K. Glad
Department of Mathematics, University of Oslo, Oslo, Norway
e-mail: glad@math.uio.no

S. Richardson
MRC Biostatistics Unit, Cambridge Institute of Public Health, University of Cambridge, Cambridge, UK
e-mail: sylvia.richardson@mrc-bsu.cam.ac.uk

M. Vannucci
Department of Statistics, Rice University, Houston, TX, USA
e-mail: marina@rice.edu

A. Frigessi et al. (eds.), *Statistical Analysis for High-Dimensional Data*,
Abel Symposia 11, DOI 10.1007/978-3-319-27099-9_1

1 High-Dimensional Inference in Regression

A large amount of research has focused over the last 15 years on estimating the parameters or selection of variables in high-dimensional models, mainly in linear and generalized linear models. See for example the monographs [16, 47] or the review article [31].

A core task of statistical frequentist inference, namely the construction of confidence intervals and hypothesis tests, is much less developed. Recently, a few methods for assigning p-values and obtaining confidence intervals for individual components β_j of a high-dimensional parameter β (e.g. the vector of regression parameters in a (generalized) linear model) have been suggested [14, 50, 63, 70, 73, 95, 107, 110, 111, 118]. Generalizations to constructing confidence intervals for low-dimensional individual parameters for undirected graphical model [49, 85], for instrumental variable models [4], or for very general models [71] have been considered as well. All of these methods use in one or another form a sparse estimator for the unknown high-dimensional parameter of interest. A prime example is the Lasso [105], but versions of it with other regularization penalties can be used as well [29, 117, 119–121]. The article in this volume by van de Geer and Stucky [108] presents some theory assuming "weak" sparsity only, in terms of the ℓ_r-norm ($0 < r < 1$) allowing for very many non-zero components. Whether the assumption of sparsity is always reasonable in real data applications remains an open question. Techniques based on random sample splitting provide some measures of stability [71, 73, 95], while other diagnostic tools would be very valuable but are largely missing so far.

Groups and Hierarchical Inference For a regression model, a major challenge for finding significant variables is due to high correlation between pairs of variables or near linear dependence among a few variables. Obviously, we cannot find a significant variable among two highly correlated variables: but we may find a significant group of variables. This basic insight leads to the concept of hierarchical inference [69]. Hierarchical clustering of the variables provides a tree with groups of correlated variables. First, on top of the hierarchy (top node of a tree), a large group of variables is tested for significance; if it turns out to be significant, one considers sequentially smaller groups (further down in the tree), unless they are not significant anymore (and thus, the method is data-driven when to stop going down the hierarchical tree). In the high-dimensional context, this procedure has been worked out [67, 70]. The article in the current volume by van de Geer and Stucky [108] considers the problem of significance testing for potentially large groups of variables in a high-dimensional linear model: the presented method is (nearly) optimal and the corresponding mathematical analysis is elegant. The method and result can be immediately used for hierarchical inference (besides its direct use for groups arising from interaction terms of factor variables or for basis expansions).

Selective Inference The theme of selective inference is to provide correct inferential statements when having chosen a (sub-)model from data. A general route to address this issue is given in [5]. Some recent work develops exact post-selection inference, where the full data is used both for selection and inference. It aims to avoid the potential inefficiency of single sample splitting, thereby restricting the focus to a class of selection procedures which are determined by affine inequalities, including the Lasso and least angle regression [33, 104]. Selective inference is a different approach to cope with the problem of high-dimensional inference: the inference is for a low-dimensional sub-model which has been selected based on high-dimensional data, in contrast to making inferential statements for the high-dimensional parameter vector in e.g. a regression model.

Software The R-package `glmnet` [34] provides a very efficient implementation of the Lasso [105] and Group Lasso [114] for generalized linear models. The R-package `glinternt` [61] is an efficient implementation for fitting linear pairwise-interaction models that satisfy a strong hierarchy. The R-package `hdi` [68] contains a collection of methods for constructing confidence intervals and p-values, including hierarchical inference, for generalized linear models: a description and overview is given in [26].

Heterogeneous Data Large-scale data often exhibit inhomogeneities, such as clusters of samples with different distributions. Approaches to deal with such potentially high-dimensional situations include high-dimensional mixed effects modeling [30, 89], high-dimensional mixture modeling [100], weighted Lasso [6] or issues with unwanted variation [36]. From a computational and statistical viewpoint, the concept of maximin estimation [72] or maximin aggregation ("magging") [15] leads to robust and meaningful estimation in presence of heterogeneous data. The article in this volume by Rothenhäusler et al. [88] develops the methodology and theory for constructing confidence intervals of the maximin effects parameters.

2 High-Dimensional Causal Inference

Causal inference is much more ambitious than estimating a measure of association from regression models [79, 99, cf.]. For a model with p covariables $X_1, \ldots, X_p$ and a response Y, the association or regression effect of a variable X_j on Y is given when conditioning on all other X_k's ($k \neq j$), i.e., when keeping these other variables X_k ($k \neq j$) fixed. In contrast, the total causal effect is a "dynamic" notion: it accounts for the fact that if we manipulate X_j, then other covariables X_k ($k \neq j$) change as well. In many scientific perturbation experiments, when manipulating a single variable, these other variables cannot be kept fixed and hence, we observe the total causal effect of a perturbation on a response of interest. For predicting such perturbation effects, before the scientific experiment, a causal inference framework is appropriate (and regression methods are fundamentally wrong).

In the high-dimensional setting, various estimation techniques have been proposed: for equivalence classes of graphs [17, 23, 25, 52, 56, 90, 99, 106], for estimating (bounds) of causal effects [28, 64], and recently for construction of confidence bounds [81].

Confirmatory inference of causal effects hinges on quite a few, non-testable assumptions, and thus, a great portion of caution should be exercised. Nevertheless, for prioritizing the next randomized experiments, high-dimensional causal inference methods seem to be useful [62, 65, 101].

Software The `R`-package `pcalg` [53] provides various methods for high-dimensional estimation of equivalence classes of graphs and for inferring bounds of causal effects.

3 Bayesian Variable Selection for High-Dimensional Analysis

Choosing a subset of variables among a set of potential explanatory variables or predictors $X_1, \ldots, X_p$ to include in a model of their relationship with a variable of interest or outcome Y is a widely studied statistical problem and a particular case of model selection, see [24, 37] and references therein. Subset selection is particularly challenging when the analysis set-up involves many more predictors than samples, the so-called large p small n paradigm, which arises commonly in the big data area, for example when modeling high-throughput genetic and genomics data. This has stimulated both methodological and algorithmic developments.

The Linear Setting The most familiar context for variable selection has been the linear model, and key properties of different Bayesian variable selection (BVS) formulations can be learned from the linear framework, [13]. The choice of prior distribution for the regression coefficients, and in particular their variance, is influential. Conjugate priors, and in particular the fully conjugate Zellner g-priors [116], have played an important role, in particular, but not solely, because of their computational advantage. They lead to feasible computations of marginal likelihoods, facilitating model comparison. Many variants of g-priors have been used, linked to different choices of mixing distributions for the variance of the regression coefficients. Properties of the resulting nonlinear Bayesian shrinkage have been thoroughly investigated by a number of authors. Depending on the choice of the hyper prior distribution for g, the shrinkage is akin to Bayesian ridge regression, Bayesian lasso or generalized versions, see discussion and additional references in [20, 40, 44, 78], and [41]. In a recent paper, Som et al. [97] show that some undesirable limiting behavior of g-priors can be avoided by using multiple values for g and introduce a block hyper-g prior. It is clear that careful thought needs to be given to the choice of prior distribution for the regression coefficients in relation to the characteristics of the context of application.

BVS Set-Up BVS formulations assume that only a subset of variables have non zero coefficients and consider a discrete model space. Priors are placed both on the model space and on the regression coefficients, with g-priors again commonly used for the regression coefficients but now restricted to the selected variables. Assuming that we stay within the linear model framework, it is common to include binary variable selection indicators γ_j indicating if variable X_j is included or not in a regression model for Y. A subset selection strategy endeavors to explore the 2^p possible models corresponding to $\boldsymbol{\gamma} = (\gamma_1, \ldots, \gamma_p)$:

$$\boldsymbol{Y} \mid \boldsymbol{\gamma} = \alpha 1_n + \boldsymbol{X}_\gamma \boldsymbol{\beta}_\gamma + \epsilon, \quad \epsilon \sim N\left(0, \sigma_\epsilon^2 I_n\right), \tag{1}$$

where $\boldsymbol{\beta}_\gamma$ is the vector of non-zero coefficients ($\gamma_j = 1$ if $\beta_j \neq 0$ and $\gamma_j = 0$ if $\beta_j = 0$), $\boldsymbol{X}_\gamma$ is the $n \times p_\gamma$ reduced design matrix with columns corresponding to $\gamma_j = 1$.

Besides the subset selection formulation (1), alternative BVS formulations rely on a mixture model approach with spike and slab priors for the regression coefficients as initially proposed by Mitchell and Beauchamp [74] and George and McCulloch [38]. As reviewed by O'Hara and Sillanpää [77], such implementations differ in the way the joint prior for (γ_j, β_j) is defined. Most of the implemented MCMC algorithms for spike and slab sample the regression coefficients via Gibbs sampling, limiting their use for large p. In the context of large p, spike and slab formulations were further discussed by Ishwaran and Rao [84] who propose a strategy of selective shrinkage of the resulting posterior mean under a re-scaled spike and slab prior. Spike and slab approaches were recently revisited by Ročková and George [87] who propose a novel computationally efficient EM algorithm to rapidly identify promising high posterior probability submodels.

Large p, Small n Framework Full Bayesian inference following (1) in the large p, small n framework requires specification of prior distributions for the regression coefficients $\boldsymbol{\beta}_\gamma$, the residual variance σ_ϵ^2 and the 2^p model space spanned by $\boldsymbol{\gamma}$. Both independent priors [46], Zellner g-prior structure with a hyper-prior on g [12] or priors translating assumptions on the total proportion of variance attributed to the variable selected [42], have been used, the latter calibrated in the context of genetic association studies. Nonlocal prior densities [51], which are identically zero when any component of β is zero, are an attractive alternative which exhibit good consistency properties. A beta binomial prior which expresses sparsity constraints on the model space is commonly used, following [91]. Associated to these different model formulations, a range of efficient stochastic algorithms aiming to explore the vast model space have been introduced, e.g. the Stochastic Shotgun (SSS) sampler [46], some inspired from population Monte Carlo, e.g. the Evolutionary Stochastic Search (ESS) sampler [9, 12]. Using parallel implementations, MCMC algorithms can be used for BVS in large model spaces such as arising in genetic association studies [11], but alternative variational inference has also been proposed in this context [19]. In order to make MCMC algorithms more feasible for large data sets, the use of adaptive schemes for variables selection has been investigated, [39, 86], but has yet to be used in practice.

Including Prior Information One of the important benefit of BVS is the ability to include prior information that could make the selection of X_j more or less likely. To integrate such information in a flexible manner, a natural extension of (1) is to specify a hierarchical model for $\{\gamma_j\}$ and use a probit or logit link for relating the underlying probabilities to external information. Stingo et al. [103] and Quintana and Conti [83] illustrate the benefit of such extensions in the genomics context. Further structural information might also be included in variable selection as proposed in [102] who generalize the model for $\{\gamma_j\}$ to a Markov Random Field in order to include prior information on network structure, see also the discussion of structured prior information in [87].

Bayesian variable selection approaches can be extended in many directions. Variable selection for multiple responses [11] can be extended to consider a large number q of responses, which are regressed in a parallel way on a large set of predictors, a common situation in integrative genomics, motivated by the so-called eQTL (expression Quantitative Trait Loci) studies. Coupling the BVS formulation with an additional hierarchical model on the $q \times p$ matrix of selection indicators allows information to be borrowed between the responses. This is particularly useful for finding key predictors controlling many responses, as shown in [10, 92] and [8].

Extensions to Other Linear Settings Spike and slab priors can be easily applied to other modeling settings where a response variable is expressed as a linear combinations of the predictors. For example, Bayesian variable selection for probit models is investigated by Sha et al. [93] and Kwon et al. [59], within the data augmentation framework of Albert and Chib [2]. Holmes and Held [48] consider logistic models—see also [82] for an alternative data augmentation scheme. Gustafson and Lefebvre [43] extend methodologies to settings where the subset of predictors associated with the propensity to belong to a class varies with the class. Sha et al. [94] consider accelerated failure time models for survival data. Extensions to the class of mixed models, that include random effects capturing heterogeneity among subjects, have also been investigated. One challenge in developing BVS approaches for random effects models is the constraint that the random effects covariance matrix needs to be semi-definite positive. Chen and Dunson [22] impose mixture priors on the regression coefficients of the fixed effects and achieve simultaneous selection of the random effects by imposing variable selection priors on the components in a special LDU decomposition of the random effects covariance. A similar approach, based on the Cholesky decomposition, is proposed by Frühwirth-Schnatter and Tüchler [35]. Cai and Dunson [18] extend the approach to generalized linear mixed models (GLMM) and [55] to logistic mixed effects models for binary data. Finally, [27, 66] and [113] consider Bayesian nonparametric approaches that use spiked Dirichlet process priors. Their approach models the unknown distribution of the regression coefficients via a Dirichlet process prior with a spike-and-slab centering distribution. This allows different predictors to have identical coefficients while performing variable selection. There, the clustering induced by the Dirichlet process is on the univariate regression coefficients and strength is borrowed across covariates. Kim et al. [54] consider similar priors in a random effects model to cluster the coefficient vectors across samples, whilst [58] consider semiparametric linear model modeling the unknown residual density through a DP mixture prior.

Regularization Priors With spike and slab priors, all possible models are embodied within a hierarchical formulation and variable selection is carried out model-wise. Regularization approaches, instead, use priors with just one continuous component and rely on the shrinkage properties of Bayesian estimators. Examples include the Laplace prior and the ridge prior. These have a singularity at the origin, which promotes an intensive shrinkage towards the zero prior mean. These priors can be expressed as scale mixture of normal distributions to facilitate computation. Popular regularized regression techniques include the Bayesian LASSO of Park and Casella [78] and Hans [44], which is equivalent to the MAP estimation under normal/exponential (Laplace) prior, and the normal scale mixture priors proposed by Griffin and Brown [40]. Casella et al.[21] propose the group LASSO and [60] the elastic net, which encourages a grouping effect in which strongly correlated predictors tend to come in or out of the model together. Lasso procedures tend to overshrink large coefficients due to the relatively light tails of the Laplace prior. To overcome the issue, [20] and [3] have proposed the horseshoe prior and generalized double Pareto shrinkage prior for linear models, respectively. The posterior summary measures (mean or median) are never zero with a positive probability, and zeroing the redundant variables out then needs to be carried out via thresholding the estimated coefficients. A solution is to augment the shrinkage priors to include a point mass at zero, see for example [45] and [112].

In summary, the Bayesian variable selection framework continues to be an active area of research both on the methodological and computational fronts. Its flexibility makes it particularly attractive for modern applications. In this brief summary, we have focused on the genomics context as one of the challenging areas where BVS is making important contributions.

4 Integration of Multiple High-Dimensional Data

Modern technologies allow measuring simultaneously many quantities of interest for a system under study: a patient in intensive care is monitored by medical equipment, which regularly collects several vital data; financial markets generate multiple time series, which describe the complex mechanisms that govern prices and rates. The joint analysis of such multiple data sets, each reflecting complementary views of the system under study, has the potential to generate power that cannot be obtained when analyzing each data component on its own. An important area, where multiple layers of data are collected, is genomics [57]. For example, in a tumor biopsy, molecular biologists measure the DNA copy number variation, mRNA gene expressions, miRNA, methylation profiles and so on, each generating between some hundreds and up to several hundred thousand measurements. In many cases, the analysis involves clinical outcomes (like survival, cancer stage, treatment response). For each data layer k, the dimension of the data is therefore n_k (number of individuals or samples where data type k has been collected) times p_k (number of variables measured), and often $p_k >> n_k$ for some of the layers k.

It is useful to distinguish three broad classes of integrative studies, which require different statistical approaches: (1) investigate the relationships between the different structures as captured by different layers of data; (2) cluster individuals into different groups, each representing different subpopulations (for example subtypes of a disease); (3) predict an outcome of the system under investigation (like survival or efficacy of therapy) for prospective new individuals, from the relevant set of data layers. This leads to supervised and non-supervised problems, with two main challenges: (1) matching the different scales of the different layers and modeling their dependence structures, and (2) selecting relevant factors and variables. We mention a few approaches which appear interesting.

In a Bayesian multiple testing set-up, Ferkingstad et al. [32] use two different data types, where the second data layer (say CNA) modulates the a priori probability that each test for a first data set is likely to be rejected, in a false discovery rate settings. The method has been used in the join analysis of Genome Wide Association Studies for various diseases [115].

Clustering methods use multiple data sources to partition the individuals (samples) into clusters which potentially represent different subtypes of the population. Shen et al. [96] suggest a way to perform the clustering of individuals using different metrics (or different noise structure) for each data type, but common latent labels among all data types, using an EM algorithm. In the likelihood, the various data types can be weighted differently. A different approach is to scale the various data layers to a common range by working with ranks [1]. We are currently testing a Bayesian Mallows model approach, to integrate various genomics type data [98].

In supervised situations, one can resort to penalized regression models, as discussed in the previous sections. After standardizing all data (scaling them into a fixed interval or transforming to mean zero and standard deviation one), one can run Lasso regression, thus treating the different molecular layers exchangeably [80]. Alternatively to plain Lasso with all covariates together in the model, and when the impact of a layer on the outcome can be assumed to be mediated through another layer (as in the case of copy number alteration (CNA), which should mostly have impact on survival of an individual via the expression of the corresponding genes), one can run weighted lasso [6, 7], where the lasso uses only one covariate type (the expression levels) while the other layer is used to modify the penalization, so that genes are penalized individually. For example, the penalization of a gene in the lasso depends on the correlation between the CNA and the outcome, so that genes with an important CNA will be penalized less in the expression analysis.

Networks are used to represent the interaction of variables in a certain system over time. The network itself is "summing up" these effects over time, and two variables are linked by an edge if they appear to interact in the process. The study of such networks has lead for example to important understanding of biological mechanisms. When there are multiple data sets, one can learn multiple networks and then compare and merge them [76] or estimate right away a consensus network [75]. Vaske and coworkers [109] exploit biological knowledge to build a hierarchical model of networks, in a genomic application.

References

1. Afsari, B., Braga-Neto, U.M., Geman, D.: Rank discriminants for predicting phenotypes from rna expression. Ann. Appl. Stat. **8**(3), 1469–1491 (2014)
2. Albert, J., Chib, S.: Bayesian analysis of binary and polychotomous response data. J. Am. Stat. Assoc. **88**, 669–679 (1993)
3. Armagan, A., Dunson, D., Lee, J.: Generalized double Pareto shrinkage. Stat. Sin. **23**, 119–143 (2013)
4. Belloni, A., Chen, D., Chernozhukov, V., Hansen, C.: Sparse models and methods for optimal instruments with an application to eminent domain. Econometrica **80**, 2369–2429 (2012)
5. Benjamini, Y., Yekutieli, D.: False discovery rate-adjusted multiple confidence intervals for selected parameters. J. Am. Stat. Assoc. **100**, 71–81 (2005)
6. Bergersen, L., Glad, I., Lyng, H.: Weighted lasso with data integration. Stat. Appl. Genet. Mol. Biol. **10**, 1–29 (2011)
7. van de Wiel, M.A., Verlaat, W., van Wieringen, W.N., Wilting, S.M.: Better prediction by use of co-data: adaptive group-regularized ridge regression. Preprint (2014). arXiv:1411.3496
8. Bhadra, A., Mallick, B.K.: Joint high-dimensional Bayesian variable and covariance selection with an application to eqtl analysis. Biometrics **69**(2), 447–457 (2013)
9. Bottolo, L., Chadeau-Hyam, M., Hastie, D.I., Langley, S.R., Petretto, E., Tiret, L., Tregouet, D., Richardson, S.: Ess++: a c++ objected-oriented algorithm for Bayesian stochastic search model exploration. Bioinformatics **27**, 587–588 (2011)
10. Bottolo, L., Petretto, E., Blankenberg, S., Cambien, F., Cook, S.A., Tiret, L., Richardson, S.: Bayesian detection of expression quantitative trait loci hot spots. Genetics **189**(4), 1449–1459 (2011)
11. Bottolo, L., Chadeau-Hyam, M., Hastie, D.I., Zeller, T., Liquet, B., Newcombe, P., Yengo, L., Wild, P.S., Schillert, A., Ziegler, A., Nielsen, S.F., Butterworth, A.S., Ho, W.K., Castagne, R., Munzel, T., Tregouet, D., Falchi, M., Cambien, F., Nordestgaard, B.G., Fumeron, F., Tybjaerg-Hansen, A., Froguel, P., Danesh, J., Petretto, E., Blankenberg, S., Tiret, L., Richardson, S.: Guess-ing polygenic associations with multiple phenotypes using a gpu-based evolutionary stochastic search algorithm. PLoS Genet. **9**, e1003657 (2013)
12. Bottolo, L., Richardson, S.: Evolutionary stochastic search. Bayesian Anal. **5**(3), 583–618 (2010)
13. Brown, P.J., Vannucci, M., Fearn, T., Multivariate Bayesian variable selection and prediction. J. R. Stat. Soc. Ser. B **60**, 627–641 (1998)
14. Bühlmann, P.: Statistical significance in high-dimensional linear models. Bernoulli **19**, 1212–1242 (2013)
15. Bühlmann, P., Meinshausen, N.: Magging: maximin aggregation for inhomogeneous large-scale data. Proc. IEEE (2015, preprint). arXiv:1409.2638
16. Bühlmann, P., van de Geer, S.: Statistics for High-Dimensional Data: Methods, Theory and Applications. Springer, New York (2011)
17. Bühlmann, P., Peters, J., Ernest, J.: CAM: causal additive models, high-dimensional order search and penalized regression. Ann. Stat. **42**, 2526–2556 (2014)
18. Cai, V., Dunson, D.B.: Bayesian covariance selection in generalized linear mixed models. Biometrics **62**, 446–457 (2006)
19. Carbonetto, P., Stephens, M.: Scalable variational inference for Bayesian variable selection in regression, and its accuracy in genetic association studies. Bayesian Anal. **7**(1), 73–108 (2012)
20. Carvalho, C.M., Polson, N.G., Scott, J.G.: The horseshoe estimator for sparse signals. Biometrika **97**, 465–480 (2010)
21. Casella, G., Ghosh, M., Gill, J., Kyung, M.: Penalized regression, standard errors, and Bayesian lassos. Bayesian Anal. **5**(2), 369–411 (2010)

22. Chen, Z., Dunson, D.B.: Random effects selection in linear mixed models. Biometrics **59**, 762–769 (2003)
23. Chickering, D.M.: Optimal structure identification with greedy search. J. Mach. Learn. Res. **3**, 507–554 (2002)
24. Clyde, M., George, E.I.: Model uncertainty. Stat. Sci. **19**, 81–94 (2004)
25. Colombo, D., Maathuis, M.H., Kalisch, M., Richardson, T.S.: Learning high-dimensional directed acyclic graphs with latent and selection variables. Ann. Stat. **40**, 294–321 (2012)
26. Dezeure, R., Bühlmann, P., Meier, L., Meinshausen, N.: High-dimensional inference: confidence intervals, p-values and R-software hdi. Stat. Sci. **30**, 533–558 (2015)
27. Dunson, D.B., Herring, A.H., Engel, S.M.: Bayesian selection and clustering of polymorphisms in functionally-related gene. J. Am. Stat. Assoc. **103**, 534–546 (2008)
28. Ernest, J., Bühlmann, P.: Marginal integration for nonparametric causal inference. Electro. J. Stat. Preprint (2014). arXiv:1405.1868
29. Fan, J., Li, R.: Variable selection via nonconcave penalized likelihood and its oracle properties. J. Am. Stat. Assoc. **96**, 1348–1360 (2001)
30. Fan, Y., Li, R.: Variable selection in linear mixed effects models. Ann. Stat. **40**, 2043–2068 (2012)
31. Fan, J., Lv, J.: A selective overview of variable selection in high dimensional feature space. Stat. Sin. **20**, 101–148 (2010)
32. Ferkingstad, E., Frigessi, A., Rue, H., Thorleifsson, G., Kong, A.: Unsupervised empirical Bayesian multiple testing with external covariates. Ann. Appl. Stat. **2**, 714–735 (2008)
33. Fithian, W., Sun, D., Taylor, J.: Optimal inference after model selection (2014, preprint). arXiv:1410.2597
34. Friedman, J., Hastie, T., Tibshirani, R.: Regularization paths for generalized linear models via coordinate descent. J. Stat. Softw. **33**, 1–22 (2010)
35. Frühwirth-Schnatter, S., Tüchler, R.: Bayesian parsimonious covariance estimation for hierarchical linear mixed models. Stat. Comput. **18**(1), 1–13 (2008)
36. Gagnon-Bartsch, J., Speed, T.: Using control genes to correct for unwanted variation in microarray data. Biostatistics **13**(3), 539–552 (2012)
37. George, E.I.: The variable selection problem. J. Am. Stat. Assoc. **95**(452), 1304–1308 (2000)
38. George, E.I., McCulloch, R.E.: Variable selection via Gibbs sampling. J. Am. Stat. Assoc. **85**, 398–409 (1993)
39. Griffin, J., Latuszynski, K.S., Steel, M.: Individual adaptation: an adaptive mcmc scheme for variable selection problems (2014, preprint). arXiv:1412.6760
40. Griffin, J.E., Brown, P.J.: Inference with normal-gamma prior distributions in regression problems. Bayesian Anal. **5**, 17–188 (2010)
41. Griffin, J.E., Brown, P.J.: Structuring shrinkage: some correlated priors for regression. Biometrika **99**(2), 481–487 (2012)
42. Guan, Y., Stephens, M.: Bayesian variable selection regression for genome-wide association studies and other large-scale problems. Ann. Appl. Stat. **5**, 1780–1815 (2011)
43. Gustafson, P., Lefebvre, G.: Bayesian multinomial regression with class-specific predictor selection. Ann. Appl. Stat. **2**, 1478–1502 (2008)
44. Hans, C.: Bayesian lasso regression. Biometrika **96**, 835–845 (2009)
45. Hans, C.: Model uncertainty and variable selection in Bayesian lasso regression. Stat. Comput. **20**, 221–229 (2010)
46. Hans, C., Dobra, A., West, M.: Shotgun stochastic search for "large p" regression. J. Am. Stat. Assoc. **102**(478), 507–516 (2007)
47. Hastie, T., Tibshirani, R., Friedman, J.: The Elements of Statistical Learning; Data Mining, Inference and Prediction, 2nd edn. Springer, New York (2009)
48. Holmes, C.C., Held, L.: Bayesian auxiliary variable models for binary and multinomial regression. Bayesian Anal. **1**, 145–168 (2006)
49. Jankova, J., van de Geer, S.: Confidence intervals for high-dimensional inverse covariance estimation. Electron. J. Stat. **9**, 1205–1229 (2015)

50. Javanmard, A., Montanari, A.: Confidence intervals and hypothesis testing for high-dimensional regression. J. Mach. Learn. Res. **15**, 2869–2909 (2014)
51. Johnson, V.E., Rossell, D.: Bayesian model selection in high-dimensional settings. J. Am. Stat. Assoc. **107**(498), 649–660 (2012)
52. Kalisch, M., Bühlmann, P.: Estimating high-dimensional directed acyclic graphs with the PC-algorithm. J. Mach. Learn. Res. **8**, 613–636 (2007)
53. Kalisch, M., Mächler, M., Colombo, D., Maathuis, M.H., Bühlmann, P.: Causal inference using graphical models with the R package pcalg. J. Stat. Softw. **47**, 1–26 (2012)
54. Kim, S., Dahl, D.B., Vannucci, M.: Spiked Dirichlet process prior for Bayesian multiple hypothesis testing in random effects models. Bayesian Anal. **4**, 707–732 (2010)
55. Kinney, S.K., Dunson, D.B.: Fixed and random effects selection in linear and logistic models. Biometrics **63**(3), 690–698 (2007)
56. Koller, D., Friedman, N.: Probabilistic Graphical Models: Principles and Techniques. MIT Press, Cambridge (2009)
57. Kristensen, V.N., Lingjærde, O.E., Russnes, H.G., Vollan, H.K.M., Frigessi, A., Børresen-Dale, A.-L.: Principles and methods of integrative genomic analyses in cancer. Nat. Rev. Cancer **14**(5), 299–313 (2014)
58. Kundu, S., Dunson, D.B.: Bayes variable selection in semiparametric linear models. J. Am. Stat. Assoc. **109**(505), 437–447 (2014)
59. Kwon, D.W., Tadesse, M.G., Sha, N., Pfeiffer, R.M., Vannucci, M.: Identifying biomarkers from mass spectrometry data with ordinal outcomes. Cancer Informat. **3**, 19–28 (2007)
60. Li, Q., Lin, v: The Bayesian elastic net. Bayesian Anal. **5**(1), 151–170 (2010)
61. Lim, M., Hastie, T.: *glinternet* (2013). R package version 0.9.0
62. Lippert, C., Listgarten, J., Liu, Y., Kadie, C.M., Davidson, R.I., Heckerman, D.: Fast linear mixed models for genome-wide association studies. Nat. Methods **8**, 833–835 (2011)
63. Lockhart, R., Taylor, J., Tibshirani, R.J., Tibshirani, R.: A significance test for the Lasso (with discussion). Ann. Stat. **42**, 413–468 (2014)
64. Maathuis, M.H., Kalisch, M., Bühlmann, P.: Estimating high-dimensional intervention effects from observational data. Ann. Stat. **37**, 3133–3164 (2009)
65. Maathuis, M.H., Colombo, D., Kalisch, M., Bühlmann, P.: Predicting causal effects in large-scale systems from observational data. Nat. Methods **7**, 247–248 (2010)
66. MacLehose, R.F., Dunson, D.B., Herring, A.H., Hoppin, J.A.: Bayesian methods for highly correlated exposure data. Epidemiology **18**(2), 199–207 (2007)
67. Mandozzi, J., Bühlmann, P.: Hierarchical testing in the high-dimensional setting with correlated variables. J. Am. Stat. Assoc. (2015, preprint). doi: 10.1080/01621459.2015.1007209. arXiv:1312.5556
68. Meier, L., Meinshausen, N., Dezeure, R.: hdi: High-Dimensional Inference (2014) R package version 0.1-2
69. Meinshausen, N.: Hierarchical testing of variable importance. Biometrika **95**, 265–278 (2008)
70. Meinshausen, N.: Group-bound: confidence intervals for groups of variables in sparse high-dimensional regression without assumptions on the design. J. R. Stat. Soc. Ser. B (2015, preprint). doi: 10.1111/rssb.12094. arXiv:1309.3489
71. Meinshausen, N., Bühlmann, P.: Stability selection (with discussion). J. R. Stat. Soc. Ser. B **72**, 417–473 (2010)
72. Meinshausen, N., Bühlmann, P.: Maximin effects in inhomogeneous large-scale data. Ann. Stat. **43**, 1801–1830 (2015)
73. Meinshausen, N., Meier, L., Bühlmann, P.: P-values for high-dimensional regression. J. Am. Stat. Assoc. **104**, 1671–1681 (2009)
74. Mitchell, T.J., Beauchamp, J.J.: Bayesian variable selection in linear regression. J. Am. Stat. Assoc. **83**, 1023–1036 (1988)
75. Oates, C.J., Mukherjee, S.: Joint structure learning of multiple non-exchangeable networks (2014, preprint). arXiv:1402.5640
76. Oates, C.J., Korkola, J., Gray, J.W., Mukherjee, S.: Joint estimation of multiple related biological networks. Ann. Appl. Stat. **8**(3), 1892–1919 (2014)

77. O'Hara, R.B., Sillanpää, M.J.: A review of Bayesian variable selection methods: What, how and which. Bayesian Anal. **4**(1), 85–118 (2009)
78. Park, T., Casella, G.: The Bayesian lasso. J. Am. Stat. Assoc. **103**(482), 681–686 (2008)
79. Pearl, J.: Causality: Models, Reasoning and Inference. Cambridge University Press, Cambridge (2000)
80. Peng, J., Zhu, J., Bergamaschi, A., Han, W., Noh, D.-Y., Pollack, J.R., Wang, P.: Regularized multivariate regression for identifying master predictors with application to integrative genomics study of breast cancer. Ann. Appl. Stat. **4**(1), 53 (2010)
81. Peters, J., Meinshausen, N., Bühlmann, P.: Causal inference using invariant prediction: identification and confidence intervals. J. R. Stat. Soc. Ser. B (2015, preprint). arXiv:1501.01332
82. Polson, N.G., Scott, J.G.: Data augmentation for non-Gaussian regression models using variance-mean mixtures. Biometrika **100**(2), 549–571 (2013)
83. Quintana, M.A., Conti, D.V.: Integrative variable selection via Bayesian model uncertainty. Stat. Med. **32**(28), 4938–4953 (2013)
84. Ishwaran, H., Rao, J.S.: Spike and slab variable selection: frequentist and Bayesian strategies. Ann. Stat. **33**, 730–773 (2005)
85. Ren, Z., Sun, T., Zhang, C.-H., Zhou, H.: Asymptotic normality and optimalities in estimation of large Gaussian graphical models. Ann. Stat. **43**, 991–1026 (2015)
86. Richardson, S., Bottolo, L., Rosenthal, J.S.: Bayesian models for sparse regression analysis of high dimensional data. Bayesian Stat. **9**, 539–569 (2010)
87. Ročková, V., George, E.I.: Emvs: the em approach to Bayesian variable selection. J. Am. Stat. Assoc. **109**(506), 828–846 (2014)
88. Rothenhäusler, D., Meinshausen, N., Bühlmann, P.: Confidence intervals for maximin effects in inhomogeneous large-scale data. In: The Abel Symposium 2014 Book, pp. 255–277 (2015)
89. Schelldorfer, J., Bühlmann, P., van de Geer, S.: Estimation for high-dimensional linear mixed-effects models using ℓ_1-penalization. Scand. J. Stat. **38**, 197–214 (2011)
90. Schmidt, M., Niculescu-Mizil, A., Murphy, K.: Learning graphical model structure using l1-regularization paths. In: Proceedings of the 22nd National Conference on Artificial Intelligence, vol. 2, pp. 1278–1283. AAAI Press/MIT Press, Menlo Park, Cambridge, MA (2007)
91. Scott, J.G., Berger, J.O.: Bayes and empirical-Bayes multiplicity adjustment in the variable-selection problem. Ann. Stat. **38**(5), 2587–2619 (2010)
92. Scott-Boyer, M.P., Imholte, G.C., Tayeb, A., Labbe, A., Deschepper, C.F., Gottardo, R.: An integrated hierarchical Bayesian model for multivariate eqtl mapping. Stat. Appl. Genet. Mol. Biol. **11**(4) (2012)
93. Sha, N., Vannucci, M., Tadesse, M.G., Brown, P.J., Dragoni, I., Davies, N., Roberts, T.C., Contestabile, A., Salmon, N., Buckley, C., Falciani, F.: Bayesian variable selection in multinomial probit models to identify molecular signatures of disease stage. Biometrics **60**(3), 812–819 (2004)
94. Sha, N., Tadesse, M.G., Vannucci, M.: Bayesian variable selection for the analysis of microarray data with censored outcome. Bioinformatics **22**(18), 2262–2268 (2006)
95. Shah, R.D., Samworth, R.J.: Variable selection with error control: another look at Stability Selection. J. R. Stat. Soc. Ser. B **75**, 55–80 (2013)
96. Shen, R., Olshen, A.B., Ladanyi, M.: Integrative clustering of multiple genomic data types using a joint latent variable model with application to breast and lung cancer subtype analysis. Bioinformatics **25**(22), 2906–2912 (2009)
97. Som, A., Hans, C.M., MacEachern, S.N.: Block hyper-g priors in Bayesian regression (2014, preprint). arXiv:1406.6419
98. Sørensen, Ø., Vitelli, V., Frigessi, A., Arjas, E.: Bayesian inference from rank data (2014, preprint). arXiv:1405.7945
99. Spirtes, P., Glymour, C., Scheines, R.: Causation, Prediction, and Search, 2nd edn. MIT Press, Cambridge (2000)

100. Städler, N., Bühlmann, P., van de Geer, S.: ℓ_1-penalization for mixture regression models (with discussion). Test **19**, 209–285 (2010)
101. Stekhoven, D.J., Moraes, I., Sveinbjörnsson, G., Hennig, L., Maathuis, M.H., Bühlmann, P.: Causal stability ranking. Bioinformatics **28**, 2819–2823 (2012)
102. Stingo, F.C., Vannucci, M.: Variable selection for discriminant analysis with Markov random field priors for the analysis of microarray data. Bioinformatics **27**(4), 495–501 (2011)
103. Stingo, F.C., Chen, Y.A., Tadesse, M.G., Vannucci, M.: Incorporating biological information in Bayesian models for the selection of pathways and genes. Ann. Appl. Stat. **5**(3), 1978–2002 (2011)
104. Taylor, J., Lockhart, R., Tibshirani, R.J., Tibshirani, R.: Exact post-selection inference for forward stepwise and least angle regression (2014, preprint). arXiv:1401.3889
105. Tibshirani, R.: Regression shrinkage and selection via the Lasso. J. R. Stat. Soc. Ser. B **58**, 267–288 (1996)
106. van de Geer, S., Bühlmann, P.: ℓ_0-penalized maximum likelihood for sparse directed acyclic graphs. Ann. Stat. **41**, 536–567 (2013)
107. van de Geer, S., Bühlmann, P., Ritov, Y., Dezeure, R.: On asymptotically optimal confidence regions and tests for high-dimensional models. Ann. Stat. **42**, 1166–1202 (2014)
108. van de Geer, S., Stucky, B.: χ^2-confidence sets in high-dimensional regression. In: The Abel Symposium 2014 Book, pp. 279–306 (2015)
109. Vaske, C.J., Benz, S.C., Sanborn, J.Z., Earl, D., Szeto, C., Zhu, J., Haussler, D., Stuart, J.M.: Inference of patient-specific pathway activities from multi-dimensional cancer genomics data using paradigm. Bioinformatics **26**(12), i237–i245 (2010)
110. Voorman, A., Shojaie, A., Witten, D.: Inference in high dimensions with the penalized score test (2014, preprint). arXiv:1401.2678
111. Wasserman, L., Roeder, K.: High dimensional variable selection. Ann. Stat. **37**, 2178–2201 (2009)
112. Xu, X., Ghosh, M.: Bayesian variable selection and estimation for group lasso. Bayesian Anal. (2015)
113. Yang, M.: Bayesian variable selection for logistic mixed model with nonparametric random effects. Comput. Stat. Data Anal. **56**, 2663–2674 (2012)
114. Yuan, M., Lin, Y.: Model selection and estimation in regression with grouped variables. J. R. Stat. Soc. Ser. B **68**, 49–67 (2006)
115. Zablocki, R.W., Schork, A.J., Levine, R.A., Andreassen, O.A., Dale, A.M., Thompson, W.K.: Covariate-modulated local false discovery rate for genome-wide association studies. Bioinformatics **30**(15), 2098–2104 (2014)
116. Zellner, A.: On assessing prior distributions and Bayesian regression analysis with g-prior distributions. In: Bayesian Inference and Decision Techniques: Essays in Honor of Bruno De Finetti, Elsevier Science Ltd. vol. 6, pp. 233–243, (1986)
117. Zhang, C.H.: Nearly unbiased variable selection under minimax concave penalty. Ann. Stat. **38**, 894–942 (2010)
118. Zhang, C.-H., Zhang, S.S.: Confidence intervals for low dimensional parameters in high dimensional linear models. J. R. Stat. Soc. Ser. B **76**, 217–242 (2014)
119. Zou, H.: The adaptive Lasso and its oracle properties. J. Am. Stat. Assoc. **101**, 1418–1429 (2006)
120. Zou, H., Hastie, T.: Regularization and variable selection via the elastic net. J. R. Stat. Soc. Ser. B **67**, 301–320 (2005)
121. Zou, H., Li, R.: One-step sparse estimates in nonconcave penalized likelihood models (with discussion). Ann. Stat. **36**, 1509–1566 (2008)

Laplace Approximation in High-Dimensional Bayesian Regression

Rina Foygel Barber, Mathias Drton, and Kean Ming Tan

Abstract We consider Bayesian variable selection in sparse high-dimensional regression, where the number of covariates p may be large relative to the sample size n, but at most a moderate number q of covariates are active. Specifically, we treat generalized linear models. For a single fixed sparse model with well-behaved prior distribution, classical theory proves that the Laplace approximation to the marginal likelihood of the model is accurate for sufficiently large sample size n. We extend this theory by giving results on uniform accuracy of the Laplace approximation across all models in a high-dimensional scenario in which p and q, and thus also the number of considered models, may increase with n. Moreover, we show how this connection between marginal likelihood and Laplace approximation can be used to obtain consistency results for Bayesian approaches to variable selection in high-dimensional regression.

1 Introduction

A key issue in Bayesian approaches to model selection is the evaluation of the marginal likelihood, also referred to as the evidence, of the different models that are being considered. While the marginal likelihood may sometimes be available in closed form when adopting suitable priors, most problems require approximation techniques. In particular, this is the case for variable selection in generalized linear models such as logistic regression, which are the models treated in this paper. Different strategies to approximate the marginal likelihood are reviewed in [7]. Our

R.F. Barber
Department of Statistics, The University of Chicago, Chicago, IL 60637, USA
e-mail: rina@uchicago.edu

M. Drton (✉)
Department of Statistics, University of Washington, Seattle, WA 98195, USA
e-mail: md5@uw.edu

K.M. Tan
Department of Biostatistics, University of Washington, Seattle, WA 98195, USA
e-mail: keanming@uw.edu

A. Frigessi et al. (eds.), *Statistical Analysis for High-Dimensional Data*,
Abel Symposia 11, DOI 10.1007/978-3-319-27099-9_2

focus will be on the accuracy of the Laplace approximation that is derived from large-sample theory; see also Sect. 4.4 in [3].

Suppose we have n independent observations of a response variable, and along with each observation we record a collection of p covariates. Write $L(\beta)$ for the likelihood function of a generalized linear model relating the response to the covariates, where $\beta \in \mathbb{R}^p$ is a vector of coefficients in the linear predictor [13]. Let $f(\beta)$ be a prior distribution, and let $\hat{\beta}$ be the maximum likelihood estimator (MLE) of the parameter vector $\beta \in \mathbb{R}^p$. Then the evidence for the (saturated) regression model is the integral

$$\int_{\mathbb{R}^p} L(\beta)f(\beta)\, d\beta,$$

and the Laplace approximation is the estimate

$$\text{Laplace} := L(\hat{\beta})f(\hat{\beta}) \left(\frac{(2\pi)^p}{\det H(\hat{\beta})} \right)^{1/2},$$

where H denotes the negative Hessian of the log-likelihood function $\log L$.

Classical asymptotic theory for large sample size n but fixed number of covariates p shows that the Laplace approximation is accurate with high probability [9]. With p fixed, this then clearly also holds for variable selection problems in which we would consider every one of the finitely many models given by the 2^p subsets of covariates. This accuracy result justifies the use of the Laplace approximation as a proxy for an actual model evidence. The Laplace approximation is also useful for proving frequentist consistency results about Bayesian methods for variable selection for a general class of priors. This is again discussed in [9]. The ideas go back to the work of Schwarz [15] on the Bayesian information criterion (BIC).

In this paper, we set out to give analogous results on the interplay between Laplace approximation, model evidence, and frequentist consistency in variable selection for regression problems that are high-dimensional, possibly with $p > n$, and sparse in that we consider only models that involve small subsets of covariates. We denote by q an upper bound on the number of active covariates. In variable selection for sparse high-dimensional regression, the number of considered models is very large, on the order of p^q. Our interest is then in bounds on the approximation error of Laplace approximations that, with high probability, hold uniformly across all sparse models. Theorem 1, our main result, gives such uniform bounds (see Sect. 3). A numerical experiment supporting the theorem is described in Sect. 4.

In Sect. 5, we show that when adopting suitable priors on the space of all sparse models, model selection by maximizing the product of model prior and Laplace approximation is consistent in an asymptotic scenario in which p and q may grow with n. As a corollary, we obtain a consistency result for fully Bayesian variable selection methods. We note that the class of priors on models we consider is the same as the one that has been used to define extensions of BIC that have consistency properties for high-dimensional variable selection problems; see, for example, [2, 4–6, 8, 11, 12, 17]. The prior has also been discussed in [16].

2 Setup and Assumptions

In this section, we provide the setup for the studied problem and the assumptions needed for our results.

2.1 Problem Setup

We treat generalized linear models for n independent observations of a response, which we denote as $Y_1, \dots, Y_n$. Each observation Y_i follows a distribution from a univariate exponential family with density

$$p_\theta(y) \propto \exp\{y \cdot \theta - \mathrm{b}(\theta)\}, \qquad \theta \in \mathbb{R},$$

where the density is defined with respect to some measure on $\mathbb{R}$. Let θ_i be the (natural) parameter indexing the distribution of Y_i, so $Y_i \sim p_{\theta_i}$. The vector $\boldsymbol{\theta} = (\theta_1, \dots, \theta_n)^T$ is then assumed to lie in the linear space spanned by the columns of a design matrix $X = (X_{ij}) \in \mathbb{R}^{n \times p}$, that is, $\boldsymbol{\theta} = X\beta$ for a parameter vector $\beta \in \mathbb{R}^p$. Our work is framed in a setting with a fixed/deterministic design X. In the language of McCullagh and Nelder [13], our basic setup uses a canonical link, no dispersion parameter and an exponential family whose natural parameter space is the entire real line. This covers, for instance, logistic and Poisson regression. However, extensions beyond this setting are possible; see, for instance, the related work of Luo and Chen [11] whose discussion of Bayesian information criteria encompasses other link functions.

We write X_i for the ith row of X, that is, the p-vector of covariate values for observation Y_i. The regression model for the responses then has log-likelihood, score, and negative Hessian functions

$$\log L(\beta) = \sum_{i=1}^{n} Y_i \cdot X_i^T\beta - \mathrm{b}(X_i^T\beta) \in \mathbb{R},$$

$$s(\beta) = \sum_{i=1}^{n} X_i \left(Y_i - \mathrm{b}'(X_i^T\beta)\right) \in \mathbb{R}^p,$$

$$H(\beta) = \sum_{i=1}^{n} X_i X_i^T \cdot \mathrm{b}''(X_i^T\beta) \in \mathbb{R}^{p \times p}.$$

The results in this paper rely on conditions on the Hessian H, and we note that, implicitly, these are actually conditions on the design X.

We are concerned with a sparsity scenario in which the joint distribution of $Y_1, \ldots, Y_n$ is determined by a true parameter vector $\beta_0 \in \mathbb{R}^p$ supported on a (small) set $J_0 \subset [p] := \{1, \ldots, p\}$, that is, $\beta_{0j} \neq 0$ if and only if $j \in J_0$. Our interest is in the recovery of the set J_0 when knowing an upper bound q on the cardinality of J_0, so $|J_0| \leq q$. To this end, we consider the different submodels given by the linear spaces spanned by subsets $J \subset [p]$ of the columns of the design matrix X, where $|J| \leq q$.

For notational convenience, we take $J \subset [p]$ to mean either an index set for the covariates or the resulting regression model. The regression coefficients in model J form a vector of length $|J|$. We index such vectors β by the elements of J, that is, $\beta = (\beta_j : j \in J)$, and we write $\mathbb{R}^J$ for the Euclidean space containing all these coefficient vectors. This way the coefficient and the covariate it belongs to always share a common index. In other words, the coefficient for the j-th coordinate of covariate vector X_i is denoted by β_j in any model J with $j \in J$. Furthermore, it is at times convenient to identify a vector $\beta \in \mathbb{R}^J$ with the vector in $\mathbb{R}^p$ that is obtained from β by filling in zeros outside of the set J. As this is clear from the context, we simply write β again when referring to this sparse vector in $\mathbb{R}^p$. Finally, $s_J(\beta)$ and $H_J(\beta)$ denote the subvector and submatrix of $s(\beta)$ and $H(\beta)$, respectively, obtained by extracting entries indexed by J. These depend only on the subvectors $X_{iJ} = (X_{ij})_{j \in J}$ of the covariate vectors X_i.

2.2 Assumptions

Recall that n is the sample size, p is the number of covariates, q is an upper bound on the model size, and β_0 is the true parameter vector. We assume the following conditions to hold for all considered regression problems:

(A1) The Euclidean norm of the true signal is bounded, that is, $\|\beta_0\|_2 \leq a_0$ for a fixed constant $a_0 \in (0, \infty)$.

(A2) There is a decreasing function $c_{\text{lower}} : [0, \infty) \to (0, \infty)$ and an increasing function $c_{\text{upper}} : [0, \infty) \to (0, \infty)$ such that for all $J \subset [p]$ with $|J| \leq 2q$ and all $\beta \in \mathbb{R}^J$, the Hessian of the negative log-likelihood function is bounded as

$$c_{\text{lower}}(\|\beta\|_2)\mathbf{I}_J \preceq \frac{1}{n} H_J(\beta) \preceq c_{\text{upper}}(\|\beta\|_2)\mathbf{I}_J.$$

(A3) There is a constant $c_{\text{change}} \in (0, \infty)$ such that for all $J \subset [p]$ with $|J| \leq 2q$ and all $\beta, \beta' \in \mathbb{R}^J$,

$$\frac{1}{n} \|H_J(\beta) - H_J(\beta')\|_{\text{sp}} \leq c_{\text{change}} \cdot \|\beta - \beta'\|_2,$$

where $\|\cdot\|_{\text{sp}}$ is the spectral norm of a matrix.

Assumption (A2) provides control of the spectrum of the Hessian of the negative log-likelihood function, and (A3) yields control of the change of the Hessian. Together, (A2) and (A3) imply that for all $\epsilon > 0$, there is a $\delta > 0$ such that

$$(1-\epsilon)H_J(\beta_0) \preceq H_J(\beta_J) \preceq (1+\epsilon)H_J(\beta_0), \tag{1}$$

for all $J \supseteq J_0$ with $|J| \leq 2q$ and $\beta_J \in \mathbb{R}^J$ with $\|\beta_J - \beta_0\|_2 \leq \delta$; see Proposition 2.1 in [2]. Note also that we consider sets J with cardinality $2q$ in (A2) and (A3) because it allows us to make arguments concerning false models, with $J \not\supseteq J_0$, using properties of the true model given by the union $J \cup J_0$.

Remark 1 When treating generalized linear models, some control of the size of the true coefficient vector β_0 is indeed needed. For instance, in logistic regression, if the norm of β_0 is too large, then the binary response will take on one of its values with overwhelming probability. Keeping with the setting of logistic regression, Barber and Drton [2] show how assumptions (A2) and (A3) hold with high probability in certain settings in which the covariates are generated as i.i.d. sample. Assumptions (A2) and (A3), or the implication from (1), also appear in earlier work on Bayesian information criteria for high-dimensional problems such as [6] or [11].

Let $\{f_J : J \subset [p], |J| \leq q\}$ be a family of probability density functions $f_J : \mathbb{R}^J \to [0,\infty)$ that we use to define prior distributions in all q-sparse models. We say that the family is log-Lipschitz with respect to radius $R > 0$ and has bounded log-density ratios if there exist two constants $F_1, F_2 \in [0,\infty)$ such that the following conditions hold for all $J \subset [p]$ with $|J| \leq q$:

(B1) The function $\log f_J$ is F_1-Lipschitz on the ball $B_R(0) = \{\beta \in \mathbb{R}^J : \|\beta\|_2 \leq R\}$, i.e., for all $\beta', \beta \in B_R(0)$, we have

$$|\log f_J(\beta') - \log f_J(\beta)| \leq F_1 \|\beta' - \beta\|_2.$$

(B2) For all $\beta \in \mathbb{R}^J$,

$$\log f_J(\beta) - \log f_J(0) \leq F_2.$$

Example 1 If we take f_J to be the density of a $|J|$-fold product of a centered normal distribution with variance σ^2, then (B1) holds with $F_1 = R/\sigma^2$ and $F_2 = 0$.

3 Laplace Approximation

This section provides our main result. For a high-dimensional regression problem, we show that a Laplace approximation to the marginal likelihood of each sparse model,

$$\text{Evidence}(J) := \int_{\mathbb{R}^J} L(\beta) f_J(\beta) d\beta \ ,$$

leads to an approximation error that, with high probability, is bounded uniformly across all models. To state our result, we adopt the notation

$$a = b(1 \pm c) \quad :\Longleftrightarrow \quad a \in [b(1-c), b(1+c)].$$

Theorem 1 *Suppose the conditions from (A1)–(A3) hold. Then, there are constants* $\nu, c_{\text{sample}}, a_{\text{MLE}} \in (0, \infty)$ *depending only on* $(a_0, c_{\text{lower}}, c_{\text{upper}}, c_{\text{change}})$ *such that if*

$$n \geq c_{\text{sample}} \cdot q^3 \max\{\log(p), \log^3(n)\},$$

then with probability at least $1 - p^{-\nu}$ *the following two statements are true for all sparse models* $J \subset [p]$, $|J| \leq q$*:*

(i) The MLE $\hat{\beta}_J$ *satisfies* $\|\hat{\beta}_J\|_2 \leq a_{\text{MLE}}$.
(ii) If additionally the family of prior densities $\{f_J : J \subset [p], |J| \leq q\}$ *satisfies the Lipschitz condition from (B1) for radius* $R \geq a_{\text{MLE}} + 1$*, and has log-density ratios bounded as in (B2), then there is a constant* $c_{\text{Laplace}} \in (0, \infty)$ *depending only on* $(a_0, c_{\text{lower}}, c_{\text{upper}}, c_{\text{change}}, F_1, F_2)$ *such that*

$$\text{Evidence}(J) = L(\hat{\beta}_J) f_J(\hat{\beta}_J) \cdot \left(\frac{(2\pi)^{|J|}}{\det H_J(\hat{\beta}_J)} \right)^{1/2} \cdot \left(1 \pm c_{\text{Laplace}} \sqrt{\frac{|J|^3 \log^3(n)}{n}} \right).$$

Proof

(i) *Bounded MLEs.* It follows from Sect. B.2 in [2][1] that, with the claimed probability, the norms $\|\hat{\beta}_J\|_2$ for true models J (i.e., $J \supseteq J_0$ and $|J| \leq 2q$) are bounded by a constant. The result makes reference to an event for which all the claims we make subsequently are true. The bound on the norm of an MLE of a true model was obtained by comparing the maximal likelihood to the likelihood at the true parameter β_0. As we show now, for false sparse models, we may argue similarly but comparing to the likelihood at 0.

Recall that a_0 is the bound on the norm of β_0 assumed in (A1) and that the functions c_{lower} and c_{upper} in (A2) are decreasing and increasing in the norm of β_0, respectively. Throughout this part, we use the abbreviations

$$c_{\text{lower}} := c_{\text{lower}}(a_0), \qquad c_{\text{upper}} := c_{\text{upper}}(a_0).$$

[1]In the proof of this theorem, we cite several results from Sect. B.2 and Lemma B.1 in [2]. Although that paper treats the specific case of logistic regression, by examining the proofs of their results that we cite here, we can see that they hold more broadly for the general GLM case as long as we assume that the Hessian conditions hold, i.e., Conditions (A1)–(A3), and therefore we may use these results for the setting considered here.

First, we lower-bound the likelihood at 0 via a Taylor-expansion using the true model J_0. For some $t \in [0, 1]$, we have that

$$\log L(0) - \log L(\beta_0) = -\beta_0^T s_{J_0}(\beta_0) - \frac{1}{2}\beta_0^T H_{J_0}(t\beta_0)\beta_0 \geq -\beta_0^T s_{J_0}(\beta_0) - \frac{1}{2} n\, a_0^2 c_{\text{upper}},$$

where we have applied (A2). Lemma B.1 in [2] yields that

$$|\beta_0^T s_{J_0}(\beta_0)| \leq \|H_{J_0}(\beta_0)^{-\frac{1}{2}} s_{J_0}(\beta_0)\|_2 \|H_{J_0}(\beta_0)^{\frac{1}{2}} \beta_0\|_2 \leq \tau_0 a_0 \sqrt{n c_{\text{upper}}},$$

where τ_0^2 can be bounded by a constant multiple of $q \log(p)$. By our sample size assumption (i.e., the existence of the constant c_{sample}), we thus have that

$$\log L(0) - \log L(\beta_0) \geq -n \cdot c_1 \tag{2}$$

for some constant $c_1 \in (0, \infty)$.

Second, we may consider the true model $J \cup J_0$ instead of J and apply (B.17) in [2] to obtain the bound

$$\log L(\hat{\beta}_J) - \log L(\beta_0) \leq \|\hat{\beta}_J - \beta_0\|_2 \cdot \left(\sqrt{n c_{\text{upper}}} \cdot \tau_{J \setminus J_0} - \frac{n c_{\text{lower}}}{4} \min \left\{ \|\hat{\beta}_J - \beta_0\|_2, \frac{c_{\text{lower}}}{2 c_{\text{change}}} \right\} \right), \tag{3}$$

where $\tau_{J \setminus J_0}^2$ can be bounded by a constant multiple of $q \log(p)$. Choosing our sample size constant c_{sample} large enough, we may deduce from (3) that there is a constant $c_2 \in (0, \infty)$ such that

$$\log L(\hat{\beta}_J) - \log L(\beta_0) \leq -n \|\hat{\beta}_J - \beta_0\|_2 c_2$$

whenever $\|\hat{\beta}_J - \beta_0\|_2 > c_{\text{lower}}/(2c_{\text{change}})$. Using the fact that $\log L(0) \leq \log(\hat{\beta}_J)$ for any model J, we may deduce from (3) that there is a constant $c_2 \in (0, \infty)$ such that

$$\log L(0) - \log L(\beta_0) \leq -n \|\hat{\beta}_J - \beta_0\|_2 c_2$$

whenever $\|\hat{\beta}_J - \beta_0\|_2 > c_{\text{lower}}/(2c_{\text{change}})$. Together with (2), this implies that $\|\hat{\beta}_J - \beta_0\|_2$ is bounded by a constant c_3. Having assumed (A1), we may conclude that the norm of $\hat{\beta}_J$ is bounded by $a_0 + c_3$.

(ii) *Laplace approximation.* Fix $J \subset [p]$ with $|J| \leq q$. In order to analyze the evidence of model J, we split the integration domain $\mathbb{R}^J$ into two regions,

namely, a neighborhood $\mathcal{N}$ of the MLE $\hat{\beta}_J$ and the complement $\mathbb{R}^J \setminus \mathcal{N}$. More precisely, we choose the neighborhood of the MLE as

$$\mathcal{N} := \left\{ \beta \in \mathbb{R}^J \ : \ \|H_J(\hat{\beta}_J)^{1/2}(\beta - \hat{\beta}_J)\|_2 \leq \sqrt{5|J|\log(n)} \right\}.$$

Then the marginal likelihood, Evidence(J), is the sum of the two integrals

$$\mathcal{I}_1 = \int_{\mathcal{N}} L(\beta) f_J(\beta) d\beta,$$

$$\mathcal{I}_2 = \int_{\mathbb{R}^J \setminus \mathcal{N}} L(\beta) f_J(\beta) d\beta.$$

We will estimate $\mathcal{I}_1$ via a quadratic approximation to the log-likelihood function. Outside of the region $\mathcal{N}$, the quadratic approximation may no longer be accurate but due to concavity of the log-likelihood function, the integrand can be bounded by $e^{-c\|\beta_J - \hat{\beta}_J\|_2}$ for an appropriately chosen constant c, which allows us to show that $\mathcal{I}_2$ is negligible when n is sufficiently large.

We now approximate $\mathcal{I}_1$ and $\mathcal{I}_2$ separately. Throughout this part we assume that we have a bound a_{MLE} on the norms of the MLEs $\hat{\beta}_J$ in sparse models J with $|J| \leq q$. For notational convenience, we now let

$$c_{\text{lower}} := c_{\text{lower}}(a_{\text{MLE}}), \qquad c_{\text{upper}} := c_{\text{upper}}(a_{\text{MLE}}).$$

(ii-a) Approximation of integral $\mathcal{I}_1$. By a Taylor-expansion, for any $\beta \in \mathbb{R}^J$ there is a $t \in [0, 1]$ such that

$$\log L(\beta) = \log L(\hat{\beta}_J) - \frac{1}{2}(\beta - \hat{\beta}_J)^T H_J \left(\hat{\beta}_J + t(\beta - \hat{\beta}_J) \right) (\beta - \hat{\beta}_J).$$

By (A3) and using that $|t| \leq 1$,

$$\left\| H_J \left(\hat{\beta}_J + t(\beta - \hat{\beta}_J) \right) - H_J(\hat{\beta}_J) \right\|_{\text{sp}} \leq n \cdot c_{\text{change}} \, \|\beta - \hat{\beta}_J\|_2.$$

Hence,

$$\log L(\beta) = \log L(\hat{\beta}_J) - \frac{1}{2}(\beta - \hat{\beta}_J)^T H_J(\hat{\beta}_J)(\beta - \hat{\beta}_J) \pm \frac{1}{2}\|\beta - \hat{\beta}_J\|_2^3 \cdot n \, c_{\text{change}}. \tag{4}$$

Next, observe that (A2) implies that

$$H_J(\hat{\beta}_J)^{-1/2} \preceq \sqrt{\frac{1}{n c_{\text{lower}}}} \cdot \mathbf{I}_J.$$

We deduce that for any vector $\beta \in \mathscr{N}$,

$$\|\beta - \hat{\beta}_J\|_2 \;\leq\; \sqrt{5|J|\log(n)}\,\|H_J(\hat{\beta}_J)^{-1/2}\|_{\mathrm{sp}} \;\leq\; \sqrt{\frac{5|J|\log(n)}{nc_{\mathrm{lower}}}}. \tag{5}$$

This gives

$$\log L(\beta) = \log L(\hat{\beta}_J) - \frac{1}{2}(\beta - \hat{\beta}_J)^T H_J(\hat{\beta}_J)(\beta - \hat{\beta}_J) \pm \sqrt{\frac{|J|^3\log^3(n)}{n}} \cdot \sqrt{\frac{125c_{\mathrm{change}}^2}{4c_{\mathrm{lower}}^3}}. \tag{6}$$

Choosing the constant c_{sample} large enough, we can ensure that the upper bound in (5) is no larger than 1. In other words, $\|\beta - \hat{\beta}_J\|_2 \leq 1$ for all points $\beta \in \mathscr{N}$. By our assumption that $\|\hat{\beta}_J\|_2 \leq a_{\mathrm{MLE}}$, the set $\mathscr{N}$ is thus contained in the ball

$$\mathscr{B} = \left\{\beta \in \mathbb{R}^J : \|\beta\|_2 \leq a_{\mathrm{MLE}} + 1\right\}.$$

Since, by (B1), the logarithm of the prior density is F_1-Lipschitz on $\mathscr{B}$, it follows from (5) that

$$\log f_J(\beta) \;=\; \log f_J(\hat{\beta}_J) \pm F_1\|\beta - \hat{\beta}_J\|_2 \;=\; \log f_J(\hat{\beta}_J) \pm F_1\sqrt{\frac{5|J|\log(n)}{nc_{\mathrm{lower}}}}. \tag{7}$$

Plugging (6) and (7) into $\mathscr{I}_1$, and writing $a = b \cdot \exp\{\pm c\}$ as a shorthand for $a \in [b \cdot e^{-c}, b \cdot e^{c}]$, we find that

$$\mathscr{I}_1 = L(\hat{\beta}_J)f_J(\hat{\beta}_J)\exp\left\{\pm\sqrt{\frac{|J|^3\log^3(n)}{n}} \cdot \left(\sqrt{\frac{5F_1^2}{nc_{\mathrm{lower}}}} + \sqrt{\frac{125c_{\mathrm{change}}^2}{4c_{\mathrm{lower}}^3}}\right)\right\} \times \int_{\mathscr{N}} \exp\left\{-\frac{1}{2}(\beta - \hat{\beta}_J)^T H_J(\hat{\beta}_J)(\beta - \hat{\beta}_J)\right\} d\beta. \tag{8}$$

In the last integral, change variables to $\xi = H_J(\hat{\beta}_J)^{1/2}(\beta - \hat{\beta}_J)$ to see that

$$\int_{\mathscr{N}} \exp\left\{-\frac{1}{2}(\beta - \hat{\beta}_J)^T H_J(\hat{\beta}_J)(\beta - \hat{\beta}_J)\right\} d\beta = \left(\det H_J(\hat{\beta}_J)\right)^{-1/2} \cdot \int_{\|\xi\|_2 \leq \sqrt{5|J|\log(n)}} \exp\left\{-\frac{1}{2}\|\xi\|_2^2\right\} d\xi$$

$$= \left(\frac{(2\pi)^{|J|}}{\det H_J(\hat{\beta}_J)} \right)^{1/2} \cdot \Pr\left\{ \chi^2_{|J|} \le 5|J|\log(n) \right\}$$

$$= \left(\frac{(2\pi)^{|J|}}{\det H_J(\hat{\beta}_J)} \right)^{1/2} \cdot \exp\{\pm 1/\sqrt{n}\}, \tag{9}$$

where we use a tail bound for the χ^2-distribution stated in Lemma 1. We now substitute (9) into (8), and simplify the result using that $e^{-x} \ge 1-2x$ and $e^x \le 1+2x$ for all $0 \le x \le 1$. We find that

$$\mathscr{I}_1 = L(\hat{\beta}_J) f_J(\hat{\beta}_J) \left(\frac{(2\pi)^{|J|}}{\det H_J(\hat{\beta}_J)} \right)^{1/2} \times \left(1 \pm 2 \left(1 + \sqrt{\frac{125 c^2_{\text{change}}}{4 c^3_{\text{lower}}}} + \sqrt{\frac{5F_1^2}{c_{\text{lower}}}} \right) \sqrt{\frac{|J|^3 \log^3(n)}{n}} \right) \tag{10}$$

when the constant c_{sample} is chosen large enough.

(ii-b) Approximation of integral $\mathscr{I}_2$. Let β be a point on the boundary of $\mathscr{N}$. It then holds that

$$(\beta - \hat{\beta}_J)^T H_J(\hat{\beta}_J)(\beta - \hat{\beta}_J) = \sqrt{5|J|\log(n)} \cdot \|H_J(\hat{\beta}_J)^{1/2}(\beta - \hat{\beta}_J)\|_2.$$

We may deduce from (6) that

$$\log L(\beta) \le \log L(\hat{\beta}_J) - \frac{\sqrt{5|J|\log(n)}}{2} \|H_J(\hat{\beta}_J)^{1/2}(\beta - \hat{\beta}_J)\|_2 + \sqrt{\frac{|J|^3 \log^3(n)}{n}} \cdot \sqrt{\frac{125 c^2_{\text{change}}}{4 c^3_{\text{lower}}}}$$

$$\le \log L(\hat{\beta}_J) - \|H_J(\hat{\beta}_J)^{1/2}(\beta - \hat{\beta}_J)\|_2 \cdot \sqrt{|J|\log(n)},$$

for $|J|^3 \log^3(n)/n$ sufficiently small, which can be ensured by choosing c_{sample} large enough. The concavity of the log-likelihood function now implies that for all $\beta \notin \mathscr{N}$ we have

$$\log L(\beta) \le \log L(\hat{\beta}_J) - \|H_J(\hat{\beta}_J)^{1/2}(\beta - \hat{\beta}_J)\|_2 \cdot \sqrt{|J|\log(n)}. \tag{11}$$

Moreover, using first assumption (B2) and then assumption (B1), we have that

$$\log f_J(\beta) \;\le\; \log f_J(0) + F_2 \;\le\; \log f_J(\hat{\beta}_J) + F_1\|\hat{\beta}_J\|_2 + F_2.$$

Since $\|\hat{\beta}_J\|_2 \le a_{\mathrm{MLE}}$, it thus holds that

$$\log f_J(\beta) \;\le\; \log f_J(\hat{\beta}_J) + F_1 a_{\mathrm{MLE}} + F_2. \tag{12}$$

Combining the bounds from (11) and (12), the integral can be bounded as

$$\mathcal{I}_2 \;\le\; L(\hat{\beta}_J) f_J(\hat{\beta}_J) e^{F_1 a_{\mathrm{MLE}} + F_2} \times \int_{\mathbb{R}^J \setminus \mathcal{N}} \exp\left\{ -\|H_J(\hat{\beta}_J)^{1/2}(\beta - \hat{\beta}_J)\|_2 \cdot \sqrt{|J|\log(n)} \right\} d\beta. \tag{13}$$

Changing variables to $\xi = H_J(\hat{\beta}_J)^{1/2}(\beta - \hat{\beta}_J)$ and applying Lemma 2, we may bound the integral in (13) as

$$\begin{aligned}
&\int_{\mathbb{R}^J \setminus \mathcal{N}} \exp\left\{ -\|H_J(\hat{\beta}_J)^{1/2}(\beta - \hat{\beta}_J)\|_2 \cdot \sqrt{|J|\log(n)} \right\} d\beta \\
&\le \left(\det H_J(\hat{\beta}_J)\right)^{-1/2} \cdot \int_{\|\xi\|_2 > \sqrt{5|J|\log(n)}} \exp\left\{ -\sqrt{|J|\log(n)} \cdot \|\xi\|_2 \right\} d\xi \\
&\le \left(\det H_J(\hat{\beta}_J)\right)^{-1/2} \cdot \frac{4(\pi)^{|J|/2}}{\Gamma\left(\frac{1}{2}|J|\right)} \frac{\sqrt{5|J|\log(n)}^{|J|-1}}{\sqrt{|J|\log(n)}} e^{-\sqrt{5}|J|\log(n)} \\
&= \left(\frac{(2\pi)^{|J|}}{\det H_J(\hat{\beta}_J)} \right)^{1/2} \cdot \frac{2\sqrt{5}}{\Gamma\left(\frac{1}{2}|J|\right)} \left(\frac{5}{2}|J|\log(n) \right)^{|J|/2-1} \cdot \frac{1}{n^{\sqrt{5}|J|}}.
\end{aligned}$$

Stirling's lower bound on the Gamma function gives

$$\frac{(|J|/2)^{|J|/2-1}}{\Gamma\left(\frac{1}{2}|J|\right)} \;=\; \frac{(|J|/2)^{|J|/2}}{\Gamma\left(\frac{1}{2}|J|+1\right)} \;\le\; \frac{1}{\sqrt{|J|\pi}} e^{|J|/2}.$$

Using this inequality, and returning to (13), we see that

$$\mathcal{I}_2 \;\le\; L(\hat{\beta}_J) f_J(\hat{\beta}_J) \left(\frac{(2\pi)^{|J|}}{\det H_J(\hat{\beta}_J)} \right)^{1/2} \times e^{F_1 a_{\mathrm{MLE}} + F_2} \cdot \frac{2e\sqrt{5}}{\sqrt{|J|\pi}} \cdot \left(\frac{5e\log(n)}{n} \right)^{|J|/2-1} \frac{1}{n^{(\sqrt{5}-1/2)\cdot|J|+1}}. \tag{14}$$

Based on this fact, we certainly have the very loose bound that

$$\mathscr{I}_2 \leq L(\hat{\beta}_J)f_J(\hat{\beta}_J)\left(\frac{(2\pi)^{|J|}}{\det H_J(\hat{\beta}_J)}\right)^{1/2} e^{F_1 a_{\text{MLE}}+F_2}\cdot\frac{1}{\sqrt{n}}, \tag{15}$$

for sufficiently large n.

(ii-c) *Combining the bounds.* From (10) and (15), we obtain that

$$\text{Evidence}(J) = \mathscr{I}_1 + \mathscr{I}_2 = L(\hat{\beta}_J)f_J(\hat{\beta}_J)\left(\frac{(2\pi)^{|J|}}{\det H_J(\hat{\beta}_J)}\right)^{1/2} \times$$
$$\left(1 \pm \left(e^{F_1 a_{\text{MLE}}+F_2} + 2 + \sqrt{\frac{125c_{\text{change}}^2}{c_{\text{lower}}^3}} + \sqrt{\frac{20F_1^2}{c_{\text{lower}}}}\right)\sqrt{\frac{|J|^3\log^3(n)}{n}}\right) \tag{16}$$

for sufficiently large n, as desired.

Remark 2 The proof of Theorem 1 could be modified to handle other situations of interest. For instance, instead of a fixed Lipschitz constant F_1 for all log prior densities, one could consider the case where $\log f_J$ is Lipschitz with respect to a constant $F_1(J)$ that grows with the cardinality of $|J|$, e.g., at a rate of $\sqrt{|J|}$ in which case the rate of square root of $|J|^3\log^3(n)/n$ could be modified to square root of $|J|^4\log^3(n)/n$. The term $e^{F_1(J)a_{\text{MLE}}}$ that would appear in (16) could be compensated using (14) in less crude of a way than when moving to (15).

4 Numerical Experiment for Sparse Bayesian Logistic Regression

In this section, we perform a simulation study to assess the approximation error in Laplace approximations to the marginal likelihood of logistic regression models. To this end, we generate independent covariate vectors $X_1, \ldots, X_n$ with i.i.d. $N(0, 1)$ entries. For each choice of a (small) value of q, we take the true parameter vector $\beta_0 \in \mathbb{R}^p$ to have the first q entries equal to two and the rest of the entries equal zero. So, $J_0 = \{1, \ldots, q\}$. We then generate independent binary responses $Y_1, \ldots, Y_n$, with values in $\{0, 1\}$ and distributed as $(Y_i|X_i) \sim \text{Bernoulli}(p_i(X_i))$, where

$$p_i(x) = \left(\frac{\exp\left(x^T\beta_0\right)}{1+\exp\left(x^T\beta_0\right)}\right) \iff \log\left(\frac{p_i(x)}{1-p_i(x)}\right) = x\cdot\beta_0,$$

based on the usual (and canonical) logit link function.

We record that the logistic regression model with covariates indexed by $J \subset [p]$ has the likelihood function

$$L(\beta) = \exp\left\{\sum_{i=1}^{n} Y_i \cdot X_{iJ}^T\beta - \log\left(1 + \exp(X_{iJ}^T\beta)\right)\right\}, \quad \beta \in \mathbb{R}^J, \tag{17}$$

where, as previously defined, $X_{iJ} = (X_{ij})_{j \in J}$ denotes the subset of covariates for model J. The negative Hessian of the log-likelihood function is

$$H_J(\beta) = \sum_{i=1}^{n} X_{iJ}X_{iJ}^T \cdot \frac{\exp(X_{iJ}^T\beta)}{\left(1 + \exp(X_{iJ}^T\beta)\right)^2}.$$

For Bayesian inference in the logistic regression model given by J, we consider as a prior distribution a standard normal distribution on $\mathbb{R}^J$, that is, the distribution of a random vector with $|J|$ independent $N(0, 1)$ coordinates. As in previous section, we denote the resulting prior density by f_J. We then wish to approximate the evidence or marginal likelihood

$$\text{Evidence}(J) := \int_{\mathbb{R}^J} L(\beta) f_J(\beta)\, d\beta.$$

As a first approximation, we use a Monte Carlo approach in which we simply draw independent samples $\beta^1, \ldots, \beta^B$ from the prior f_J and estimate the evidence as

$$\text{MonteCarlo}(J) = \frac{1}{B}\sum_{b=1}^{B} L(\beta^b),$$

where we use $B = 50{,}000$ in all of our simulations. As a second method, we compute the Laplace approximation

$$\text{Laplace}(J) := L(\hat{\beta}_J) f_J(\hat{\beta}_J) \left(\frac{(2\pi)^{|J|}}{\det H_J(\hat{\beta}_J)}\right)^{1/2},$$

where $\hat{\beta}_J$ is the maximum likelihood estimator in model J. For each choice of the number of covariates p, the model size q, and the sample size n, we calculate the Laplace approximation error as

$$\max_{J \subset [p],\, |J| \le q} \left|\, \log \text{MonteCarlo}(J) - \log \text{Laplace}(J) \,\right|.$$

We consider $n \in \{50, 60, 70, 80, 90, 100\}$ in our experiment. Since we wish to compute the Laplace approximation error of every q-sparse model, and the number of possible models is on the order of p^q, we consider $p = n/2$ and $q \in \{1, 2, 3\}$.

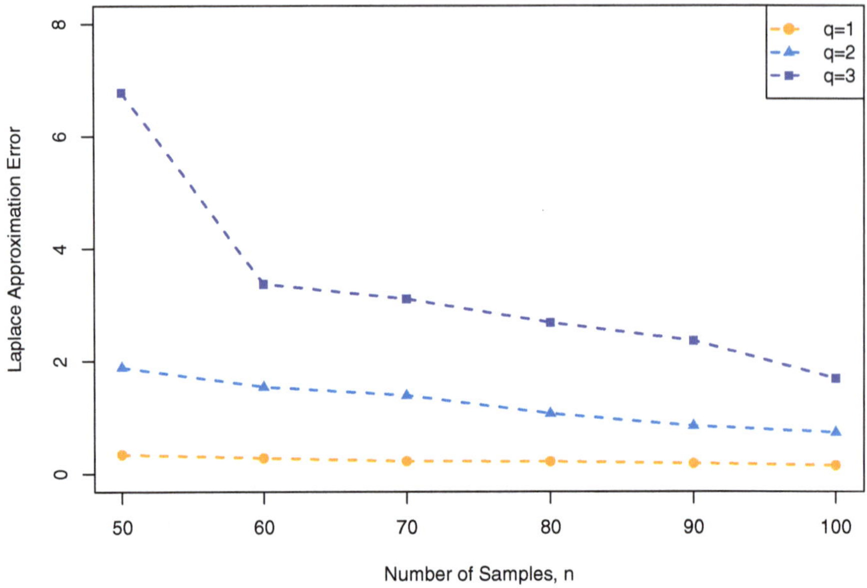

Fig. 1 Maximum Laplace approximation error, averaged over 100 data sets, as a function of the sample size n. The number of covariates is $n/2$, and the number of active covariates is bounded by $q \in \{1, 2, 3\}$

The Laplace approximation error, averaged across 100 independent simulations, is shown in Fig. 1. We remark that the error in the Monte Carlo approximation to the marginal likelihood is negligible compared to the quantity plotted in Fig. 1. With two independent runs of our Monte Carlo integration routine, we found the Monte Carlo error to be on the order of 0.05.

For each $q = 1, 2, 3$, Fig. 1 shows a decrease in Laplace approximation error as n increases. We emphasize that p and thus also the number of considered q-sparse models increase with n. As we increase the number of active covariates q, the Laplace approximation error increases. These facts are in agreement with Theorem 1. This said, the scope of this experiment is clearly limited by the fact that only small values of q and moderate values of p and n are computationally feasible.

5 Consistency of Bayesian Variable Selection

In this section, we apply the result on uniform accuracy of the Laplace approximation (Theorem 1) to prove a high-dimensional consistency result for Bayesian variable selection. Here, consistency refers to the property that the probability of choosing the most parsimonious true model tends to one in a large-sample limit. As discussed in Sect. 1, we consider priors of the form

$$P_\gamma(J) \propto \binom{p}{|J|}^{-\gamma} \cdot \mathbb{1}\{|J| \leq q\}, \qquad J \subset [p], \tag{18}$$

where $\gamma \geq 0$ is a parameter that allows one to interpolate between the case of a uniform distribution on models ($\gamma = 0$) and a prior for which the model cardinality $|J|$ is uniformly distributed ($\gamma = 1$).

Bayesian variable selection is based on maximizing the (unnormalized) posterior probability

$$\mathrm{Bayes}_\gamma(J) := \binom{p}{|J|}^{-\gamma} \mathrm{Evidence}(J) \tag{19}$$

over $J \subset [p]$, $|J| \leq q$. Approximate Bayesian variable section can be based on maximizing instead the quantity

$$\mathrm{Laplace}_\gamma(J) := \binom{p}{|J|}^{-\gamma} \mathrm{Laplace}(J). \tag{20}$$

We will identify asymptotic scenarios under which maximization of $\mathrm{Laplace}_\gamma$ yields consistent variable selection. Using Theorem 1, we obtain as a corollary that fully Bayesian variable selection, i.e., maximization of Bayes_γ, is consistent as well.

To study consistency, we consider a sequence of variable selection problems indexed by the sample size n, where the n-th problem has p_n covariates, true parameter $\beta_0(n)$ with support $J_0(n)$, and signal strength

$$\beta_{\min}(n) = \min_{j \in J_0(n)} |(\beta_0(n))_j|.$$

In addition, let q_n be the upper bound on the size of the considered models. The following consistency result is similar to the related results for extensions of the Bayesian information criterion; see, for instance, [2, 6].

Theorem 2 *Suppose that $p_n = n^\kappa$ for $\kappa > 0$, that $q_n = n^\psi$ for $0 \leq \psi < 1/3$, that $\beta_{\min}(n) = n^{-\phi/2}$ for $0 \leq \phi < 1 - \psi$, and that $\kappa > \psi$. Assume that (A1) holds for a fixed constant a_0 and that there a fixed functions c_{lower} and c_{upper} with respect to which the covariates satisfy the Hessian conditions (A2) and (A3) for all $J \supseteq J_0(n)$ with $|J| \leq 2q_n$. Moreover, assume that for the considered family of prior densities $\{f_J(\cdot) : J \subset [p_n], |J| \leq q_n\}$ there are constants $F_3, F_4 \in (0, \infty)$ such that, uniformly for all $|J| \leq q_n$, we have*

$$\sup_\beta f_J(\beta) \leq F_3 < \infty, \qquad \inf_{\|\beta\|_2 \leq a_{\mathrm{MLE}}} f_J(\beta) \geq F_4 > 0,$$

where a_{MLE} *is the constant from Theorem 1(i). Then, for any* $\gamma > 1 - \frac{1-2\psi}{2(\kappa-\psi)}$, *model selection with* $\mathrm{Laplace}_\gamma$ *is consistent in the sense that the event*

$$J_0(n) = \arg\max\{\mathrm{Laplace}_\gamma(J) : J \subset [p_n], |J| \leq q_n\}$$

has probability tending to one as $n \to \infty$.

Together with Theorem 1, the proof of Theorem 2, which we give below, also shows consistency of the fully Bayesian procedure.

Corollary 1 *Under the assumptions of Theorem 2, fully Bayesian model selection is consistent, that is, the event*

$$J_0(n) = \arg\max\{\mathrm{Bayes}_\gamma(J) : J \subset [p_n], |J| \leq q_n\}$$

has probability tending to one as $n \to \infty$.

Proof (Proof of Theorem 2) Our scaling assumptions for p_n, q_n and $\beta_{\min}(n)$ are such that the conditions imposed in Theorem 2.2 of [2] are met for n large enough. This theorem and Theorem 1(i) in this paper then yield that there are constants $\nu, \epsilon, C_{\mathrm{false}}, a_{\mathrm{MLE}} > 0$ such that with probability at least $1 - p_n^{\nu}$ the following three statements hold simultaneously:

(a) For all $|J| \leq q_n$ with $J \supseteq J_0(n)$,

$$\log \mathrm{L}(\hat{\beta}_J) - \log \mathrm{L}(\hat{\beta}_{J_0(n)}) \;\leq\; (1+\epsilon)(|J \backslash J_0(n)| + \nu)\log(p_n)\,. \tag{21}$$

(b) For all $|J| \leq q_n$ with $J \not\supseteq J_0(n)$,

$$\log \mathrm{L}(\hat{\beta}_{J_0}(n)) - \log \mathrm{L}(\hat{\beta}_J) \;\geq\; C_{\mathrm{false}}\, n\, \beta_{\min}(n)^2\,. \tag{22}$$

(c) For all $|J| \leq q_n$ and some constant $a_{\mathrm{MLE}} > 0$,

$$\|\hat{\beta}_J\|_2 \leq a_{\mathrm{MLE}}. \tag{23}$$

In the remainder of this proof we show that these three facts, in combination with further technical results from [2], imply that

$$J_0(n) = \arg\max\{\mathrm{Laplace}_\gamma(J) : J \subset [p_n], |J| \leq q_n\}. \tag{24}$$

For simpler notation, we no longer indicate explicitly that p_n, q_n, β_0 and derived quantities vary with n. We will then show that

$$\log \frac{\text{Laplace}_\gamma(J_0)}{\text{Laplace}_\gamma(J)} =$$

$$(\log P(J_0) - \log P(J)) + \left(\log L(\hat{\beta}_{J_0}) - \log L(\hat{\beta}_J)\right) - |J\backslash J_0| \log \sqrt{2\pi}$$

$$+ \left(\log f_{J_0}(\hat{\beta}_{J_0}) - \log f_J(\hat{\beta}_J)\right) + \frac{1}{2}\left(\log\det H_J(\hat{\beta}_J) - \log\det H_{J_0}(\hat{\beta}_{J_0})\right) \tag{25}$$

is positive for any model given by a set $J \neq J_0$ of cardinality $|J| \leq q$. We let

$$c_{\text{lower}} := c_{\text{lower}}(a_{\text{MLE}}), \qquad c_{\text{upper}} := c_{\text{upper}}(a_{\text{MLE}}).$$

We note that this definition of c_{lower} and c_{upper} differs from the one used in the proof of Theorem 1.

False Models If $J \not\supseteq J_0$, that is, if the model is false, we observe that

$$\log P(J_0) - \log P(J) = -\gamma \log \binom{p}{|J_0|} + \gamma \log \binom{p}{|J|} \geq -\gamma \log \binom{p}{|J_0|} \geq -\gamma q \log p.$$

Moreover, by (A2) and (23),

$$\log\det H_J(\hat{\beta}_J) - \log\det H_{J_0}(\hat{\beta}_{J_0}) \geq |J| \cdot \log(n c_{\text{lower}}) - |J_0| \cdot \log(n c_{\text{upper}})$$
$$\geq -q \log\left(n \frac{c_{\text{upper}}}{\min\{c_{\text{lower}}, 1\}}\right).$$

Combining the lower bounds with (22), we obtain that

$$\log \frac{\text{Laplace}_\gamma(J_0)}{\text{Laplace}_\gamma(J)}$$
$$\geq C_{\text{false}} n \beta_{\min}^2 - |J\backslash J_0| \log(\sqrt{2\pi}) - q \log\left(p^\gamma n \frac{c_{\text{upper}}}{\min\{c_{\text{lower}}, 1\}}\right) + \log\left(\frac{F_4}{F_3}\right)$$
$$\geq C_{\text{false}} n \beta_{\min}^2 - q \log\left(\frac{c_{\text{upper}}}{\min\{c_{\text{lower}}, 1\}} \cdot \sqrt{2\pi} n p^\gamma\right) + \log\left(\frac{F_4}{F_3}\right).$$

By our scaling assumptions, the lower bound is positive for sufficiently large n.

True Models It remains to resolve the case of $J \supsetneq J_0$, that is, when model J is true. We record that from the proof of Theorem 2.2 in [2], it holds on the considered event of probability at least $1 - p^{-\nu}$ that for any $J \supseteq J_0$,

$$\|\hat{\beta}_J - \beta_0\|_2 \le \frac{4\sqrt{c_{\text{upper}}}}{\sqrt{n}c_{\text{lower}}}\tau_{|J\backslash J_0|}, \tag{26}$$

where

$$\tau_r^2 = \frac{2}{(1-\epsilon')^3} \cdot \left[(J_0 + r)\log\left(\frac{3}{\epsilon'}\right) + \log(4p^\nu) + r\log(2p)\right].$$

Under our scaling assumptions on p and q, it follows that $\|\hat{\beta}_J - \beta_0\|_2$ tends to zero as $n \to \infty$.

We begin again by considering the prior on models, for which we have that

$$\begin{aligned}
\log P(J_0) - \log P(J) &= \gamma \log \frac{|J_0|!(p-|J_0|)!}{|J|!(p-|J|)!} \\
&\ge -\gamma |J\backslash J_0| \log q + \gamma |J\backslash J_0| \log(p-q) \\
&\ge -\gamma |J\backslash J_0| \log q + \gamma |J\backslash J_0| (1-\tilde{\epsilon}) \log p
\end{aligned}$$

for all n sufficiently large. Indeed, we assume that $p = n^\kappa$ and $q = n^\psi$ with $\kappa > \psi$ such that $p - q \ge p^{1-\tilde{\epsilon}}$ for any small constant $\tilde{\epsilon} > 0$ as long as p is sufficiently large relative to q.

Next, if $J \supsetneq J_0$, then (A2) and (A3) allow us to relate $H_J(\hat{\beta}_J)$ and $H_{J_0}(\hat{\beta}_{J_0})$ to the respective Hessian at the true parameter, i.e., $H_J(\beta_0)$ and $H_{J_0}(\beta_0)$. We find that

$$\begin{aligned}
\log\left(\frac{\det H_J(\hat{\beta}_J)}{\det H_{J_0}(\hat{\beta}_{J_0})}\right) &\ge \log\left(\frac{\det H_J(\beta_0)}{\det H_{J_0}(\beta_0)}\right) + |J| \log\left(1 - \frac{c_{\text{change}}}{c_{\text{lower}}}\|\hat{\beta}_J - \beta_0\|_2\right) \\
&\quad - |J_0| \log\left(1 + \frac{c_{\text{change}}}{c_{\text{lower}}}\|\hat{\beta}_{J_0} - \beta_0\|_2\right).
\end{aligned}$$

Note that by assuming n large enough, we may assume that $\|\hat{\beta}_J - \beta_0\|_2$ is small enough for the logarithm to be well defined; recall (26). Using that $x \ge \log(1+x)$ for all $x > -1$ and $\log(1 - \frac{x}{2}) \ge -x$ for all $0 \le x \le 1$, we see that

$$\begin{aligned}
\log\left(\frac{\det H_J(\hat{\beta}_J)}{\det H_{J_0}(\hat{\beta}_{J_0})}\right) &\ge \log\left(\frac{\det H_J(\beta_0)}{\det H_{J_0}(\beta_0)}\right) - 2|J|\frac{c_{\text{change}}}{c_{\text{lower}}}\|\hat{\beta}_J - \beta_0\|_2 \\
&\quad - |J_0|\frac{c_{\text{change}}}{c_{\text{lower}}}\|\hat{\beta}_{J_0} - \beta_0\|_2.
\end{aligned}$$

Under our scaling assumptions, $q^3\log(p) = o(n)$, and thus applying (26) twice shows that

$$-2|J|\frac{c_{\text{change}}}{c_{\text{lower}}}\|\hat{\beta}_J - \beta_0\|_2 - |J_0|\frac{c_{\text{change}}}{c_{\text{lower}}}\|\hat{\beta}_{J_0} - \beta_0\|_2$$

is larger than any small negative constant for n large enough. For simplicity, we take the lower bound as -1. By (A2), it holds that

$$\log\left(\frac{\det H_J(\beta_0)}{\det H_{J_0}(\beta_0)}\right) = \log\det\left(H_{J\setminus J_0}(\beta_0) - H_{J_0,J\setminus J_0}(\beta_0)^T H_{J_0}(\beta_0)^{-1} H_{J_0,J\setminus J_0}(\beta_0)\right)$$
$$\geq |J\setminus J_0|\log(n) + |J\setminus J_0|\log(c_{\text{lower}}),$$

because the eigenvalues of the Schur complement of $H_J(\beta_0)$ are bounded the same way as the eigenvalues of $H_J(\beta_0)$; see, e.g., Chap. 2 of [18]. Hence, for sufficiently large n, the following is true for all $J \supsetneq J_0$:

$$\log\det H_J(\hat{\beta}_J) - \log\det H_{J_0}(\hat{\beta}_{J_0}) \;\geq\; |J\setminus J_0|\log(n) + |J\setminus J_0|\log(c_{\text{lower}}) - 1. \quad (27)$$

Combining the bound for the model prior probabilities with (21) and (27), we have for any true model $J \supsetneq J_0$ that

$$\log\frac{\text{Laplace}_\gamma(J_0)}{\text{Laplace}_\gamma(J)} \geq -(1+\epsilon)(|J\setminus J_0| + \nu)\log(p) + \gamma|J\setminus J_0|(1-\tilde{\epsilon})\log(p)$$
$$+\frac{1}{2}|J\setminus J_0|\log(n) - \gamma|J\setminus J_0|\log(q) + \frac{1}{2}|J\setminus J_0|\left(\log\frac{c_{\text{lower}}}{2\pi}\right) + \log\left(\frac{F_4}{F_3}\right) - 1.$$

Collecting terms and using that $|J\setminus J_0| \geq 1$, we obtain the lower bound

$$\log\frac{\text{Laplace}_\gamma(J_0)}{\text{Laplace}_\gamma(J)} \geq \frac{1}{2}|J\setminus J_0|\Bigg\{\log(n) - \log q^{2\gamma}$$
$$+2\left[(1-\tilde{\epsilon})\gamma - (1+\epsilon)(1+\nu)\right]\log(p) + \log\left(\frac{c_{\text{lower}}}{2\pi}\right)\Bigg\} + \log\left(\frac{F_4}{F_3}\right) - 1.$$

This lower bound is positive for all n large because our assumption that $p = n^\kappa$, $q = n^\psi$ for $0 \leq \psi < 1/3$, and

$$\gamma > 1 - \frac{1-2\psi}{2(\kappa-\psi)}$$

implies that

$$\lim_{n\to\infty}\frac{\sqrt{n}}{p^{(1+\epsilon)(1+\nu)-\gamma(1-\tilde{\epsilon})}q^\gamma} = \infty \quad (28)$$

provided the constants ϵ, ν, and $\tilde{\epsilon}$ are chosen sufficiently small.

6 Discussion

In this paper, we showed that in the context of high-dimensional variable selection problems, the Laplace approximation can be accurate uniformly across a potentially very large number of sparse models. We also demonstrated how this approximation result allows one to give results on the consistency of fully Bayesian techniques for variable selection.

In practice, it is of course infeasible to evaluate the evidence or Laplace approximation for every single sparse regression model, and some search strategy must be adopted instead. Some related numerical experiments can be found in [5, 6, 17], and [2], although that work considers BIC scores that drop some of the terms appearing in the Laplace approximation.

Finally, we emphasize that the setup we considered concerns generalized linear models without dispersion parameter and with canonical link. The conditions from [11] could likely be used to extend our results to other situations.

7 Technical Lemmas

This section provides two lemmas that were used in the proof of Theorem 1.

Lemma 1 (Chi-Square Tail Bound) *Let χ^2_k denote a chi-square random variable with k degrees of freedom. Then, for any $n \geq 3$,*

$$\mathbb{P}\left\{\chi^2_k \leq 5k\log(n)\right\} \geq 1 - \frac{1}{n^k} \geq \exp\{-1/\sqrt{n}\}.$$

Proof Since $\log(n) \geq 1$ when $n \geq 3$, we have that

$$k + 2\sqrt{k \cdot k\log(n)} + 2k\log(n) \;\leq\; 5k\log(n).$$

Using the chi-square tail bound in [10], it thus holds that

$$\begin{aligned}\mathbb{P}\left\{\chi^2_k \leq 5k\log(n)\right\} &\geq \mathbb{P}\left\{\chi^2_k \leq k + 2\sqrt{k \cdot k\log(n)} + 2k\log(n)\right\}\\ &\geq 1 - e^{-k\log(n)}.\end{aligned}$$

Finally, for the last step, by the Taylor series for $x \mapsto e^x$, for all $n \geq 3$ we have

$$\exp\{-1/\sqrt{n}\} \leq 1 - \frac{1}{\sqrt{n}} + \frac{1}{2} \cdot \frac{1}{n} \leq 1 - \frac{1}{n}.$$

Lemma 2 *Let $k \geq 1$ be any integer, and let $a, b > 0$ be such that $ab \geq 2(k-1)$. Then*

$$\int_{\|\xi\|_2 > a} \exp\{-b\|\xi\|_2\} d\xi \;\leq\; \frac{4(\pi)^{k/2}}{\Gamma\left(\frac{1}{2}k\right)} \frac{a^{k-1}}{b} e^{-ab},$$

where the integral is taken over $\xi \in \mathbb{R}^k$.

Proof We claim that the integral of interest is

$$\int_{\|\xi\|_2 > a} \exp\{-b\|\xi\|_2\} d\xi = \frac{2(\pi)^{k/2}}{b^k \Gamma\left(\frac{1}{2}k\right)} \int_{r=ab}^{\infty} r^{k-1} e^{-r} dr. \tag{29}$$

Indeed, in $k = 1$ dimension,

$$\int_{\|\xi\|_2 > a} \exp\{-b\|\xi\|_2\} d\xi = 2 \int_{r=a}^{\infty} e^{-br} dr = \frac{2}{b} e^{-ab},$$

which is what (29) evaluates to. If $k \geq 2$, then using polar coordinates (see Exercises 7.1–1.3 in [1]), we find that

$$\begin{aligned} \int_{\|\xi\|_2 > a} \exp\{-b\|\xi\|_2\} d\xi &= 2\pi \int_{r=a}^{\infty} r^{k-1} e^{-br} dr \cdot \prod_{i=1}^{k-2} \int_{-\pi/2}^{\pi/2} \cos^i(\theta_i) d\theta_i \\ &= 2\pi \int_{r=a}^{\infty} r^{k-1} e^{-br} dr \cdot \prod_{i-1}^{k-2} \frac{\sqrt{\pi}\, \Gamma\left(\frac{1}{2}(i+1)\right)}{\Gamma\left(\frac{1}{2}(i+2)\right)}, \end{aligned}$$

which again agrees with the formula from (29).

Now, the integral on the right-hand side of (29) defines the upper incomplete Gamma function and can be bounded as

$$\Gamma(k, ab) = \int_{r=ab}^{\infty} r^{k-1} e^{-r} dr \leq 2e^{-ab}(ab)^{k-1}$$

for $ab \geq 2(k-1)$; see inequality (3.2) in [14]. This gives the bound that was to be proven.

References

1. Anderson, T.W.: An Introduction to Multivariate Statistical Analysis. Wiley Series in Probability and Statistics, 3rd edn. Wiley-Interscience, Hoboken, NJ (2003)
2. Barber, R.F., Drton, M.: High-dimensional Ising model selection with Bayesian information criteria. Electron. J. Stat. **9**, 567–607 (2015)

3. Bishop, C.M.: Pattern Recognition and Machine Learning. Information Science and Statistics. Springer, New York (2006)
4. Bogdan, M., Ghosh, J.K., Doerge, R.: Modifying the Schwarz Bayesian information criterion to locate multiple interacting quantitative trait loci. Genetics **167**(2), 989–999 (2004)
5. Chen, J., Chen, Z.: Extended Bayesian information criteria for model selection with large model spaces. Biometrika **95**(3), 759–771 (2008)
6. Chen, J., Chen, Z.: Extended BIC for small-n-large-P sparse GLM. Stat. Sinica **22**(2), 555–574 (2012)
7. Friel, N., Wyse, J.: Estimating the evidence—a review. Statistica Neerlandica **66**(3), 288–308 (2012)
8. Frommlet, F., Ruhaltinger, F., Twaróg, P., Bogdan, M.: Modified versions of Bayesian information criterion for genome-wide association studies. Comput. Stat. Data Anal. **56**(5), 1038–1051 (2012)
9. Haughton, D.M.A.: On the choice of a model to fit data from an exponential family. Ann. Stat. **16**(1), 342–355 (1988)
10. Laurent, B., Massart, P.: Adaptive estimation of a quadratic functional by model selection. Ann. Stat. **28**(5), 1302–1338 (2000)
11. Luo, S., Chen, Z.: Selection consistency of EBIC for GLIM with non-canonical links and diverging number of parameters. Stat. Interface **6**(2), 275–284 (2013)
12. Luo, S., Xu, J., Chen, Z.: Extended Bayesian information criterion in the Cox model with a high-dimensional feature space. Ann. Inst. Stat. Math. **67**(2), 287–311 (2015)
13. McCullagh, P., Nelder, J.A.: Generalized Linear Models. Monographs on Statistics and Applied Probability, 2nd edn. Chapman & Hall, London (1989)
14. Natalini, P., Palumbo, B.: Inequalities for the incomplete gamma function. Math. Inequal. Appl. **3**(1), 69–77 (2000)
15. Schwarz, G.: Estimating the dimension of a model. Ann. Stat. **6**(2), 461–464 (1978)
16. Scott, J.G., Berger, J.O.: Bayes and empirical-Bayes multiplicity adjustment in the variable-selection problem. Ann. Stat. **38**(5), 2587–2619 (2010)
17. Żak-Szatkowska, M., Bogdan, M.: Modified versions of the Bayesian information criterion for sparse generalized linear models. Comput. Stat. Data Anal. **55**(11), 2908–2924 (2011)
18. Zhang, F. (ed.): The Schur Complement and Its Applications. Numerical Methods and Algorithms, vol. 4. Springer, New York (2005)

Preselection in Lasso-Type Analysis for Ultra-High Dimensional Genomic Exploration

Linn Cecilie Bergersen, Ismaïl Ahmed, Arnoldo Frigessi, Ingrid K. Glad, and Sylvia Richardson

Abstract We address the issue of variable preselection in high-dimensional penalized regression, such as the lasso, a commonly used approach to variable selection and prediction in genomics. Preselection—to start with a manageable set of covariates—is becoming increasingly necessary for enabling advanced analysis tasks to be carried out on data sets of huge size created by high throughput technologies. Preselection of features to be included in multivariate analyses based on simple univariate ranking is a natural strategy that has often been implemented despite its potential bias. We demonstrate this bias and propose a way to correct it. Starting with a sequential implementation of the lasso with increasing lists of predictors, we exploit a property of the set of corresponding cross-validation curves, a pattern that we call "freezing". The ranking of the predictors to be included sequentially is based on simple measures of associations with the outcome, which can be pre-computed in an efficient way for ultra high dimensional data sets externally to the penalized regression implementation. We demonstrate by simulation that our sequential approach leads in a vast majority of cases to a safe and

---

Authors Ingrid K. Glad, Sylvia Richardson contributed equally.

L.C. Bergersen • I.K. Glad (✉)
Department of Mathematics, University of Oslo, Oslo, Norway
e-mail: linncecilieb@gmail.com; glad@math.uio.no

I. Ahmed
INSERM, CESP Center for Research in Epidemiology and Population Health, Paris, France
e-mail: ismail.ahmed@inserm.fr

A. Frigessi
Oslo Centre for Biostatistics and Epidemiology, University of Oslo, Oslo, Norway
e-mail: frigessi@medisin.uio.no

S. Richardson
MRC Biostatistics Unit, Cambridge Institute of Public Health, University of Cambridge, Cambridge, UK
e-mail: sylvia.richardson@mrc-bsu.cam.ac.uk

A. Frigessi et al. (eds.), *Statistical Analysis for High-Dimensional Data*,
Abel Symposia 11, DOI 10.1007/978-3-319-27099-9_3

efficient way of focusing the lasso analysis on a smaller and manageable number of predictors. In situations where the lasso performs well, we need typically less than 20 % of the variables to recover the same solution as if using the full set of variables. We illustrate the applicability of our strategy in the context of a genome-wide association study and on microarray genomic data where we need just 2.5 % and 13 % of the variables respectively. Finally we include an example where 260 million gene-gene interactions are ranked and we are able to recover the lasso solution using only 1 % of these. Freezing offers great potential for extending the applicability of penalized regressions to current and upcoming ultra high dimensional problems in bioinformatics. Its applicability is not limited to the standard lasso but is a generic property of many penalized approaches.

1 Introduction

Regression with a number P of covariates, which is much larger than the number n of independent samples, is becoming a recurrent situation in science and biomedicine. While there is often a design constraint to the number of samples (e.g. due to cost and availability of patients), measurement technologies and storing capacity allow the recording of huge amounts of characteristics of each unit/sample. This information is very often in excess, in the sense that only a very small part of the collected covariates plays a role in the biological mechanisms under study. When a sparsity assumption can be made, it is often of great interest to detect the important covariates for prediction, data compression, or classification. Since the cardinal paper by Tibshirani [17], l_1-norm regularization has played a fundamental role in $P > n$ regression and has been widely applied to facilitate knowledge discovery. The most popular method is the lasso [17], and its many variants and relatives [14, 19, 23–25]. Lasso has become a reference tool in genomic analyses [20, 21].

The lasso belongs to the penalized regression family in which a regularization parameter λ governs the level of shrinkage. A key issue is to find the optimal value for λ, which in practice is determined by K-fold cross-validation. There are several efficient algorithms that find the lasso solution, including LARS [7] and coordinate descent [10], in the R package `glmnet`. The computational complexity of these algorithms to compute the entire solution path as a function of λ is $O(P^3 + nP^2)$, which is computationally demanding when P is large [11]. With the advent of high throughput technologies, it is often not possible to use them directly on the full dataset because it becomes cumbersome to even load all covariates into standard statistical softwares like R or Matlab. For example, a typical genomic application can have $P = 30{,}000$ covariates, here gene expressions, or more than one million SNPs in genome-wide association studies (GWAS). In addition, there is a growing interest in investigating more complex mechanisms, for example accounting for gene by environment and epistatic interactions. For the latter, even if reduced to pair or triplet as in [3, 5, 22], the incorporation of epistatic interaction terms in multivariate models becomes rapidly prohibitive. Therefore, it is often necessary to reduce the number of covariates prior to the analysis, by performing preselection.

Preselection of covariates has been done in practice very frequently [6, 16, 21], and often without recognizing that the preselection may have an important effect on the solution. To preselect the most promising variables, it is common to use simple univariate regression. This is however dangerous: it is known, and we document this aspect further in this paper, that such a preselection will very often lead to overfitting and preselection bias, depending on the number of preselected variables [1, 13]. The problem is that preselection often will encourage the wrong amount of regularization in the cross-validation, which in the end gives a lasso solution with too many selected features as compared to the solution that would be obtained when implementing the lasso on the whole data. To overcome this problem, we give conditions for the existence of a specific behavior of the lasso in combination with cross-validation, which we call *freezing*. In recent years, an important literature has grown, proposing various preselection [9].

In particular, covariate elimination rules for the lasso have been successfully developed, [8, 18]. These rules allow to exclude many variables which are clearly not relevant for the regression for given values of λ, leading to significant speed-up of `glmnet`. Nevertheless, the issue of being able to perform such analysis on ultra-high data set remains.

In this paper we propose a new, simple and computationally feasible, preselection rule for $P > n$ sparse regression, which typically needs only to process a small fraction of the data. Our approach works in combination with cross-validation for any implementation of lasso regression. While the subset of the covariates ultimately selected is not theoretically guaranteed to produce the same solution as the cross-validated optimal lasso solution, we argue why it will most often succeed to do so. In an extensive simulation study explicitly constructed to challenge its reliability, we show that our algorithm almost always reaches the optimal lasso solution for the full data set using only a small fraction of the covariates. Note that our rule operates externally to the lasso loop by selecting potentially relevant variables for successive inclusion in a lasso procedure, as well as simultaneously deciding the optimal amount of penalization for prediction. This makes it possible to analyze data of ultra high-dimension as illustrated in our last data example. The fact that we operate outside the lasso loop, means that we in addition profit from tools for computational efficiency already implemented within the lasso, such as the sequentially strong selection rules in `glmnet` [18].

We conclude this section with a review of the standard lasso procedure and how to determine the optimal value of λ through cross-validation. Thereafter we give an example of preselection bias and illustrate the concept of freezing. The rest of the paper is organized as follows. In Sect. 2, we define freezing and outline a practical implementations of our algorithm. In Sect. 3 we present an extensive simulation study that illustrates the reliability of the new algorithm and the reduced number of variables it allows to operate with. We apply the preselection rule to genomic data, including two ultra high-dimensional data sets where the global lasso solution for the full data set is not possible to obtain with a software like R in standard mode. Final considerations and extensions are given in Sect. 4.

1.1 Illustrating Preselection Bias and Freezing

Consider a high-dimensional regression problem with n observations, P covariates organized in a design matrix $\boldsymbol{X}$, a response vector $\boldsymbol{y}$ and where some preselection rule is needed to reduce dimensionality prior to a lasso analysis. Although our rule will apply in combination with a range of lasso-type methods, our illustrating example is the standard lasso where the solution is computed through a cyclical coordinate descent algorithm as in the `glmnet` package [10]. Extension to other regression models, such as logistic regression, is also straightforward. An example of this type is considered in Sect. 3.

Suppose all predictors are standardized to have mean zero and variance one. Let β_0 be the intercept, $\boldsymbol{\beta}$ the coefficient vector for all covariates and $l(\beta_0, \boldsymbol{\beta})$ the log-likelihood function. The lasso estimator $(\hat{\beta}_0, \hat{\boldsymbol{\beta}})$ is obtained by adding a l_1-penalty to the negative log-likelihood to be minimized:

$$(\hat{\beta}_0, \hat{\boldsymbol{\beta}}) = \underset{\beta_0, \boldsymbol{\beta}}{\operatorname{argmin}} \{-l(\beta_0, \boldsymbol{\beta}) + \lambda ||\boldsymbol{\beta}||_1\}. \tag{1}$$

Here, the penalty parameter λ controls the amount of penalization, and is most commonly chosen by K-fold cross-validation. This involves minimization of a cross-validation criterion $CV(\lambda)$ depending on an appropriate loss function.

For linear regression the lasso estimates can be obtained by minimizing the penalized residual sum of squares;

$$\hat{\boldsymbol{\beta}} = \underset{\boldsymbol{\beta} \in \mathbb{R}^P}{\operatorname{argmin}} \left\{ \frac{1}{2} ||\boldsymbol{y} - \boldsymbol{X}\boldsymbol{\beta}||_2^2 + \lambda ||\boldsymbol{\beta}||_1 \right\}, \tag{2}$$

and the optimal λ for prediction can for example be obtained by minimizing the cross-validated prediction mean squared error

$$CV(\lambda) = \frac{1}{n} \sum_{k=1}^{K} \sum_{i \in f_k} (y_i - \hat{y}_i^{-k}(\lambda))^2;$$

here K is the number of folds, f_k is the set of indices of the samples in fold k, and $\hat{y}_i^{-k}(\lambda)$ is the fitted predicted value for observation i when fold k involving observation i, is left out of the estimation.

We illustrate the property of freezing in an example based on a random simulation run from the experiments described in Sect. 3. The top black curve in Fig. 1a is the cross-validation curve for the full data set with all covariates. The global minimum of this curve is located in λ^* and we call the selected variables using λ^*, the global solution. Based on a procedure using a smaller number of covariates, we aim at tracking enough of this curve to nevertheless reveal the global optimum in λ^* and hence the global solution.

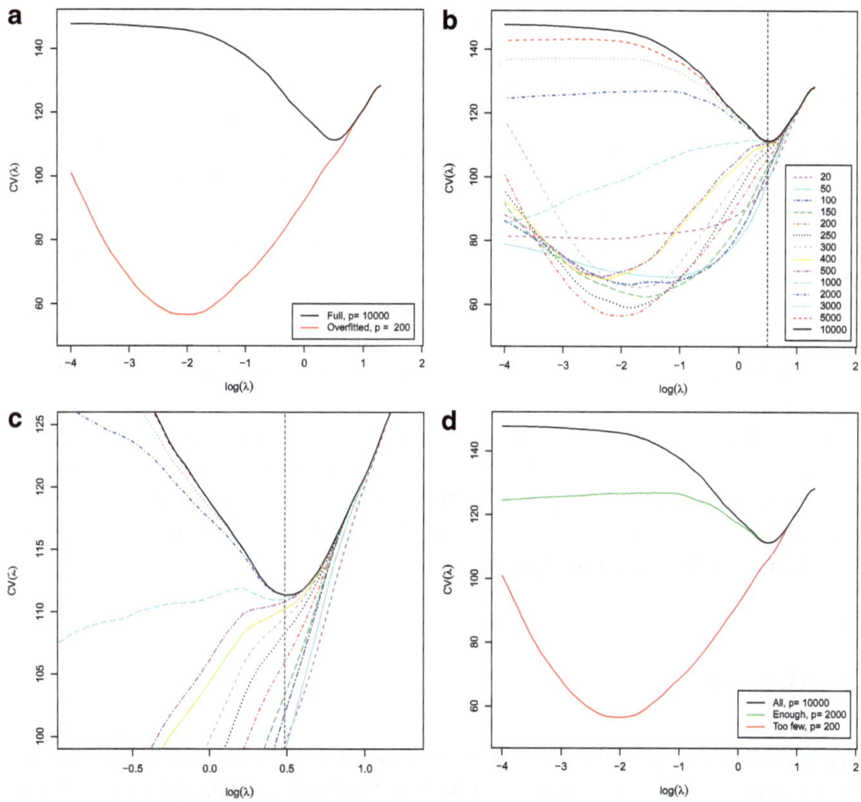

Fig. 1 Illustration of preselection bias. (**a**) Illustration of preselection bias when 200 correlation ranked variables are used instead of the full set of 10,000 variables. The *black curve* is the cross-validation curve when lasso uses all variables. The *red curve* is the cross-validation curve when only the 200 variables most correlated to $\boldsymbol{y}$ are used. Comparing the two minima shows that the preselection leads to less penalization and hence more selected variables. (**b**) Illustration of the freezing phenomenon. The *vertical line* indicates the cross-validation optimal solution. We see that the cross-validation curves based on an increasing set of p covariates are equal to the full cross-validation curve (in *black*) for smaller and smaller λ when p increases. (**c**) Enlarged detail of (**b**). (**d**) Illustration of a typical situation for which preselecting 2000 variables will lead to the same optimal value of λ and the same lasso solution as with the whole data. Note that the x-axis of λ is in log-scale and decreasing from right to left, with strongest penalization in the right end

The red curve in Fig. 1a shows a typical example of preselection bias. This curve is obtained using a subset of the covariates, namely the p (here $p = 200$) top ranked variables based on univariate correlation of each variable with the response. This is a commonly employed strategy to reduce the dimension of the problem. It is obvious from Fig. 1a that preselection of variables based on the univariate ranking may lead to a completely different and smaller optimal value of λ and hence to a model of higher dimensionality. In this particular example, lasso based on the top 200 preselected variables selects 98 variables, while the number of variables selected in the optimal lasso solution based on all variables is only 33.

However, when we fit several lasso models, for a suitable grid of λ, using subsets with an increasing number p of covariates ordered on the basis of univariate analyses, an interesting feature appears. When increasing p, we see in Fig. 1b, c that the cross-validation curves, corresponding to lasso estimation based on increasing subsets, start to coincide more and more for smaller values on the λ scale. Indeed the cross-validation curve, as a function of λ and p, stabilizes from large to smaller values of λ and increasing p. We say that the cross-validation curves are freezing in the λ-p space. Freezing allows to learn parts of the curve corresponding to less and less strong penalization as the number of covariates included in the subsets is increased. More importantly, it allows to identify the value of λ which would turn out to be optimal by cross-validation if all variables were used, our λ^*, based only on a smaller subset of the covariates. This property is exploited by our preselection algorithm.

Figure 1d illustrates the three scenarios of having all, enough or too few variables for the curve to be frozen up to the global optimal value of λ and slightly more. For the green curve corresponding to $p = 2000$ instead of the full 10,000, we see how the true minimum and the solution for the full set of covariates can be discovered based on a smaller subset of the data.

2 Methods

We begin with making the concept of freezing of cross-validation curves precise. The purpose is to find the smallest preselected set so that running lasso on this set gives the same cross-validated solution as if lasso is run on all variables.

2.1 *Cross-Validation Freezing*

Let $\boldsymbol{x}_1, \ldots, \boldsymbol{x}_P$ be a set of P ordered covariate vectors, $\boldsymbol{x}_p \in \mathbb{R}^n$, and let $C_F = \{1, \ldots, P\}$, F for "full", and $C_p = \{1, \ldots, p\}$ with $1 \leq p \leq P$. Let $S_F(\lambda)$ be the set of indices of the nonzero coefficients corresponding to the lasso solution of (2) with penalty λ using the full set of covariates in C_F. Recall that we denote by λ^* the optimal penalty corresponding to the global solution based on the full set. $S_p(\lambda)$ is the set of indices of the nonzero coefficients when running the lasso with penalty λ using only the covariates in C_p. We denote by $\hat{\beta}_{j,C_p}(\lambda), j = 1, \ldots, p$, the estimated regression coefficients when running the lasso with penalty λ only on the subset of covariates in C_p.

(a) The first simple point to note is that, as soon as the preselected set C_{p_1} (for some index p_1) includes all the variables that would ultimately be chosen by the lasso run on all covariates for a particular value of λ, then running a lasso on C_{p_1} or any larger set C_{p_2} with $p_2 > p_1$, will always result in the same set of regression coefficients. More precisely, for fixed λ, let $p_0(\lambda)$ be the smallest index p for which $S_F(\lambda) \subseteq C_p$. Then it is easy to prove that

$$S_p(\lambda) = S_F(\lambda) \quad \forall p \geq p_0(\lambda), \text{and} \tag{3a}$$

$$\forall p \geq p_0(\lambda), \text{it holds that } \hat{\beta}_{j,C_p}(\lambda) = \hat{\beta}_{j,C_F}(\lambda), \quad \forall j \in C_p. \tag{3b}$$

(b) Next consider a grid Λ spanning the range of penalty parameters from λ_{min} up to λ_{max}, $\Lambda = \{\lambda_1 = \lambda_{min}, \lambda_2, \ldots, \lambda_L = \lambda_{max}\}$. For every $p \in \{1, 2, \ldots, P\}$ there exists a smallest $l \in \{1, 2, \ldots, L\}$, with $l = l(p)$, such that $S_F(\lambda_k) \subseteq C_p$ for all $k = l, l+1, \ldots, L$. Hence for a given subset C_p there is an interval on the λ-axis, given by the set $[\lambda_{l(p)}, \lambda_{l(p)+1}, \ldots, \lambda_{max}]$, for which solving the lasso with all covariates or only with the top p in C_p is the same: it will give the same active sets and estimated coefficients. It also follows that $l(p_2) \leq l(p_1)$ if $p_2 > p_1$. When increasing p, the set of λ values where we find the full solution using only C_p grows. This monotonicity is the second important property that we will exploit in our sequential strategy.
(c) Consider now the cross-validation curve in λ, for a subset C_p of the covariates, given by

$$CV_{C_p}(\lambda) = \frac{1}{n} \sum_{k=1}^{K} \sum_{i \in f_k} (y_i - \hat{y}^{-k}_{i,C_p}(\lambda))^2.$$

Here $\hat{y}^{-k}_{i,C_p}(\lambda)$ is the fitted value for observation i from lasso with penalty λ using covariates given by C_p when fold $k = k(i)$ involving observation i is left out of the estimation and K is the number of folds. That is,

$$\hat{y}^{-k}_{i,C_p}(\lambda) = \sum_{j \in C_p} x_{ij} \hat{\beta}^{-k}_{j,C_p}(\lambda), \quad \text{for} \quad k = k(i),$$

where x_{ij} is the covariate value for sample i and variable j, and $\hat{\beta}^{-k}_{j,C_p}(\lambda)$, $\forall j \in C_p$, are the estimated regression coefficients from the cross-validation training set when the kth fold is left out and using covariates in C_p only. Similarly $CV_{C_F}(\lambda)$ is the cross-validation curve using all covariates in C_F. We also define $S_F^{-k}(\lambda)$ to be the set of indices of nonzero coefficients in the lasso with penalty λ and the full set of covariates, but when the kth fold is left out. Similarly $S_p^{-k}(\lambda)$ is the set of indices of nonzero coefficients when running the lasso with penalty λ on covariates in C_p and the kth fold left out. Hence, $\hat{\beta}_{j,C_p}^{-k}(\lambda) = 0$ for $j \notin S_p^{-k}(\lambda)$.

(d) Finally, we need to combine information from all K folds. For every fold k and fixed λ, there is a $p_{0,k}(\lambda)$ which is the smallest p such that $S_F^{-k}(\lambda) \subseteq C_p$. If we let

$$p_{0,cv}(\lambda) = \max_{k=1,\dots,K} p_{0,k}(\lambda), \tag{4}$$

then $\forall p \geq p_{0,cv}(\lambda)$, the cross-validation curves satisfy

$$CV_{C_p}(\lambda) = CV_{C_F}(\lambda). \tag{5}$$

Our algorithm is aimed at detecting $p_{0,cv}(\lambda)$ and is based on the concept of freezing.

Freezing We say that the cross-validation curve has frozen in (λ, p) if

$$CV_{C_{p'}}(\lambda') = CV_{C_F}(\lambda'), \quad \forall \lambda' \geq \lambda \quad \forall p' \geq p.$$

Given λ, for each fold k there exists a $p_k(\lambda)$ such that $S_F^{-k}(\lambda') \subseteq C_{p_k(\lambda)}$, $\forall k, \forall \lambda' > \lambda$, and we say that the cross-validation curve is frozen in $(\lambda, \max_k p_k(\lambda))$. To be of practical interest, we describe an algorithm to detect freezing, which allows using in most cases only a small fraction of the variables. The simple proofs of statements in this section are collected in Appendix 1.

2.2 *Using Freezing to Guide Preselection*

Our goal is to track the part of the cross-validation curve, which would be obtained when using all covariates, while just using a smaller number of these. Define a grid set Λ of penalty parameter values from λ_{min} to λ_{max}, choose an appropriate rule to order the covariates and an increasing sequence of subset sizes $0 < p_1 < \dots < p_M = P$, with subsets of covariates C_{p_m}. We will discuss later on how to choose this sequence, typically we will use a fixed increment.

To detect potential freezing points, in the first part of our algorithm we increase the number of variables successively from p_m to p_{m+1} and run the lasso, until two successive curves are identical from λ_{max} down and beyond a minimum in $\lambda_{p_m}^*$ of the curves. We will show in experiments that simple orderings most frequently lead to $p_m \ll P$, that is a substantial reduction in dimension of the problem. There is however no 'guarantee' that at this point $S_F(\lambda^*) \subseteq C_{p_m}$, nor that $\lambda^*_{p_m} = \lambda^*$ though, in our experience, this first step works well in most cases. To control for rare occurrences where this first part does not return the true value of λ^*, we design a second part to our algorithm.

Algorithm Part 1 : Single Ordering

---

(1) Compute $CV_{C_{p_m}}(\lambda)$, for all $\lambda \in \Lambda$, for $m = 1, 2, 3, \ldots$, until

$$CV_{C_{p_{m+1}}}(\lambda) = CV_{C_{p_m}}(\lambda) \quad \forall \lambda \in \tilde{\Lambda},$$

where $\tilde{\Lambda} = [\tilde{\lambda}, \lambda_{max}]$ contains a minimum of $CV_{C_{p_m}}(\lambda)$ in $\lambda^*_{p_m} > \tilde{\lambda}$.

(2) Solve the lasso problem in $\lambda^*_{p_m}$ using only C_{p_m} and return the solution $\hat{\boldsymbol{\beta}}_{C_{p_m}}$.

The idea of part 2 is very simple and based on *sequential reordering*: once we have found a first "local point of freezing" we compute residuals using the current coefficients $\hat{\boldsymbol{\beta}}_{C_{p_m}}(\lambda^*_{p_m})$ and take these as outcomes, instead than the original $\boldsymbol{y}$, to reorder the non-selected variables $C_F \setminus C_{p_m}$. Based on this new ordering, consider the top ranked $A_{\tilde{p}}$ variables and run lasso on these variables $A_{\tilde{p}} \cup C_{p_m}$. If the freezing point is confirmed, stop and return the solution C_{p_m}. Otherwise this was a false freezing point (as $A_{\tilde{p}}$ included again a useful variable) and we continue until we find a new freezing point, which is again checked using new residuals. See Appendix 2 for more details.

Algorithm Part 2 : Repeated Ordering

---

(1) Run Algorithm Part 1 until it stops in C_{p_m}.

(2) Compute residuals

$$\boldsymbol{r} = \boldsymbol{y} - \boldsymbol{X}_{C_{p_m}} \hat{\boldsymbol{\beta}}_{C_{p_m}},$$

where $\hat{\boldsymbol{\beta}}_{C_{p_m}} = \hat{\boldsymbol{\beta}}_{C_{p_m}}(\lambda^*_{p_m})$ and $\boldsymbol{X}_{C_{p_m}}$ is the reduced matrix of variables in C_{p_m} only.

(3) Reorder the unused variables in $C_F \setminus C_{p_m}$ based on $|\boldsymbol{r}^T \boldsymbol{x}_j|$. Define $A_{\tilde{p}}$ as the $\tilde{p}$ top ranked covariates.

(4) Compute a new $CV_{\tilde{C}_{p_{m+1}}}(\lambda)$, where now $\tilde{C}_{p_{m+1}} = C_{p_m} + A_{\tilde{p}}$.

(5) **If** $CV_{\tilde{C}_{p_{m+1}}}(\lambda) = CV_{C_{p_m}}(\lambda) \quad \forall \lambda \in \tilde{\Lambda}$, where $\tilde{\Lambda} = [\tilde{\lambda}, \lambda_{max}]$ contains the minimum of $CV_{C_{p_m}}(\lambda)$ in $\lambda^*_{p_m} > \tilde{\lambda}$, then stop and return the solution $\hat{\boldsymbol{\beta}}_{C_{p_m}}$.
Else go to 1: Continue running Algorithm Part 1 using the new order from (3).

When reordering the unused variables given the currently selected variables $S_{p_m}(\lambda^*_{p_m})$, one could apply the Karush-Kuhn-Tucker (KKT) conditions to determine new variables that should enter the solution in $\lambda^*_{p_m}$. Using the KKT condition in this setting means checking if $|\boldsymbol{r}^T\boldsymbol{x}_j| > \lambda^*_{p_m}$. The additional set $A_{\tilde{p}}$ should at least contain the variables for which this is true. As we are not necessarily interested in the solution in $\lambda^*_{p_m}$, we should choose $\tilde{p}$ such that we include more variables than what is implied by the KKT conditions. Note that the algorithm is not theoretically guaranteed to be safe, though in our extensive simulations it failed only three times, as we will see in Sect. 3.

It is of course obvious that the sequence of subset sizes $p_1 < p_2 < p_3 < \ldots$ and the increment $\tilde{p}$ in the algorithm are very important. To simplify, we will typically consider regularly spaced sequences. Too small increments may lead Part 1 of the algorithm to stop too early and therefore requires many reorderings. Too large increments will rapidly lead to using most variables. In this paper we do not optimize the sequence of cardinalities, but rather investigate several fixed increments (+100, +200, +500, +1000), and illustrate their impact in Sect. 3. Intuitively, it appears important to choose increments, such that the successive set $C_{p_{m+1}}$ has a high chance to include a new variable (not present in C_{p_m}) in its lasso set $S_{p_{m+1}}(\lambda^*_{p_m})$. In many applications, the covariates can be thought to be correlated in blocks, but independent between blocks. In GWAS, a block would be a series of variables (here SNPs) in linkage disequilibrium. Typically this would mean up to 50 SNPs, on current platforms. In these cases the increments should be significantly larger than the expected block size. It has been proved [9] that under certain strong conditions on the covariates, univariate correlation ranking is such that the top $o(n)$ variables include the active set with high probability, indicating an increment of order n.

Note that in cases where the cross-validation curve for the full data is multimodal, our algorithm may choose a local minimum between λ^* and λ_{max}. This would give a more parsimonious solution compared to the solution in λ^*. It is easy to change the stopping rule for example by continuing beyond the found minimum, to investigate if there is a change in the sign of the curvature soon after.

3 Results and Discussion

In the following two subsections, we study preselection and investigate the performances of our heuristics to find the optimal lasso solution and the possible gain in terms of the number of variables actually used. We first do this by simulation, and then turn to three genomic datasets of varying types and dimensions.

3.1 Simulation Study

In all experiments, we fit linear regression models with l_1 penalty using the R-package `glmnet` [10] and use tenfold cross-validation. Response data $\boldsymbol{y}$ were generated from $\boldsymbol{y} = \boldsymbol{X}\boldsymbol{\beta} + \boldsymbol{\epsilon}$, with $P = 10{,}000$ covariates for $n = 200$ samples and $\boldsymbol{\epsilon} \sim N(0, \sigma^2\boldsymbol{I})$. Unless otherwise stated, we chose ten variables uniformly at random and assigned half of them coefficient values equal to 2 and half of them coefficient values equal to -2. Two typical levels for the signal to noise ratio were considered; $SNR = 0.5$ and $SNR = 2$. As initial ranking we use the univariate correlation between each variable and the outcome.

The covariate data $\boldsymbol{X}$ were generated in various ways with different correlation structures. For each setting A–F a total of 100 simulations of $\boldsymbol{y}$ were generated for each $\boldsymbol{X}$:

A *Independent features.* Covariates were simulated independently from the standard normal distribution.

B *Blocks of Toeplitz correlated features.* The covariates were simulated according to a multivariate standard normal distribution with variables correlated in blocks of 100 covariates. Within each block the pairwise correlation between the jth and the kth covariate is given by $\rho^{|j-k|}$ with $\rho = 0.9$. Between blocks we simulated independently.

C *Blocks of equally correlated features.* The covariates were simulated in blocks of 500 covariates. Each block was simulated according to a multivariate standard normal distribution with an equal pairwise correlation 0.6 within each block and independent between blocks. The nonzero regression coefficients are this time assigned to variables in ten different blocks.

D *SNP-like features.* We used $P = 10{,}000$ SNPs (each taking three values) from a real GWAS-study to maintain a realistic correlation structure in $\boldsymbol{X}$.

E *Two equal blocks of equally correlated features.* Covariates were simulated in two blocks of 5000 covariates. Each block was generated according to a multivariate standard normal distribution with an equal pairwise correlation 0.6 within each block and independent between the two blocks. Five variables from one block were assigned nonzero coefficient values of magnitude 0.2 and five variables from the other block were assigned coefficient values of magnitude 2

F *Two unequal blocks.* The covariate data $\boldsymbol{X} = (\boldsymbol{X}_a, \boldsymbol{X}_b)$, where $\boldsymbol{X}_a$ is an $n \times p_a$ matrix, and $\boldsymbol{X}_b$ is an $n \times p_b$ matrix with $p_a = 5$ and $p_b = 9995$ were generated according to

$$\boldsymbol{X}_a \sim N(\boldsymbol{0}, \boldsymbol{\Sigma}^a), \quad \text{with} \quad \boldsymbol{\Sigma}^a_{jk} = 0 \quad \forall j \neq k, \quad \boldsymbol{\Sigma}_{jj} = 1,$$

$$\boldsymbol{X}_b \sim N(\boldsymbol{0}, \boldsymbol{\Sigma}^b), \quad \text{with} \quad \boldsymbol{\Sigma}^b_{jk} = 0.6 \quad \forall j \neq k, \quad \boldsymbol{\Sigma}_{jj} = 1,$$

and independency between the two blocks $\boldsymbol{X}_a$ and $\boldsymbol{X}_b$. The vector of regression coefficients is $\boldsymbol{\beta} = (\boldsymbol{\beta}_a, \boldsymbol{\beta}_b)$, where $\boldsymbol{\beta}_a = (0.2, 0.2, 0.2, 0.2, 0.2)$ and $\boldsymbol{\beta}_b = (2, 2, 2, 2, 2, 0, \ldots, 0)$.

The unrealistic situations E and F are constructed in order to induce stopping of Algorithm Part 1 in a wrong minimum. Situations B and D mimic most realistic genomic examples.

3.1.1 How Many Variables Are Needed to Avoid Preselection Bias?

In this section we study when freezing happens, i.e. when the cross-validation curves are frozen down and beyond the global minimum in λ^*. We present the results for Scenario B and $SNR = 0.5$, while the results for some of the other scenarios are given in the Appendix 3.

Figure 2 shows that the optimal number of variables selected from the full data by the lasso with cross-validation, varied from 0 to 264 in 100 simulations of $\boldsymbol{y}$ for the same $\boldsymbol{X}$, while the true number of nonzero coefficients was actually only 10. As expected, the smallest number of variables needed for freezing in λ^*, increases in parallel with the number of variables selected by the lasso. The reason is that when the number of variables in the lasso solution increases, we have to go further down on the list of ranked variables to include all of them in a C_p set, see Table 1. To clarify this, we divided the simulation runs into three groups based on the analysis of the full data sets: the lasso selects few, ≤ 20, the lasso selects many $(20, 80)$, the lasso selects very many, ≥ 80. When the lasso selects few variables (38 out of 100 experiments), on average only less than 3 % of the 10,000 covariates are required to be frozen in the true optimal value λ^*.

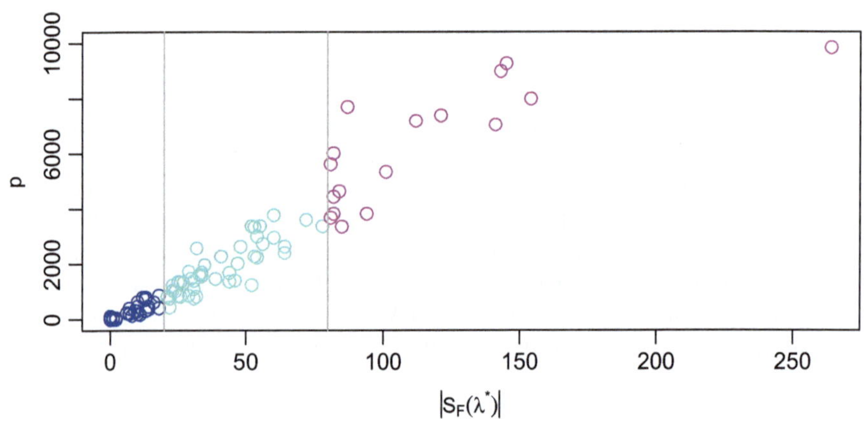

Fig. 2 Relation between size of lasso solution and smallest freezing size. Plot of the number of nonzero regression coefficients in the lasso vs. the smallest freezing size p in λ^* for 100 simulations for the same one $\boldsymbol{X}$ in Scenario B. We see that the number of variables needed increases with the size of the lasso set $S_F(\lambda^*)$. Situations where the lasso selects few (≤ 20), many (between 20 and 80 variables) or very many (≥ 80) are indicated by the *vertical lines*

Table 1 Results for 100 experiments of Fig. 2

Group	# exp.	$\# \hat{\beta} \neq 0$	% of data needed
≤20	38	6.13 (6.10)	2.54 (2.61)
[21, 79]	45	40.33 (14.96)	18.68 (9.07)
≥80	17	114.06 (46.75)	62.51 (21.08)

The number of experiments in each group is reported together with the average number of covariates selected by the lasso, and the gain of our method, reported as the percentage of the data (number of variables) needed before the cross-validation curve is frozen in λ^*. The latter two columns report averages within each group with standard deviations given in parentheses

In the second group of experiments (45 out of 100 simulation runs) all runs have a nicely behaved unimodal cross-validation curve for the full solution and freezing needs on average only 19 % of the variables. When the lasso selects very many variables (17 out of 100 experiments), the cross-validation curves need more variables to be frozen in the global minimum at λ^* (on average 63 % as in Table 1), and in some few situations we must include almost all of the covariates before it would be frozen in λ^*.

The results for the other scenarios given in Appendix 3 are similar, indicating a strong dependence between the smallest number of variables needed for the curves to be frozen in λ^* and how many variables the lasso would select on the full set.

3.1.2 Detecting Freezing: Performance of Algorithm

In this section we investigate how our algorithm finds the optimal full lasso solution that would have been obtained using all variables, based on a smaller number of preselected covariates. Unless otherwise stated, we use increments of 1000 variables in both the sequence of p and for $\tilde{p}$ in the algorithm.

The output $(\lambda^*_{p_m}, \hat{\boldsymbol{\beta}}_{C_{pm}})$ of the algorithm is either (a) the correct full solution or (b) it corresponds to a local minimum of the full cross-validation curve, or (c) it is a false solution caused by erroneous stopping of the algorithm. We report how frequent each such type of solution is in each scenario. If the minimum of the full cross-validation curve is in λ_{max}, or if the cross-validation curves do not freeze far enough before all variables are included, all variables will be included before the algorithm stops. For each situation A–F, in Tables 2 and 3 we report results as follows:

Column 3 number of simulations with λ_{max} (empty model) as optimal for the full data set, correctly identified by the algorithm.

Column 4 number of simulations for which the cross-validation curves do not freeze until $p = P$; no preselection possible with our ranking.

Table 2 Results using the single ordering Algorithm Part 1 based on 100 independent simulations in each scenario

Scenario	SNR	Min. in λ_{max}	No freezing before $p = P$	Stops in first local minimum	Correct solution	False solution
A	0.5	40	0	2	57	1
	2	0	0	2	94	4
B	0.5	13	0	11	76	0
	2	0	6	5	85	4
C	0.5	0	24	3	68	5
	2	0	54	4	37	5
D	0.5	11	1	2	85	1
	2	0	1	1	91	7
E	0.5	0	0	0	2	98
	2	0	17	3	9	71
F	0.5	0	0	7	23	70
	2	0	6	7	21	66

Table 3 Results using the repeated ordering Algorithm Part 2 based on 100 independent simulations in each scenario

Scenario	SNR	Min. in λ_{max}	No freezing before $p = P$	Stops in first local min.	Correct solution	False solution
A	0.5	40	0	2	57	1
	2	0	0	2	97	1
B	0.5	13	1	11	75	0
	2	0	11	5	84	0
C	0.5	0	24	3	73	0
	2	0	60	3	37	0
D	0.5	11	1	2	85	1
	2	0	4	1	95	0
E	0.5	0	6	9	85	0
	2	0	28	6	66	0
F	0.5	0	0	11	89	0
	2	0		13	81	0

Column 5 number of simulations for which the algorithm stops in a local minimum of the cross-validation curves, instead than in λ^*.
Column 6 number of simulations for which the algorithm stops in the correct optimal full lasso solution, using less than P variables.
Column 7 number of simulations for which the algorithm stops in a false solution, leading to preselection bias.

We first consider the Algorithm Part 1. Table 2 shows that for the four first scenarios A–D, the full global solution is obtained in the majority of cases and the naive Algorithm Part 1 commits errors quite rarely. In contrast, for the two last settings E and F, the naive algorithm stops erroneously frequently. This is as expected because the data are explicitly constructed in order to provoke situations where Algorithm Part 1 would erroneously stop in a false solution. In general, when there are strong correlations within submatrices of the data matrix $\boldsymbol{X}$, the initial ranking based on marginal correlation with $\boldsymbol{y}$ typically does not capture quickly the active variables $S_F(\lambda^*)$ as these are often intermixed in the ordered list with correlated variables that are not relevant. If the increments in the sequence of p are smaller than the typical dimension of such blocks, the likelihood that Algorithm Part 1 will stop erroneously increases. For Scenario E and F, we have very large blocks of correlated variables such that including 1000 new variables in each step of Algorithm Part 1 is not enough and often causes the algorithm to stop in the wrong solution. It is not easy to find examples where erroneous stopping of Algorithm Part 1 happens frequently, without considering situations like E and F where there is a strong degree of linear dependency within large submatrices of the design matrix. Indeed these settings represent situations where the irrepresentable condition [4] on the design matrix $\boldsymbol{X}$ is violated, and therefore lasso in itself is not consistent.

Now we consider the full algorithm with repeated ordering, see Table 3. Erroneous stopping of Algorithm Part 1 is what we want to avoid by the reordering step in Algorithm Part 2. Comparing Table 2 with Table 3 we observe that all erroneous stoppings in scenarios E and F are avoided, while only three occurrences of erroneous stopping remain (out of 1200 in total). These are probably a consequence of the choice of increments in the sequence for p, for which there is always a trade-off between the gain in efficiency of the algorithm and its safety. With larger increments in the sequence p_m we seldom commit mistakes, while small steps will decrease the number of variables needed though with larger chance of committing errors. In practice, large increments in the sequence of p_m will protect against false stopping of our Algorithm Part 2 and in most cases the naive Algorithm Part 1 will be sufficient to avoid preselection bias.

In Fig. 3 we study the impact of the increments in the sequence of p_m for the algorithm, applied to Scenario B. We choose increments equal to $+100$, $+200$, $+500$ and $+1000$. In the left panels the number of variables needed for the full algorithm to stop is plotted vs. the number of variables $|S_{p_m}(\lambda^*_{p_m})|$ that are selected. We color each simulation run as blue when the solution is correct, light green when the solution corresponds just to a local minimum and red when the solution is erroneous. We observe that the smaller the increments are, the earlier the algorithm stops and less variables are used. However, when the increments are small, the errors also become more frequent.

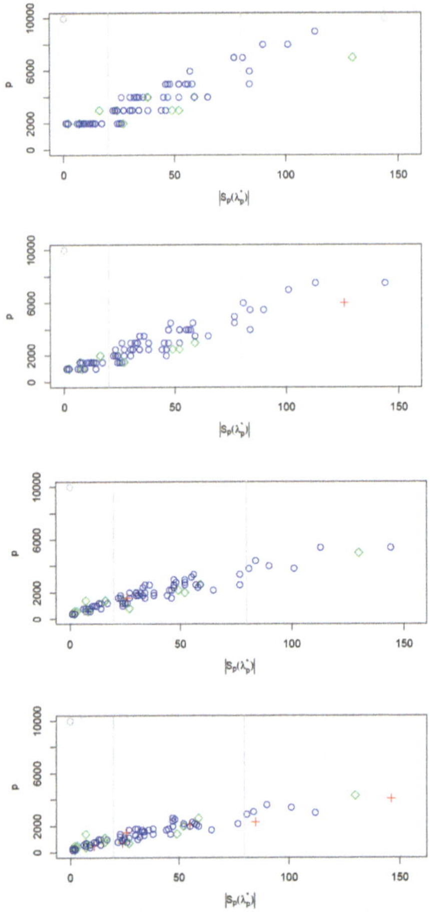

Step size in p-scheduling: 1000

	$[1, 20]$	$[21, 79]$	≥ 80
# exp.	28	51	8
% of variables needed	20.71 (2.62)	37.25 (11.68)	75.00 (16.04)

# of runs where false freezing occurs: 0

Step size in p-scheduling: 500

	$[1, 20]$	$[21, 79]$	≥ 80
# exp.	30	49	8
% of variables needed	12.67 (3.14)	28.78 (8.93)	61.25 (11.88)

# of runs where false freezing occurs: 1

Step size in p-scheduling: 200

	$[1, 20]$	$[21, 79]$	≥ 80
# exp.	31	49	7
% of variables needed	8.13 (3.26)	20.94 (6.18)	45.43 (7.18)

# of runs where false freezing occurs: 1

Step size in p-scheduling: 100

	$[1, 20]$	$[21, 79]$	≥ 80
# exp.	31	48	8
% of variables needed	6.19 (3.02)	16.04 (5.23)	33.38 (6.57)

# of runs where false freezing occurs: 6

Fig. 3 Performance of Algorithm Part 2 in Scenario B. Results using Algorithm Part 2 with reordering in Scenario B. *Left panel*: the number of nonzero regression coefficients returned by the Algorithm Part 2 vs. the number of covariates needed before our algorithm stops, is plotted for increments +1000, +500, +200 and +100 respectively. The type of minimum found is indicated: correct full solution (*blue circle*), full local solution (*green diamond*), false solution (*red plus symbol*) or no solution (*black circle*). *Vertical lines* indicate situations where few ($\leq$20), many (between 20 and 80 variables) or very many ($\geq$80) variables were selected. *Right panel*: The number of experiments in each group, the number of covariates needed with standard deviations given in parenthesis and the number of false solutions. Runs where lasso on all covariates has empty solution are omitted (13 cases)

3.2 Genomic Case Studies

In this section we illustrate the suggested preselection strategy on the analysis of three genomic data sets. The first example illustrates our approach in a standard high-dimensional linear regression setting with approximately 22,000 predictors, where the aim is to find a predictive signature. The second example is an example of a GWAS analysis where the covariate matrix is of even higher dimensions, with 800,000 predictors, 4000 patients and a binary response. The third example is a truly ultra-high dimensional situation where we have included all pairwise gene-gene interactions, resulting in more than 260 million predictors. In the last two cases, we are not able to obtain the full lasso solution using standard implementations.

3.2.1 Bone Biopsy Data: Body Mass Index

In this example we demonstrate our approach on data previously studied in [15]. The data contain gene expression measurements of 22,815 genes for 84 women's trans-iliacal bone biopsies. The data were already normalized as described in [15]. As response we consider the body mass index (BMI) which is continuous, calling for linear regression and the marginal correlation is used to order the gene expressions.

The cross-validation curves for subsets constructed based on the initial ranking are plotted in Fig. 4. Applying the Algorithm Part 1, a minimum is found at $\log(\lambda) \approx$

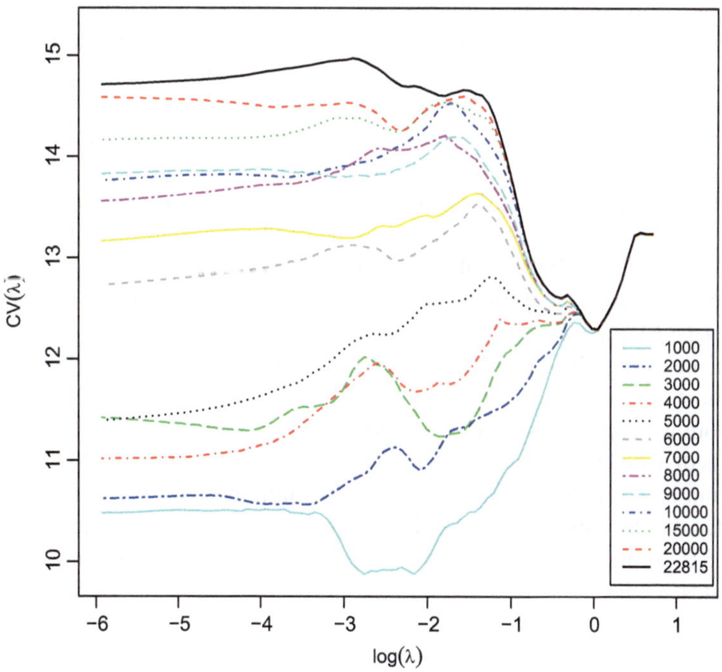

Fig. 4 Curves for example 1, Bone biopsy data—BMI response. Cross-validation curves for the bone biopsy example with 22,815 covariates and BMI response. The cross-validation criterion is the prediction mean squared error and the curves correspond to subsets determined from the initial ranking based on marginal correlation with the response and with fixed increments +1000. The *black curve* is the cross-validation curve for the full data set. We see that the curves for $p = 2000$ and $p = 3000$ are identical in an interval which includes the minimum at $\log(\lambda) \approx 0.05$ and this minimum is also confirmed by the repeated ordering as in Part 2 of the algorithm

0.05 for $p = 2000$ and $p = 3000$ covariates. The same minimum is also found after reordering according to Algorithm Part 2 and since we can run lasso on all covariates in this case, we can confirm that the solution was the correct one. Thus, we obtain the same lasso solution, with nine nonzero coefficients, as for all of the data, by using only 13 % of the covariates.

3.2.2 Parkinson's Disease Data

This example is an illustration of our approach to preselection in the logistic regression setting with a binary response, where $l(\beta_0, \boldsymbol{\beta})$ in (1) is replaced by the log-likelihood function for the logistic regression model and the binomial deviance is used as criterion in the cross-validation.

We consider the publicly available dataset of a recent genome-wide association study (GWAS) performed on 2000 individuals with Parkinson's disease and 1986 controls [12] (http://www.ncbi.nlm.nih.gov/gap, dbGaP Study Acc: phs000196.v2.p1). The genetic data contained initially a list of 1,012,895 single nucleotide polymorphisms (SNPs). This list was further reduced to 811,917 SNPs by applying standard quality controls criteria: SNPs with a minor allele frequency less than 0.01, a genotype call rate less than 99 % or in Hardy Weinberg disequilibrium ($p < 10^{-6}$) were excluded from the analysis.

The plot in Fig. 5 shows the cross-validation curves for eight increasing subsets of the covariates when they are initially ordered based on p-values testing univariate association of each covariate with the response. Applying our algorithm, the minimum at $log(\lambda) \approx -3.61$ is found already for $p = 20{,}000$. This corresponds to 103 variables selected by the lasso and the solution is confirmed after reordering and adding $\tilde{p} = 5000$ variables as in the Algorithm Part 2. Note that since we use the logistic regression model the variables are reordered according to $|[\boldsymbol{y} - \{p(\hat{\beta}_0, \hat{\boldsymbol{\beta}})\}]^T \boldsymbol{x}_j|$ when $p(\hat{\beta}_0, \hat{\boldsymbol{\beta}})$ is the logistic function with the current estimated coefficients, using the covariates in $C_{20{,}000}$, inserted. More than 800,000 covariates for almost 4000 samples cannot be processed in a straightforward manner in R. Therefore we compare with $p = 400{,}000$, which is easily treated when $n = 4000$. It seems that we have learned enough of the data already at $p = 20{,}000$ and that this minimum is likely to coincide with the global minimum for the full data set. This indicates that by using our approach, we are able to analyze the data based on less than 2.5 % of the covariates only, to recover the likely lasso solution of all 811,917 covariates, a huge gain.

3.2.3 Bone Biopsy Data with Interactions: Bone Mineral Density

In order to demonstrate how the freezing approach works for truly ultra huge data sets, we use the 22,815 gene expressions of the first example, and include all pairwise interactions in addition to main effects in the design matrix. This results in more than 260 million predictors in the linear regression model, a situation

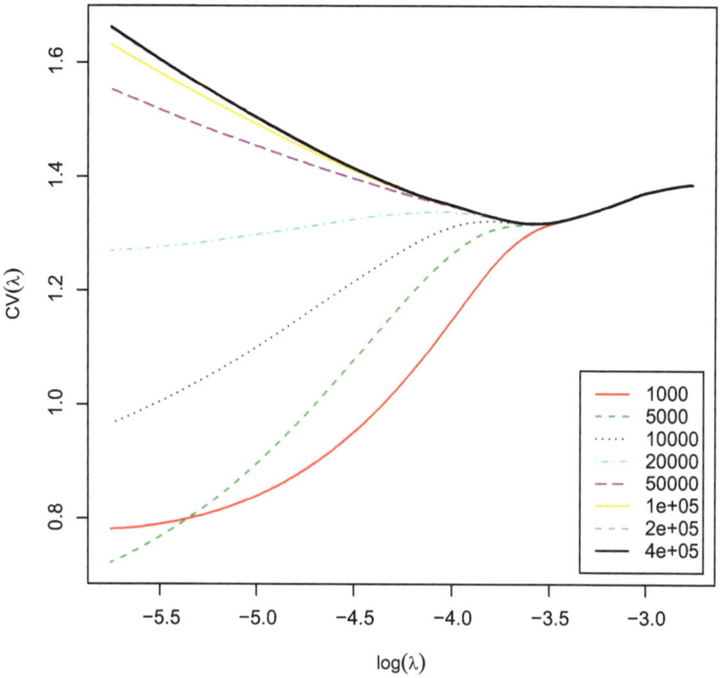

Fig. 5 Curves for example 2, Parkinson's disease data. Cross-validation curves for the big data example with 811,917 SNPs and a binary response. All of the curves in the figure correspond to subsets constructed based on the initial ranking. The *black curve* is the cross-validation curve for 400,000 covariates, which is approximately the maximum number we are able to run for in our standard R implementation. The criterion used in the cross-validation is the binomial deviance. We see that the curves coincide down and beyond a minimum already from $p = 20{,}000$. Here 103 variables are selected by the lasso. The full algorithm with repeated ordering confirms this minimum

that cannot be handled with any existing lasso software without some preselection procedure. The response in this example is bone mineral density (BMD), measured as explained in [15].

To make a simple ordering of both the main effects and pairwise interactions, we calculated the correlation of each of these predictors with the response. This gives an ordered list of more than 260 million elements. In this illustration we do not impose that main effects are selected together with the corresponding interaction terms as in [3]. Applying the Algorithm Part 1 to a sequence of top elements of this list, it seems that the cross-validation curves freeze already for three million elements. The cross-validation curves are plotted in Fig. 6. The solution for this minimum is a selected set of 30 interactions. We have run the algorithms up to ten million predictors. Due to memory limitations of R we cannot run the lasso on all the predictors in this case and thus check that this is the correct lasso solution. However, based on our extensive experiments, it is very likely that by using these preselected

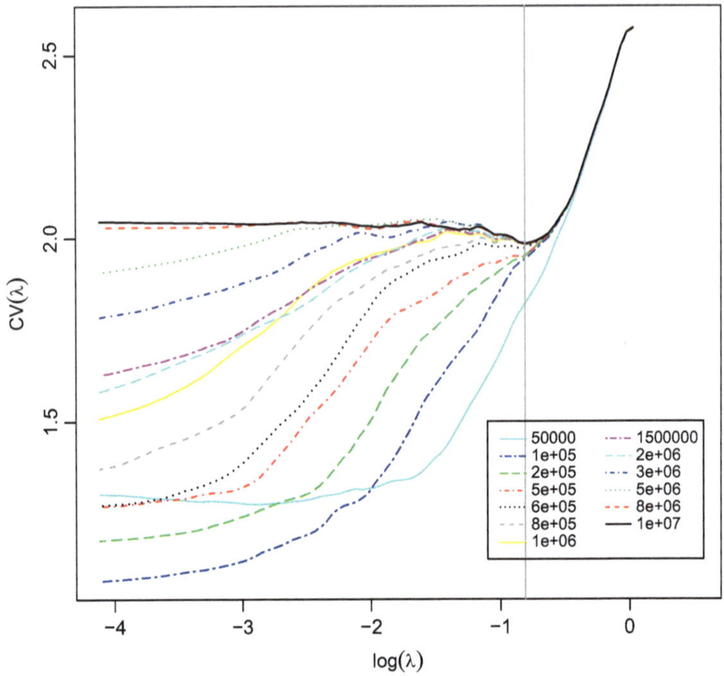

Fig. 6 Curves for example 3, Bone biopsy data—BMD response. Cross-validation curves for the bone biopsy example with more than 260 million predictors (22,815 covariates and all pairwise interactions) and BMD response. The cross-validation criterion is the prediction mean squared error and the curves correspond to subsets determined from the initial ranking based on marginal correlation of each predictor with the response and with increments as indicated in the *box*. The *black curve* is the cross-validation curve for ten million predictors. We see that the curves for $p = 2$ million and $p = 3$ million are identical in an interval which includes a minimum at and this minimum is also confirmed by the repeated ordering as in Part 2 of the algorithm

1.1 % of the 260 million predictors, we have found a close solution. In such an ultra high dimensional case, where some kind of preselection is mandatory, the concept of freezing is especially useful and powerful.

4 Conclusions

We propose a new approach to avoid preselection bias, based on an algorithm which exploits freezing of cross-validation curves and univariate orderings of the covariates. We discuss why our procedure will typically lead to the full lasso solution in a variety of genomic applications, also supported by extensive simulations.

The possible gain is impressive with less than 1.1 and 2.5 % of the variables needed in the huge genomic data examples in Sect. 3. Simulation results also show that we are able to reduce the number of covariates significantly, for example for Situation B we use typically about 20 % of the variables depending on the increments in the algorithm. Our algorithm exploits a simple property of the cross-validation curves, freezing, that has not been discussed before to the best of our knowledge. Freezing can be identified by successive reordering of the variables, and our sequential scheme stops in the vast majority of cases at the right solution if the step size in the p sequence is not too small.

In the simulation experiments, we saw that when the cross-validation curve is multimodal, very flat in an interval around the minimum or keeps decreasing when $\lambda \to 0$, the advantage of our approach is reduced. Other aspects that affect efficiency of our method are the sample size, and how the samples are allocated to the different folds in the cross-validation. It is important to make sure that samples are randomly allocated to the folds and to check if different splittings lead to different results. As this is a general issue of cross-validation we have not studied this in further detail, but stress that the division into folds, the number of folds and the sample size n influence performance. This is because all variables that are active within each single training set of the cross-validation are needed in the subset of covariates C_p before the curve is frozen.

The usefulness of our preselection rule relies on an initial ordering of the variables such that all covariates active in the cross-validation folds, for an interval of λ that reveals the minimum, are included in C_p for a small p. An optimal ordering would be one reflecting the lasso behavior; in practice we look for an approximation of such a ranking based on simple univariate computations. In the case of linear regression we used $|\boldsymbol{y}^T\boldsymbol{x}_j|$ or inner product with partial residuals. For generalized linear models, variables can be ranked based on p-values testing univariate association between the covariates and the response. The univariate sorting of the P covariates has a worst case computational complexity of $O(P \log P)$. Preselection based on the univariate association between outcome and covariates has been used often previously. For example it has been suggested to use it as a preliminary step to supervised principal components analysis [2] or in marginal regression thresholding [11].

Our approach computes a level of preselection which is likely to avoid bias. It is also well defined for cross-validation curves based on deviance and area under the roc curve (AUC) and suitable for methods like the relaxed lasso [14], the first step of the adaptive lasso [4, 24], elastic net [25] and the group lasso [23], among others.

In summary, we have demonstrated that a simple external preselection scheme based on univariate ordering of the variables and the freezing patterns of cross-validation curves in λ and p, can be used to recover the lasso solution based on all covariates. This is an important step in the feasible implementation of penalized regression for ultra high-dimensional data.

Software Availability

An R code is available at http://folk.uio.no/glad/cvfreezing/.

Acknowledgements This research was supported by grant number 204664 from the Norwegian Research Council (NRC) and by Statistics for Innovation $(\text{sfi})^2$, a centre for research based innovation funded by NRC. SR and LCB spent a research period in Paris at Inserm UMRS937, and SR has an adjunct position at $(\text{sfi})^2$. IA was funded by a grant from the Agence Nationale de la Recherche (ANR Maladies neurologiques et maladies psychiatriques) as part of a project on the relation between Parkinson's disease and genes involved in the metabolism and transport of xenobiotics (PI: Alexis Elbaz, Inserm) for which access to GWAS data was obtained through dbGAP; this work utilized in part data from the NINDS DbGaP database from the CIDR:NGRC PARKINSONS DISEASE STUDY (Accession: phs000196.v2.p1). Sjur Reppe at Ullevaal University Hospital provided the Bone biopsy data.

Appendix 1

Proof 1 (Proof of (3a) and (3b)) Fix λ, and drop it from the notation for simplicity. Let

$$f_{C_p}(\boldsymbol{\beta}_{C_p}) = \sum_{i=1}^{n}(y_i - \sum_{j\in C_p} x_{ij}\beta_{j,C_p})^2 + \lambda \sum_{j\in C_p} |\beta_{j,C_p}|,$$

and similarly for $f_{C_F}(\boldsymbol{\beta}_{C_F})$. Given $\boldsymbol{\beta}_{C_p}$, we can form the vector in $\mathbb{R}^P$ with $|C_F \setminus C_p|$ zeros as $(\boldsymbol{\beta}_{C_p}, \boldsymbol{\beta}_{C_F\setminus C_p} = \mathbf{0})$. For such a vector it holds

$$f_{C_p}(\boldsymbol{\beta}_{C_p}) = f_{C_F}(\boldsymbol{\beta}_{C_p}, \boldsymbol{\beta}_{C_F\setminus C_p} = \mathbf{0}). \tag{6}$$

Next we show that the nonzero components of

$$\underset{\boldsymbol{\beta}_{C_p}}{\text{argmin}} f_{C_p}(\boldsymbol{\beta}_{C_p})$$

are the same as the nonzero components of

$$\underset{\boldsymbol{\beta}_{C_F}}{\text{argmin}} f_{C_F}(\boldsymbol{\beta}_{C_F})$$

when $S_F \subseteq C_p$. In fact, because $S_F \subseteq C_p$, we first have

$$\underset{\boldsymbol{\beta}_{C_p}}{\text{argmin}} f_{C_p}(\boldsymbol{\beta}_{C_p}) = \underset{\boldsymbol{\beta}_{S_F}, \boldsymbol{\beta}_{C_p\setminus S_F}}{\text{argmin}} f_{C_p}(\boldsymbol{\beta}_{S_F}, \boldsymbol{\beta}_{C_p\setminus S_F}).$$

Now we add some zero coefficients, such that

$$f_{C_p}(\boldsymbol{\beta}_{S_F}, \boldsymbol{\beta}_{C_p \setminus S_F}) = f_{C_F}(\boldsymbol{\beta}_{S_F}, \boldsymbol{\beta}_{C_p \setminus S_F}, \boldsymbol{\beta}_{C_F \setminus C_p} = \mathbf{0})$$

by (6). Hence

$$\underset{\boldsymbol{\beta}_{C_p}}{\operatorname{argmin}} f_{C_p}(\boldsymbol{\beta}_{C_p}) = \underset{\boldsymbol{\beta}_{S_F}, \boldsymbol{\beta}_{C_p \setminus S_F}}{\operatorname{argmin}} f_{C_F}(\boldsymbol{\beta}_{S_F}, \boldsymbol{\beta}_{C_p \setminus S_F}, \boldsymbol{\beta}_{C_F \setminus C_p} = \mathbf{0}). \tag{7}$$

When we minimize $f_{C_F}(\boldsymbol{\beta}_{C_F})$, we know that for the solution $\hat{\boldsymbol{\beta}}_{C_F \setminus C_p} = \mathbf{0}$. Hence we can drop the constraint that $\boldsymbol{\beta}_{C_F \setminus C_p} = \mathbf{0}$ in (7) and minimize over $\boldsymbol{\beta}_{C_F \setminus C_p}$ also, without making any difference. We obtain that the nonzero components of

$$\underset{\boldsymbol{\beta}_{C_p}}{\operatorname{argmin}} f_{C_p}(\boldsymbol{\beta}_{C_p})$$

are the same as the nonzero components of

$$\underset{\boldsymbol{\beta}_{S_F}, \boldsymbol{\beta}_{C_p \setminus S_F}, \boldsymbol{\beta}_{C_F \setminus C_p}}{\operatorname{argmin}} f_{C_F}(\boldsymbol{\beta}_{S_F}, \boldsymbol{\beta}_{C_p \setminus S_F}, \boldsymbol{\beta}_{C_F \setminus C_p}) = \underset{\boldsymbol{\beta}_{C_F}}{\operatorname{argmin}} f_{C_F}(\boldsymbol{\beta}_{C_F}).$$

Let

$$\hat{\boldsymbol{\beta}}_{C_F} = \underset{\boldsymbol{\beta}_{C_F}}{\operatorname{argmin}} f_{C_F}(\boldsymbol{\beta}_{C_F}).$$

Then for $j \in S_F$, $\hat{\boldsymbol{\beta}}_{j,C_F} \neq 0$. Therefore since the nonzero components of

$$\underset{\boldsymbol{\beta}_{C_p}}{\operatorname{argmin}} f_{C_p}(\boldsymbol{\beta}_{C_p})$$

are the same as the nonzero components of

$$\underset{\boldsymbol{\beta}_{C_F}}{\operatorname{argmin}} f_{C_F}(\boldsymbol{\beta}_{C_F})$$

when $S_F \subseteq C_p$, also $\hat{\boldsymbol{\beta}}_{j,C_p} \neq 0$. The opposite is also true: if $\hat{\boldsymbol{\beta}}_{j,C_p} \neq 0$, then $j \in S_F$ and $\hat{\boldsymbol{\beta}}_{j,C_F} \neq 0$. Similarly for $j \notin S_F$. This proves that

(a) $S_p(\lambda) = S_F(\lambda) \quad \forall p \geq p_0(\lambda)$,
(b) $\hat{\beta}_{j,C_p}(\lambda) = \hat{\beta}_{j,C_F}(\lambda), \quad \forall p \geq p_0(\lambda), \forall j$.

Proof 2 (Proof of (4) and (5)) For fixed λ we have that if

$$p_1 \geq p_{0,cv}(\lambda) = \max_{k=1,\ldots,K} p_{0,k}(\lambda),$$

then

$$p_1 \geq p_{0,k}(\lambda) \quad \forall k.$$

By (3a) and (3b) it follows that for all $p_2 > p_1 \geq p_{0,k}(\lambda)$ and $\forall k$

$$S_{p_1}^{-k}(\lambda) = S_{p_2}^{-k}(\lambda) = S_F^{-k}(\lambda) \tag{8}$$

and

$$\hat{\beta}_{j,C_{p_1}}^{-k}(\lambda) = \hat{\beta}_{j,C_{p_2}}^{-k}(\lambda), \quad \forall j \in S_F^{-k}(\lambda). \tag{9}$$

Then

$$\begin{aligned}
\hat{y}_{i,C_{p_2}}^{-k}(\lambda) &= \sum_{j \in C_{p_2}} x_{ij} \hat{\beta}_{j,C_{p_2}}^{-k}(\lambda) \\
&= \sum_{j \in S_{p_2}^{-k}(\lambda)} x_{ij} \hat{\beta}_{j,C_{p_2}}^{-k}(\lambda) + \sum_{j \notin S_{p_2}^{-k}(\lambda)} x_{ij} \hat{\beta}_{j,C_{p_2}}^{-k}(\lambda) \qquad (10) \\
&= \sum_{j \in S_{p_2}^{-k}(\lambda)} x_{ij} \hat{\beta}_{j,C_{p_2}}^{-k}(\lambda) \\
&= \sum_{j \in S_{p_1}^{-k}(\lambda)} x_{ij} \hat{\beta}_{j,C_{p_2}}^{-k}(\lambda) \qquad (11) \\
&= \sum_{j \in S_{p_1}^{-k}(\lambda)} x_{ij} \hat{\beta}_{j,C_{p_1}}^{-k}(\lambda), \qquad (12)
\end{aligned}$$

because the last term in (10) is zero and the two last equalities in (11) and (12) follows from (8) and (9) respectively. Similarly we have

$$\hat{y}_{i,C_{p_1}}^{-k}(\lambda) = \sum_{j \in S_{p_1}^{-k}(\lambda)} x_{ij} \hat{\beta}_{j,C_{p_1}}^{-k}(\lambda),$$

so that $\hat{y}_{i,C_{p_1}}^{-k}(\lambda) = \hat{y}_{i,C_{p_2}}^{-k}(\lambda)$ holds $\forall i$. Finally this implies $CV_{C_{p_1}}(\lambda) = CV_{C_{p_2}}(\lambda) = CV_{C_F}(\lambda)$ and hereby (5).

Appendix 2

We collect here some further arguments which lead to the reordering of the Part 2 of our algorithm. Consider two consecutive cross-validation curves for C_{p_m} and $C_{p_{m+1}}$, and assume that the two curves coincide in an interval $\tilde{\Lambda} = [\tilde{\lambda}, \lambda_{max}]$ which includes a minimum in $\lambda^*_{p_m} > \tilde{\lambda}$. Part 1 of our algorithm would stop with p_m variables and return the solution $S_{p_m}(\lambda^*_{p_m})$. By definition of freezing, if $S^{-k}_{p_{m+1}}(\lambda) \subseteq C_{p_m}$ for all folds k and for all $\lambda \in \tilde{\Lambda}$, then the two curves for C_{p_m} and $C_{p_{m+1}}$ are identical in $\lambda^*_{p_m}$ and in all other values of $\lambda \in \tilde{\Lambda}$. Nevertheless $S_F(\lambda^*)$ might not be included in C_{p_m}, and hence $S_{p_m}(\lambda^*_{p_m})$ is not the correct solution for the full data set. If on the contrary, there are some variables that are active in the cross-validation for $C_{p_{m+1}}$ that are not in C_{p_m}, that is for any k, $S^{-k}_{p_{m+1}}(\lambda^*_{p_m}) \not\subset C_{p_m}$, then the two curves would not coincide down and beyond $\lambda^*_{p_m}$ and hence the algorithm would not erroneously stop. Therefore the sequence of preselected sets should be such that, while waiting for $S_F(\lambda^*)$ to be included in a C_{p_m} (at which point the curves cannot change anymore in the minimum), the new active set $S_{p_{m+1}}(\lambda^*_{p_m})$ in the current minimum $\lambda^*_{p_m}$ includes typically some new variables which were not in the previous set C_{p_m}. This leads to the idea of *sequential reordering* once we have found a first "local point of freezing". The idea of Part 2 of our algorithm follows this line, and greedily constructs the new next set $C_{p_{m+1}}$ by introducing new variables which have a high chance to be in $S_{p_{m+1}}(\lambda^*_{p_m})$. This is done by reordering the unused variables based on the residuals $\boldsymbol{r}$, computed using the selected variables $S_{p_m}(\lambda^*_{p_m})$.

Appendix 3

Further details from the simulation studies are summarized here. First, we consider the linear regression model as described in the main manuscript, while results from experiments using a logistic regression model are reported thereafter.

Linear Regression Model

The results are reported for Scenario A, B and D and the data are generated as described in Sect. 3 in the main manuscript. We investigate how many variables are needed to avoid the preselection bias.

Comparing Scenario A, B and D, we see that freezing can be very useful not only in situations with no correlation among the covariates, but also in situations where the covariates are correlated. The results are quite similar, with a small advantage when the covariates are generated independently. This is possibly because the marginal correlation ranking captures the true nonzero coefficients earlier when there is little correlation among the covariates.

For all three scenarios, we observe that when models of less noise are considered (*SNR* $\approx$ 2), there are practically no situations for which the lasso selects less than 20 variables. When *SNR* $\approx$ 0.5 there are more situations where the cross-validation curves have well-defined minima leading to a smaller number of selected variables, hence there is a greater advantage of using our approach in these situations. For example for the situations where the lasso selects less than 80 variables, the largest gain is observed when *SNR* $\approx$ 0.5, where the average % of data needed to recover the optimal solution is not more than 15 %, 19 % and 15 % for the three different scenarios respectively.

Scenario A (Table 4 and Fig. 7)

Table 4 Results from 100 experiments of Scenario A

	$P = 10{,}000$					
	SNR 0.5			SNR 2		
Group	# exp.	# $\hat{\beta} \neq 0$	Data needed (%)	# exp.	# $\hat{\beta} \neq 0$	Data needed (%)
≤20	72	3.38 (5.38)	1.45 (2.06)	0	– (–)	– (–)
[21, 79]	22	43.60 (17.41)	14.04 (11.70)	31	62.94 (10.23)	24.45 (7.72)
≥80	6	139.83 (51.67)	42.89 (24.99)	69	110.29 (20.40)	46.98 (12.78)

The number of experiments in each group is reported together with the average number of covariates selected by the lasso and the percentage of the data needed before the cross-validation curves are frozen down and below the global minimum. The latter two measures are reported as averages within each group with standard deviations given in parentheses

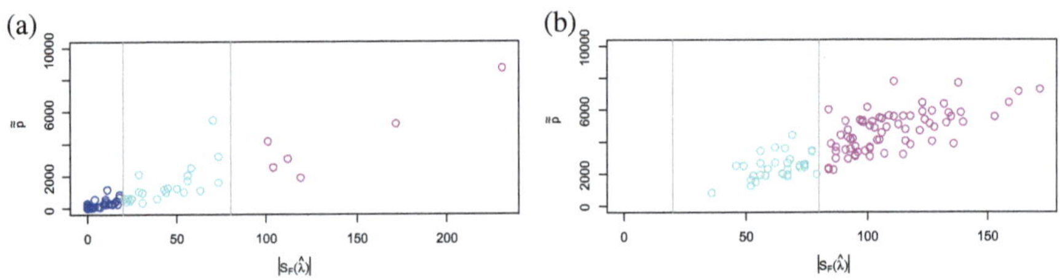

Fig. 7 Scenario A: Plot of number of nonzero regression coefficients in the lasso vs. $\tilde{\tilde{p}}$, where $\tilde{\tilde{p}}$ is the smallest p for which the curves are frozen in the optimal λ denoted by $\hat{\lambda}$. The results are for 100 replications and different choices of *SNR*, and situations where the lasso selects few (≤20), many (between 20 and 80 variables) or very many (≥80) are indicated by the *grey vertical lines*. (**a**) $P = 10{,}000$, $SNR = 0.5$; (**b**) $P = 10{,}000$, $SNR = 2$

Scenario B (Table 5 and Fig. 8)

Table 5 Results from 100 experiments of Scenario B

	$P = 10{,}000$					
	SNR 0.5			SNR 2		
Group	# exp.	# $\hat{\beta} \neq 0$	Data needed (%)	# exp.	# $\hat{\beta} \neq 0$	Data needed (%)
$\leq$20	38	6.13 (6.10)	2.54 (2.61)	0	– (–)	– (–)
[21, 79]	45	40.33 (14.96)	18.68 (9.07)	54	64.04 (12.20)	50.23 (14.00)
$\geq$80	17	114.06 (46.75)	62.51 (21.08)	46	108.83 (31.36)	79.06 (13.82)

The number of experiments in each group is reported together with the average number of covariates selected by the lasso and the percentage of the data needed before the cross-validation curves are frozen down and below the global minimum. The latter two measures are reported as averages within each group with standard deviations given in parentheses

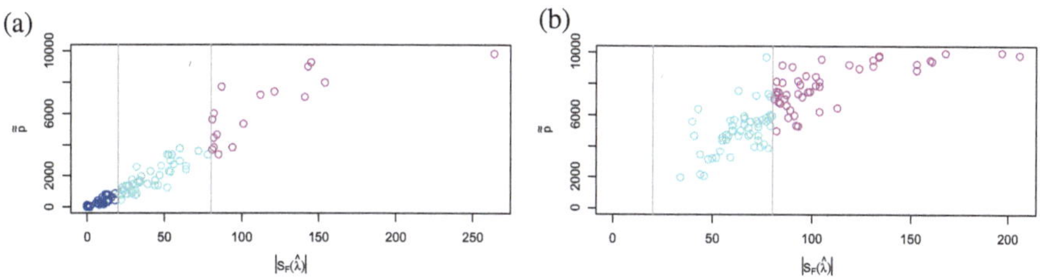

Fig. 8 Scenario B: Plot of number of nonzero regression coefficients in the lasso vs. $\tilde{\tilde{p}}$, where $\tilde{\tilde{p}}$ is the smallest p for which the curves are frozen in the optimal λ denoted by $\hat{\lambda}$. The results are for 100 replications and different choices of *SNR*, and situations where the lasso selects few ($\leq$20), many (between 20 and 80 variables) or very many ($\geq$80) are indicated by the *grey vertical lines*. (**a**) $P = 10{,}000$, $SNR = 0.5$; (**b**) $P = 10{,}000$, $SNR = 2$

Scenario D (Table 6 and Fig. 9)

Table 6 Results from 100 experiments of Scenario D

	$P = 10{,}000$					
	SNR 0.5			SNR 2		
Group	# exp.	# $\hat{\beta} \neq 0$	Data needed (%)	# exp.	# $\hat{\beta} \neq 0$	Data needed (%)
$\leq$20	45	7.64 (6.84)	3.90 (6.24)	0	– (–)	– (–)
[21, 79]	48	39.10 (14.76)	14.38 (8.41)	60	55.52 (14.20)	39.09 (14.76)
>80	7	123.29 (42.32)	46.34 (22.51)	40	109.60 (27.62)	71.80 (16.94)

The number of experiments in each group is reported together with the average number of covariates selected by the lasso and the percentage of the data needed before cross-validation curves are frozen down and below the global minimum. The latter two measures are reported as averages within each group with standard deviations given in parentheses

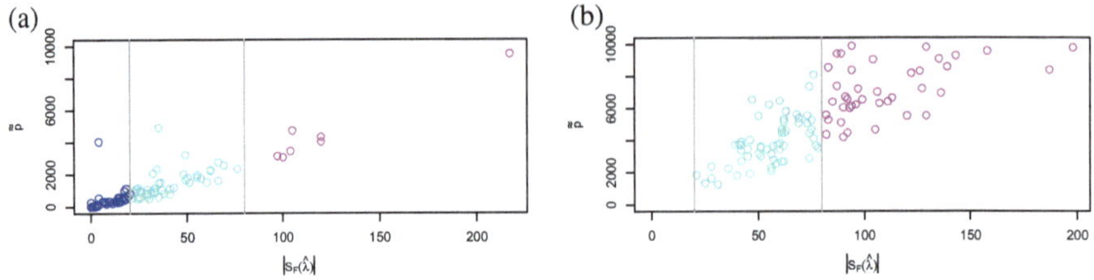

Fig. 9 Scenario D: Plot of number of nonzero regression coefficients in the lasso vs. $\tilde{\tilde{p}}$, where $\tilde{\tilde{p}}$ is the smallest p for which the curves are frozen in the optimal λ denoted by $\hat{\lambda}$. The results are for 100 replications and different choices of *SNR*, and situations where the lasso selects few (≤20), many (between 20 and 80 variables) or very many (≥80) are indicated by the *grey vertical lines*. (**a**) $P = 10{,}000$, $SNR = 0.5$; (**b**) $P = 10{,}000$, $SNR = 2$

Table 7 Results from 100 experiments with continuous correlated features in a logistic regression model with a binary response

	$P = 10{,}000$		
Group	# exp.	# $\hat{\beta} \neq 0$	Data needed (%)
≤20	0	– (–)	– (–)
(21,79)	57	60.74 (13.65)	46.09 (16.47)
≥80	43	90.91 (6.89)	67.05 (17.98)

The number of experiments in each group is reported together with the average number of covariates selected by the lasso and the percentage of the data needed before cross-validation curves are frozen down and below the global minimum. The latter two measures are reported as averages within each group with standard deviation given in parentheses

Logistic Regression Model

Finally we do one experiment of 100 replications with a binary response. For simplicity, in this experiment we only consider the covariate matrix generated as in Scenario B and with $P = 10{,}000$. Results are summarized in Table 7 and Fig. 10. Here we also observe situations where the cross-validated optimal solution is not well-defined and the lasso selects very many. Nevertheless in 57 out of 100 experiments the curves will be frozen down and below the minimum in λ^* for less than 50 % of the data. In several cases it happens already for 20–30 % of the data.

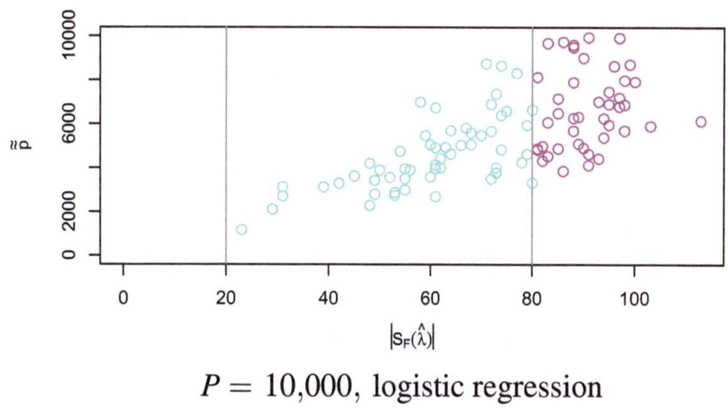

Fig. 10 Plot of number of nonzero regression coefficients in the lasso vs. $\tilde{\tilde{p}}$, where $\tilde{\tilde{p}}$ is the smallest p for which the curves are frozen in the optimal λ denoted by $\hat{\lambda}$, in the example using logistic regression. The results are reported for 100 replications, and situations where the lasso selects few ($\leq$20), many (between 20 and 80 variables) or very many ($\geq$80) are indicated by the *grey vertical lines*

References

1. Ambroise, C., McLachlan, G.J.: Selection bias in gene extraction on the basis of microarray gene-expression data. Proc. Natl. Acad. Sci. **99**(10), 6562–6566 (2002)
2. Bair, E., Hastie, T., Paul, D., Tibshirani, R.: Prediction by supervised principal components. J. Am. Stat. Assoc. **101**(473), 119–137 (2006)
3. Bien, J., Taylor, J., Tibshirani, R.: A lasso for hierarchical testing of interactions. Ann. Stat. **41**(3), 1111–1141 (2013)
4. Bühlmann, P., van de Geer, S.: Statistics for High-Dimensional Data: Methods, Theory and Applications. Springer Series in Statistics. Springer, Berlin (2011)
5. Cantor, R.M., Lange, K., Sinsheimer, J.S.: Prioritizing GWAS results: a review of statistical methods and recommendations for their application. Am. J. Hum. Genet. **86**(1), 6–22 (2010)
6. Cho, S., Kim, K., Kim, Y.J., Lee, J.-K., Cho, Y.S., Lee, J.-Y., Han, B.-G., Kim, H., Ott, J., Park, T.: Joint identification of multiple genetic variants via elastic-net variable selection in a genome-wide association analysis. Ann. Hum. Genet. **74**(5), 416–428 (2010)
7. Efron, B., Hastie, T., Johnstone, I., Tibshirani, R.: Least angle regression. Ann. Stat. **32**, 407–499 (2004)
8. El Ghaoui, L., Viallon, V., Rabbani, T.: Safe feature elimination for the lasso and sparse supervised learning problems. ArXiv e-prints 1009.4219 (2011)
9. Fan, J., Lv, J.: Sure independence screening for ultrahigh dimensional feature space. J. R. Stat. Soc. Ser. B (Stat. Methodol.) **70**(5), 849–911 (2008)
10. Friedman, J., Hastie, T., Tibshirani, R.: Regularization paths for generalized linear models via coordinate descent. J. Stat. Softw. **33**(1), 1–22 (2010)
11. Genovese, C.R., Jin, J., Wasserman, L., Yao, Z.: A comparison of the lasso and marginal regression. J. Mach. Learn. Res. **13**(1), 2107–2143 (2012)
12. Hamza, T.H., Zabetian, C.P., Tenesa, A., Laederach, A., Montimurro, J., Yearout, D., Kay, D.M., Doheny, K.F., Paschall, J., Pugh, E., Kusel, V.I., Collura, R., Roberts, J., Griffith, A., Samii, A., Scott, W.K., Nutt, J., Factor, S.A., Payami, H.: Common genetic variation in the HLA region is associated with late-onset sporadic parkinsons disease. Nat. Genet. **42**(9), 781–785 (2010)

13. Hastie, T., Tibshirani, R., Friedman, J.: The Elements of Statistical Learning: Data Mining, Inference, and Prediction, 2nd edn. Springer Series in Statistics. Springer, New York (2009)
14. Meinshausen, N.: Relaxed lasso. Comput. Stat. Data Anal. **52**(1), 374–393 (2007)
15. Reppe, S., Refvem, H., Gautvik, V.T., Olstad, O.K., Høvring, P.I., Reinholt, F.P., Holden, M., Frigessi, A., Jemtland, R., Gautvik, K.M.: Eight genes are highly associated with BMD variation in postmenopausal caucasian women. Bone **46**(3), 604–612 (2010)
16. Simon, R.M., Korn, E.L., McShane, L.M., Radmacher, M.D., Wright, G.W., Zhao, Y.: Design and analysis of DNS microarray investigations. In: Statistics for Biology and Health. Springer, New York (2004)
17. Tibshirani, R.: Regression shrinkage and selection via the lasso. J. R. Stat. Soc. **58**, 267–288 (1996)
18. Tibshirani, R., Bien, J., Friedman, J., Hastie, T., Simon, N., Taylor, J., Tibshirani, R.J.: Strong rules for discarding predictors in lasso-type problems. J. R. Stat. Soc. Ser. B (Stat. Methodol.) **74**(2), 245–266 (2012)
19. van de Geer, S., Bühlmann, P., Zhou, S.: The adaptive and the thresholded lasso for potentially misspecified models (and a lower bound for the lasso). Electron. J. Stat. **5**, 688–749 (2011)
20. Waldmann, P., Mészáros, G., Gredler, B., Fuerst, C., Sölkner, J.: Evaluation of the lasso and the elastic net in genome-wide association studies. Frontiers in Genetics, **4**, 270. http://doi.org/10.3389/fgene.2013.00270 (2013)
21. Waldron, L., Pintilie, M., Tsao, M.-S., Shepherd, F.A., Huttenhower, C., Jurisica, I.: Optimized application of penalized regression methods to diverse genomic data. Bioinformatics **27**(24), 3399–3406 (2011)
22. Yang, C., Wan, X., Yang, Q., Xue, H., Yu, W.: Identifying main effects and epistatic interactions from large-scale snp data via adaptive group lasso. BMC Bioinf. **11**(Suppl. 1), S18 (2010)
23. Yuan, M., Lin, Y.: Model selection and estimation in regression with grouped variables. J. R. Stat. Soc. Ser. B **68**(1), 49–67 (2006)
24. Zou, H.: The adaptive lasso and its oracle properties. J. Am. Stat. Assoc. **101**(476), 1418–1429 (2006)
25. Zou, H., Hastie, T.: Regularization and variable selection via the elastic net. J. R. Stat. Soc. Ser. B (Stat. Methodol.) **67**(2), 301–320 (2005)

Spectral Clustering and Block Models: A Review and a New Algorithm

Sharmodeep Bhattacharyya and Peter J. Bickel

Abstract We focus on spectral clustering of unlabeled graphs and review some results on clustering methods which achieve weak or strong consistent identification in data generated by such models. We also present a new algorithm which appears to perform optimally both theoretically using asymptotic theory.

1 Introduction

Since its introduction in [14], spectral analysis of various matrices associated to groups has become one of the most widely used clustering techniques in statistics and machine learning.

In the context of unlabeled graphs, a number of methods, all of which come under the broad heading of spectral clustering have been proposed. These methods based on spectral analysis of adjacency matrices or some derived matrix such as one of the Laplacians [26, 27, 29, 30, 32] have been studied in connection with their effectiveness in identifying members of blocks in exchangeable graph block models. In this paper after introducing the methods and models, we intend to review some of the literature. We relate it to the results of Mossel et al. [24] and Massoulié [22], where it is shown that for very sparse models, there exists a phase transition below which members cannot be identified better than chance and also showed that above the phase transition one can do better using rather subtle methods. In [5] we develop a spectral clustering method based on the matrix of geodesic distances between nodes which can achieve the goals of the work we cited and in fact behaves well for all unlabeled networks, sparse, semi-sparse and dense. We give a statement and sketch the proof of these claims in [5] but give a full argument for the sparse case considered by the above authors only in this paper. We give the necessary

S. Bhattacharyya (✉)
Department of Statistics, Oregon State University, 44 Kidder Hall, Corvallis, OR, USA
e-mail: bhattash@science.oregonstate.edu

P.J. Bickel
Department of Statistics, University of California at Berkeley, 367 Evans Hall, Berkeley, CA, USA
e-mail: bickel@stat.berkeley.edu

A. Frigessi et al. (eds.), *Statistical Analysis for High-Dimensional Data*,
Abel Symposia 11, DOI 10.1007/978-3-319-27099-9_4

preliminaries in Sect. 2, more history in Sect. 3 and show the theoretical properties of the method in Sect. 4.

2 Preliminaries

There are many standard methods of clustering based on numerical similarity matrices which are discussed in a number of monographs (e.g., Hartigan [18], Leroy and Rousseeuw [28]). We shall not discuss these further. Our focus is on unlabeled graphs of n vertices characterized by adjacency matrices, $A = ||a_{ij}||$ for n data points, with $a_{ij} = 1$ if there is an edge between i and j and $a_{ij} = 0$ otherwise. The natural assumption then is, $A = A^T$. Our basic goal is to divide the points in K sets such that on some average criterion the points in a given subset are more similar to each other than to those of other subsets. Our focus is on methods of clustering based on the spectrum (eigenvalues and eigenvectors) of A or related matrices.

2.1 Notation and Formal Definition of Stochastic Block Model

Definition 1 A graph $G^K(B, (P, \boldsymbol{\pi}))$ generated from the **stochastic block model** (SBM) with K blocks and parameters $P \in (0, 1)^{K \times K}$ and $\boldsymbol{\pi} \in (0, 1)^K$ can be defined in following way—each vertex of graph G_n is assigned to a community $\boldsymbol{c} \in \{1, \ldots, K\}$. The $(c_1, \ldots, c_n)$ are independent outcomes of multinomial draws with parameter $\boldsymbol{\pi} = (\pi_1, \ldots, \pi_K)$, where $\pi_i > 0$ for all i. Conditional on the label vector $\boldsymbol{c} \equiv (c_1, \ldots, c_n)$, the edge variables A_{ij} for $i < j$ are independent Bernoulli variables with

$$\mathbb{E}[A_{ij}|\boldsymbol{c}] = P_{c_i c_j} = \min\{\rho_n B_{c_i c_j}, 1\}, \tag{1}$$

where $P = [P_{ab}]$ and $B = [B_{ab}]$ are $K \times K$ symmetric matrices. We call P the **connection probability** matrix and B the **kernel** matrix for the connection. So, we have $P_{ab} \leq 1$ for all $a, b = 1, \ldots, K$, $P\mathbf{1} \leq \mathbf{1}$ and $\mathbf{1}^T P \leq \mathbf{1}$ element-wise.

By definition $A_{ji} = A_{ij}$, and $A_{ii} = 0$ (no self-loops).

This formulation is a reparametrization due to Bickel and Chen [6] of the definition of Holland and Leinhardt [19]. It permits separate consideration asymptotically of the density of the graph and its structure as follows:

$$\mathrm{P}\,(\text{Vertex 1 belongs to block } a \text{ and vertex 2 to block } b \text{ and are connected}) = \pi_a \pi_b P_{ab}$$

with P_{ab} depending on n. $P_{ab} = \rho_n \min(B_{ab}, 1/\rho_n)$. We can interpret ρ_n as the unconditional probability of an edge and B_{ab} essentially as

$$\text{P}\left(\text{Vertex 1 belongs to } a \text{ and vertex 2 belongs to } b | \text{ an edge between 1 and 2}\right).$$

Set $\Pi = \text{diag}(\pi_1, \ldots, \pi_K)$.

1. Define the matrices as $M = \Pi B$ and $S = \Pi^{1/2} B \Pi^{1/2}$.
2. Note that the eigenvalues of M are the same as the symmetric matrix S and in particular are real-valued.
3. The eigenvalues of the expected adjacency matrix $\bar{A} \equiv \mathbb{E}(A)$ are also the same as those of S but with multiplicities. We denote the eigenvalues by their absolute order, $\lambda_1 \geq |\lambda_2| \geq \cdots \geq |\lambda_K|$.

Let us denote $(\varphi_1, \ldots, \varphi_K)$, $\varphi_i \in \mathbb{R}^K$, as the eigenvectors of S corresponding to the eigenvalues $\lambda_1, \ldots, \lambda_K$. If a set of λ_j's are equal to λ, we choose eigenvectors from the eigenspace corresponding to the λ as appropriate. Then, we have, $\phi_i = \Pi^{-1/2}\varphi_i$ and $\psi_i = \Pi^{1/2}\varphi_i$ as the left and right eigenvectors of M. Also, $\langle \phi_i, \phi_j \rangle_\pi = \sum_{k=1}^K \pi_k \phi_{ik} \phi_{jk} = \delta_{ij}$. The spectral decomposition of M, S and B are

$$B = \sum_{k=1}^K \lambda_k \phi_k \phi_k^T, \quad S = \sum_{k=1}^K \lambda_k \varphi_k \varphi_k^T, \quad M = \sum_{k=1}^K \lambda_k \psi_k \phi_k^T.$$

2.2 *Spectral Clustering*

The basic goal of community detection is to infer the node labels $\boldsymbol{c}$ from the data. Although we do not explicitly consider parameter estimation, they can be recovered from $\hat{\boldsymbol{c}}$, an estimate of $(c_1, \ldots, c_n)$ by

$$\hat{P}_{ab} \equiv \frac{1}{O_{ab}} \sum_{i=1}^n \sum_{j=1}^n A_{ij} \mathbf{1}\left(\hat{\boldsymbol{c}}_i = a, \hat{\boldsymbol{c}}_j = b\right), \quad 1 \leq a, b \leq K, \tag{2}$$

where,

$$O_{ab} \equiv \begin{cases} n_a n_b, & 1 \leq a, b \leq K, a \neq b \\ n_a(n_a - 1), & 1 \leq a \leq K, a = b \end{cases}, \; n_a \equiv \sum_{i=1}^n \mathbf{1}\left(\hat{\boldsymbol{c}}_i = a\right), \; 1 \leq a \leq K$$

There are a number of approaches for community detection based on modularities [6, 17], maximum likelihood and variational likelihood [7, 10] and approximations such as semidefinite programming approaches [2], pseudolikelihood [3] but these all tend to be computationally intensive and/or require good initial assignments of blocks. The methods which have proved both computationally effective and asymptotically correct in a sense we shall discuss are related to spectral analysis of the adjacency or related matrices.They differ in important details.

Given an $n \times n$ symmetric matrix M based on A, the algorithms are of the form:

1. Using the spectral decomposition of M or a related generalized eigenproblem.
2. Obtain an $n \times K$ matrix of K $n \times 1$ vectors.
3. Apply K means clustering to the n K-dimensional row vectors of the matrix of Step 2.
4. Identify the indices of the rows belonging to cluster j ,$j = 1, \ldots, K$ with vertices belonging to block j.

In addition to A, three graph Laplacian matrices discussed by von Luxburg [31], have been considered extensively, as well as some others we shall mention briefly below and the matrix we shall show has optimal asymptotic properties and discuss in greater detail. The matrices popularly considered are:

- $L = D - A$: the graph Laplacian.
- $L_{\mathrm{rw}} = D^{-1}A$: the random walk Laplacian.
- $L_{\mathrm{sym}} = D^{-1/2}AD^{-1/2}$: the symmetric Laplacian.

Here $D = \mathrm{diag}(A\mathbf{1})$, the diagonal matrix whose diagonal is the vector of row sums of A. She considers optimization problems which are relaxed versions of combinatorial problems which implicitly define clusters as sets of nodes with more internal than external edges. L and L_{sym} appear in two of these relaxations.

The form of step 2 differs for L and Lsym with the K vectors of the L problem corresponding to the top K eigenvalues of the generalized eigenvalue problem $Lv = \lambda Dv$, while the n K-dimensional vectors of the L_{sym} problem are obtained by normalizing the rows of the matrix of K eigenvectors corresponding to the top K eigenvalues of L_{sym}. Their relation to the K block model is through asymptotics.

Why is spectral clustering expected to work? Given A generated by a K-block model, let $\boldsymbol{c} \leftrightarrow (n_1, \ldots, n_K)$ where, n_a is the number of vertices assigned to type a. Then we can write,

$$\mathbb{E}(A|\boldsymbol{c}) = PQP^T$$

where, P is a permutation matrix and $Q_{n \times n}$ has successive blocks of n_1 rows, n_2 rows and so on with all the vectors in each row the same. Thus $\mathrm{rank}(\mathbb{E}(A|\boldsymbol{c})) = K$. The same is true of the asymptotic limit of L given $\boldsymbol{c}$.

If asymptotics as $n \to \infty$ justify concentration of A or L around their expectations then we expect all eigenvalues other than the largest K in absolute value are small. It follows that the n rows of the K eigenvectors associated with the top K eigenvalues should be resolvable into K clusters in $\mathbb{R}^K$ with cluster members identified with rows of $A_{n \times n}$, see [27, 30] for proofs.

2.3 Asymptotics

Now we can consider several asymptotic regimes as $n \to \infty$. Let $\lambda_n = n\rho_n$ be the average degree of the graph.

(I) The *dense* regime: $\lambda_n = \Omega(n)$.
(II) The *semi dense* regime: $\lambda_n / log(n) \to \infty$.
(III) The *semi sparse* regime: Not semidense but $\lambda_n \to \infty$.
(IV) The *sparse* regime: $\lambda_n = O(1)$.

Here are some results in the different regimes. We define a method of vertex assignment to communities as a random map $\delta : \{1, \ldots, n\} \to \{1, \ldots, K\}$ where randomness comes through the dependence of delta on A as a function. Thus spectral clustering using the various matrices which depend on A is such a δ.

Definition 2 δ is said to be *strongly consistent* if

$$\mathrm{P}(i \text{ belongs to } a \text{ and } \delta(i) = a \text{ for all } i, a) \to 1 \text{ as } n \to \infty.$$

Note that the blocks are only determined up to permutation.

Bickel and Chen [6] show that in the (semi) dense regime a method called profile likelihood is strongly consistent under minimal identifiability conditions and later this result was extended [7] to fitting by maximum likelihood or variational likelihood. In fact, in the (semi) dense regime, the block model likelihood asymptotically agrees with the joint likelihood of A and vertex block identities so that efficient estimation of all parameters is possible. It is easy to see that the result cannot hold in the (semi)sparse regime since isolated points then exist with probability 1.

Unfortunately all of these methods are computationally intensive. Although spectral clustering is not strongly consistent, a slight variant, reassigning vertices in any cluster a which are maximally connected to another cluster b rather than a, is strongly consistent.

Definition 3 δ is said to be *weakly consistent* if and only if

$$W \equiv n^{-1} \sum_{i=1}^{n} \mathrm{P}\left(i \in a, \delta(i) \neq a | \forall i, a\right) = o(1)$$

Spectral clustering applied to A [30] or the Laplacians ([27] in the manner we have described) has been shown to be weakly consistent in the semi dense to dense regimes. Even weak consistency fails for parts of the sparse regime [1]. The best that can be hoped for is $W < \frac{1}{2}$. A sharp problem has been posed and eventually resolved in a series of papers, Decelle et al. [13], Mossel et al. [25]. These writers considered the case $K = 2, \pi_1 = \pi_2, B_{11} = B_{22}$. First, Decelle et al. [13] argued on physical grounds that if, $F = (B_{11} - B_{12})^2 / 2(B_{11} + B_{12}) \leq 1$, then $W \geq 1/2$ for any method and parameters are unestimable from the data even if they satisfy the minimal identifiability conditions given below. On the other hand Mossel et al. [25] and independently Massoulié et al. [22], devised admittedly slow methods such that if $F > 1$ then $W < 1/2$ and parameters can be estimated consistently.

We now present a fast spectral clustering method given in greater detail in [5] which yields weak consistency for the semisparse regime on and also has the properties of the Mossel et al. and Massoulie methods. In fact, it reaches the phase transition threshold for all K not just K=2, but still restricted to $\pi_j = 1/K$, all j and $B_{aa} + 2\sum[B_{ab} : b \neq a]$ independent of a for all a.

We note that Zhao et al. [16] exhibit a two-stage algorithm which exhibits the same behavior but its properties in sparse case are unknown. The algorithm given in the next section involves spectral clustering of a new matrix, that of all geodesic distances between i and j.

3 Algorithm

As usual let G_n, an undirected graph on n vertices be the data, denote the vertex set by $V(G_n) \equiv \{v_1, \ldots, v_n\}$ and the edge set by $E(G_n) \equiv \{e_1, \ldots, e_m\}$ with cardinalities $|V(G_n)| = n$ and $E(G_n)| = m$.

As usual a path between vertices u and v is a set of edges $\{(u, v_1), (v_1, v_2), \ldots, (v_{\ell-1}, v)\}$ and the length of such a path is ℓ.

The algorithm we propose depends on the graph distance or geodesic distance between vertices in a graph.

Definition 4 The **Graph** or **Geodesic distance** between two vertices i and j of graph G is given by the length of the shortest path between the vertices i and j, if they are connected. Otherwise, the distance is infinite.

So, for any two vertices $u, v \in V(G)$, graph distance, d_g is defined by

$$d_g(u, v) = \begin{cases} \min\{\ell | \exists \text{ path of length } \ell \text{ between } u \text{ and } v\}, \\ \infty, \text{ if } u \text{ and } v \text{ are not connected} \end{cases}$$

For implementation, we can replace ∞ by $n + 1$, when, u and v are not connected, since any path with loops can not be a geodesic. The main steps of the algorithm are as follows

1. Find the graph distance matrix $D = [d_g(v_i, v_j)]_{i,j=1}^n$ for a given network but with distance upper bounded by $k \log n$. Assign non-connected vertices an arbitrary high value.
2. Perform hierarchical clustering to identify the giant component G^C of graph G. Let $n_C = |V(G^C)|$.
3. Normalize the graph distance matrix on G^C, D^C by
$$\bar{D}^C = -\left(I - \frac{1}{n_C}\mathbf{1}\mathbf{1}^T\right)(D^C)^2\left(I - \frac{1}{n_C}\mathbf{1}\mathbf{1}^T\right)$$
4. Perform eigenvalue decomposition on $\bar{D}^C$.
5. Consider the top K eigenvectors of normalized distance matrix $\bar{D}^C$ and $\tilde{\mathbf{W}}$ be the $n \times K$ matrix formed by arranging the K eigenvectors as columns in $\tilde{\mathbf{W}}$. Perform

K-means clustering on the rows $\tilde{\mathbf{W}}$, that means, find an $n \times K$ matrix $\mathbf{C}$, which has K distinct rows and minimizes $||\mathbf{C} - \tilde{\mathbf{W}}||_F$.
6. (Alternative to 5.) Perform Gaussian mixture model based clustering on the rows of $\tilde{\mathbf{W}}$, when there is an indication of highly-varying average degree between the communities.
7. Let $\hat{\mathbf{c}} : V \mapsto [K]$ be the block assignment function according to the clustering of the rows of $\tilde{\mathbf{W}}$ performed in either Step 5 or 6.

Here are some important observations about the implementation of the algorithm:

(a) There are standard algorithms for graph distance finding in the algorithmic graph theory literature. In the algorithmic graph theory literature the problem is known as the **all pairs shortest path** problem. The two most popular algorithms are Floyd-Warshall [15, 33] and Johnson's algorithm [20].
(b) Step 3 of the algorithm is nothing but the classical multi-dimensional scaling (MDS) of the graph distance matrix.
(c) In the Step 5 of the algorithm K-means clustering is appropriate if the expected degree of the blocks are equal. However, if the expected degree of the blocks are different, this leads to multi scale behavior in the eigenvectors of the normalized distance matrix and bad behavior in practice. So, we perform Gaussian Mixture Model (GMM) based clustering instead of K-means to take into account that.

General theoretical results on the algorithm will be given in [5]. In this paper, we first restrict to the sparse regime. We do so because the arguments in the sparse regime are essentially different from the others. Curiously, it is in the sparse and part of the semi-sparse regime only that the matrix $\bar{D}^C$ concentrates to an $n \times n$ matrix with K distinct types of row vectors as for the other methods of spectral clustering. It does not concentrate in the dense regime, while the opposite is true of A and L. They do not concentrate outside the semidense regime. That the geodesic matrix does not concentrate in the dense regime can easily be seen since asymptotically all geodesic paths are of constant length. But the distributions of path lengths differs from block to block ensuring that the spectral clustering works. But we do not touch this further here.

4 Theoretical Results

Throughout this section we take $\rho_n = \frac{1}{n}$ and specialize to the case

$$B = (p - q)\mathrm{I}_{K\times K} + q\mathbf{1}\mathbf{1}^T$$

where, I is the identity and $\mathbf{1} = (1, \ldots, 1)^T$. That is, all K blocks have the same probability p of connecting two block members and probability q of connecting members of two different blocks and $p > q$. We also assume that $\pi_a = \frac{1}{K}$, $a = 1, \ldots, K$, all blocks are asymptotically of the same size. We restrict ourselves to this model here because it is the one treated by Mossel et al. [25] and already subtle technical details are not obscured. Here is the result we prove.

Theorem 1 *For the given model, if*

$$(p-q)^2 > K(p+(K-1)q), \tag{3}$$

and our algorithm is applied, $\hat{\mathbf{c}}$ *results and* $\mathbf{c}$ *is the true assignment function, then,*

$$\left[\frac{1}{n}\sum_{i=1}^{n}\mathbf{1}\left(\mathbf{c}(v_i)\neq\hat{\mathbf{c}}(v_i)\right)<\frac{1}{2}\right]\to 1 \tag{4}$$

Notes:

1. Equation (3) marks the phase transition conjectured by Decelle et al. [13].
2. A close reading of our proof shows that as $(p-q)^2/K(p+(K-1)q)\to\infty$, $\frac{1}{n}\sum_{i=1}^{n}\mathbf{1}\left(\mathbf{c}(v_i)\neq\hat{\mathbf{c}}(v_i)\right)\xrightarrow{P}0$.

We conjecture that our conclusion in fact holds under the following conditions,

(A1) We consider $\lambda_1 > 1$, $\lambda_1 > \max_{j\geq 2}\lambda_j$, $1\leq j\leq K$ and $\lambda_K > 0$. For M, there exists a k such that $(M^k)_{ab} > 0$ for all $a,b=1,\ldots,K$. Also, $\pi_j > 0$, for $j=1,\ldots,K$.

(A2) Each vertex has the same asymptotic average degree $\alpha > 1$, that is,

$$\alpha=\sum_{k=1}^{K}\pi_k B_{ak}=\sum_{k=1}^{K}M_{ak},\quad \text{for all } a\in\{1,\ldots,K\}$$

(A3) We assume that

$$\lambda_K^2 > \lambda_1$$

or alternatively, there exists real positive t, such that,

$$\sum_{k=1}^{K}\phi_k(a)\lambda_k^t\phi_k(b)\leq n,\quad \text{for all } a,b=1,\ldots,K$$

Note that (A1)–(A3) all hold for the case we consider. In fact, under our model,

$$\lambda_1=\frac{p+(K-1)q}{K},\quad \lambda_2=\frac{p-q}{K},\quad \lambda_2=\lambda_3=\cdots=\lambda_K$$

with (A3) being the condition of the theorem.

Our argument will be stated in a form that is generalizable and we will indicate revisions in intermediate statements as needed, pointing in particular to a lemma whose conclusion only holds if an implication of (A3) we conjecture is valid.

The theoretical analysis of the algorithm has two main parts:

I. Finding the limiting distribution of graph distance between two typical vertices of type a and type b (where, $a, b = 1, \ldots, K$). This part of the analysis is highly dependent on results from multi-type branching processes and their relation with stochastic block models. The proof techniques and results are borrowed from [4, 8] and [9].
II. Finding the behavior of the top K eigenvectors of the graph distance matrix D using the limiting distribution of the typical graph distances. This part of analysis is highly dependent on perturbation theory of linear operators. The proof techniques and results are borrowed from [11, 21] and [30].

We will state two theorems corresponding to I and II above.

Theorem 2 *Under our model, the graph distance $d_G(u, v)$ between two uniformly chosen vertices of type a and b respectively, conditioned on being connected, satisfies the following asymptotic relation:*

(i) If $a = b$, for any $\varepsilon > 0$, as $n \to \infty$,

$$\mathrm{P}\left[(1-\varepsilon)\tau_1 \leq d_G(u, v) \leq (1+\varepsilon)\tau_1\right] = 1 - o(1) \tag{5}$$

where, τ_1 is the minimum real positive t, which satisfies the relation below,

$$\left[\lambda_2^t + \frac{\lambda_1^t - \lambda_2^t}{K}\right] = n \tag{6}$$

(ii) If $a \neq b$, for any $\varepsilon > 0$, as $n \to \infty$,

$$\mathrm{P}\left[(1-\varepsilon)\tau_2 \leq d_G(u, v) \leq (1+\varepsilon)\tau_2\right] = 1 - o(1) \tag{7}$$

where, τ_2 is the minimum real positive t, which satisfies the relation below,

$$\left[\frac{\lambda_1^t - \lambda_2^t}{K}\right] = n \tag{8}$$

In Theorem 2 we have a point-wise result. To use matrix perturbation theory for part II we need the following.

Theorem 3 *Let $\mathbb{D}_B$ be the restriction of the geodesic matrix to vertices in the big component of G_n. Then, under our model,*

$$\mathrm{P}\left[\left\|\frac{\mathbf{D}}{\log n} - \mathbb{D}\right\|_F \leq o(n)\right] = 1 - o(1)$$

where, $\mathbb{D}_{ij} \equiv \sigma_1 = \tau_1/\log n$*, if* v_i *and* v_j *have same type and* $\mathbb{D}_{ij} \equiv \sigma_2 = \tau_2/\log n$*, otherwise, where,* τ_1 *and* τ_2 *are solutions t in Eqs.* (6) *and* (8) *respectively.*

To generalize Theorem 1, we need appropriate generalizations of Theorem 2 and 3. Heuristically, it may be argued that the generalizations (τ_{sb}), $a, b = 1, \ldots, K$ should satisfy the equations,

$$\sum_{k=1}^{K} \phi_k(a)\lambda_k^t \phi_k(b) = (S^t)_{ab} = n, \quad \text{for } a \leq b \in [K] \tag{9}$$

Our conjecture is that (A1)–(A3) imply that the equations have asymptotic solutions and that the statements of Theorem 2 and 3 hold with obvious modifications.

Note that in Theorem 2, since $\lambda_j = \lambda_2$, $2 \leq j \leq K$ there are effectively only two equations and modifications are also needed for other degeneracies in the parameters. We next turn to a branching process result in [9] which we will use heavily.

4.1 A Key Branching Process Result

As others have done we link the network formed by SBM with the tree network generated by multi-type Galton-Watson branching process. In our case, the Multi-type branching process (MTBP) has type space $S = \{1, \ldots, K\}$, where a particle of type $a \in S$ is replaced in the next generation by a set of particles distributed as a Poisson process on S with intensity $(B_{ab}\pi_b)_{b=1}^K = (M_{ab})_{b=1}^K$. Recall the definitions of B, M and S from Sect. 2.1. We denote this branching process, started with a single particle of type a, by $\mathscr{B}_{B,\pi}(a)$. We write $\mathscr{B}_{B,\pi}$ for the same process with the type of the initial particle random, distributed according to $\boldsymbol{\pi}$. According to Theorem 8.1 of Chapter 1 of [23], the branching process has a positive survival probability if $\lambda_1 > 1$, where, λ_1 is the Perron-Frobenius eigenvalue of M, a positive regular matrix. Recall that for our special M, $\lambda_1 = \frac{p-q}{K} + 1$.

Definition 5

(a) Define $\rho(B, \pi; a)$ as the probability that the branching process, $\mathscr{B}_{B,\pi}(a)$, survives for eternity.
(b) Define,

$$\rho \equiv \rho(B, \pi) \equiv \sum_{a=1}^{K} \rho(B, \pi; a)\pi_a \tag{10}$$

as the **survival probability** of the branching process $\mathscr{B}_{B,\pi}$ given that its initial distribution is $\boldsymbol{\pi}$

We denote $Z_t = (Z_t(a))_{a=1}^{K}$ as the population of particles of K different types, with $Z_t(a)$ denoting particles of type a, at generation t for the Poisson multi-type branching process $\mathscr{B}_{B,\pi}$, with B and π as defined in Sect. 4. From Theorem 24 of [9], we get that

Theorem 4 ([9]) *Let $\beta > 0$ and $Z_0 = x \in \mathbb{N}^K$ be fixed. There exists $C = C(x, \beta) > 0$ such that with probability at least $1 - n^{-\beta}$, for all $k \in [K]$, all $s, t \geq 0$, with $0 \leq s < t$,*

$$|\langle \phi_k, Z_s \rangle - \lambda_k^{s-t} \langle \phi_k, Z_t \rangle| \leq C(t+1)^2 \lambda_1^{s/2} (\log n)^{3/2} \tag{11}$$

Remark The above stated theorem is a special case of the general theorem stated in [9]. The general theorem is required for generalizing Theorem 1. The general version of the theorem is

Theorem 5 ([9]) *Let $\beta > 0$ and $Z_0 = x \in \mathbb{N}^K$ be fixed. There exists $C = C(x, \beta) > 0$ such that with probability at least $1 - n^{-\beta}$, for all $k \in [K_0]$ (where, K_0 is the largest integer such that $\lambda_k^2 > \lambda_1$ for all $k \leq K_0$), all $s, t \geq 0$, with $0 \leq s < t$,*

$$|\langle \phi_k, Z_s \rangle - \lambda_k^{s-t} \langle \phi_k, Z_t \rangle| \leq C(t+1)^2 \lambda_1^{s/2} (\log n)^{3/2} \tag{12}$$

and for all $k \in [K] \backslash [K_0]$, for all $t \geq 0$,

$$|\langle \phi_k, Z_t \rangle| \leq C(t+1)^2 \lambda_1^{t/2} (\log n)^{3/2} \tag{13}$$

Finally, for all $k \in [K] \backslash [K_0]$, all $t \geq 0$, $\mathbb{E}|\langle \phi_k, Z_t \rangle|^2 \leq C(t+1)^3 \lambda_1^t$.

4.2 The Neighborhood Exploration Process

The neighborhood exploration process of a vertex v in graph G generated from an SBM gives us a handle on the link between local structures of a graph from SBM and multi-type branching process. Recall the definitions of SBM parameters from Sect. 2.1 and the definitions of Poisson multi-type branching process from Sect. 4.1. We assume all vertices of graph G_n generated from a stochastic block model has been assigned a community or type ξ_i (say) for vertex $v_i \in V(G_n)$.

The *neighborhood exploration process*, $(G, v)_L$, of a vertex v in graph G_n, generates a *spanning tree* of the induced subgraph of G_n consisting of vertices of at most L-distance from v. The spanning tree is formed from the exploration process which starts from a vertex v as the *root* in the random graph G_n generated from stochastic block model. The set of vertices of type a of the random graph G_n that are neighbors of v and has not been previously explored are called $\Gamma_{1,a}(v)$ and $N_{1,a}(v) = |\Gamma_{1,a}(v)|$ for $a = 1, \ldots, K$ and $N_1(v) = (N_{1,1}(v), \ldots, N_{1,K}(v))$. So, $\Gamma_1(v) = \{\Gamma_{1,1}(v), \ldots, \Gamma_{1,K}(v)\}$ are the children of the root v at step $\ell = 1$

in the spanning tree of the neighborhood exploration process. The neighborhood exploration process is repeated at second step by looking at the neighbors of type a of the vertices in $\Gamma_1(v)$ that has not been previously explored and the set is called $\Gamma_{2,a}(v)$ and $N_{2,a}(v) = |\Gamma_{2,a}(v)|$ for $a = 1, \ldots, K$. Similarly, $\Gamma_2(v) = \{\Gamma_{2,1}(v), \ldots, \Gamma_{2,K}(v)\}$ are the children of vertices $\Gamma_1(v)$ at step $\ell = 2$ in the spanning tree of the neighborhood exploration process. The exploration process is continued until step $\ell = L$. Note that the process stops when all the vertices in G_n has been explored. So, if G_n is connected, then, $L \leq$ the diameter of the graph G_n.

Since, we either consider G_n connected or only the giant component of G_n, the neighborhood exploration process will end in a finite number of steps but the number of steps may depend on n and is equal to the diameter, L, of the connected component of the graph containing the root v. It follows from Theorem 14.11 of [8] that

$$L/\log_{\lambda_1}(n) \xrightarrow{P} 1. \tag{14}$$

Now, we find a coupling relation between the *neighborhood exploration process* of a vertex of type a in stochastic block model and a multi-type Galton-Watson process, $\mathscr{B}(a)$ starting from a vertex of type a. The Lemma is based on Proposition 31 of [9].

Lemma 1 *Let $w(n)$ be a sequence such that $w(n) \to \infty$ and $w(n)/n \to 0$. Let (T, v) be the random rooted tree associated with the Poisson multi-type Galton-Watson branching process defined in Sect. 2.1 started from $Z_0 = \delta_{c_v}$ and (G, v) be the spanning tree associated with neighborhood exploration process of random SBM graph G_n starting from v. For $\ell \leq \tau$, where τ is the number of steps required to explore $w(n)$ vertices in (G, v), the total variation distance, d_{TV}, between the law of $(G, v)_\ell$ and $(T, v)_\ell$ at step ℓ goes to zero as $O\left(n^{-\frac{1}{2}} \vee w(n)/n\right) = o(1)$.*

Proof Let us start the neighborhood exploration process starting with vertex v of a graph generated from an SBM model with parameters $(P, \pi) = (B/n, \pi)$. Correspondingly the multi-type branching process starts from a single particle of type $\boldsymbol{c}_v$, where, $\boldsymbol{c}_v$ is the type or class of vertex v in SBM.

Let t be such that $0 \leq t < \tau$, where, τ is defined in the Lemma statement. Now, for such a $t \geq 0$, let $(x_{t+1}(1), \ldots, x_{t+1}(K))$ be leaves of (T, v) at time t starting from a vertex v_t generated by step t of class $\boldsymbol{c}_{v_t} = a$. Let $(y_{t+1}(1), \ldots, y_{t+1}(K))$ be the vertices exposed at step t of the exploration process starting from a vertex of class a, where, $a \in [K]$. Now, if $\boldsymbol{c}_{v_t}$ is of type a, then, we have $x_{t+1}(b)$ follows $\text{Bin}(n_t(b), B_{ab}/n)$ and $y_{t+1}(b)$ follows $\text{Poi}(\pi_b B_{ab})$ for $b = 1, \ldots, K$, where, $n_t(b)$ is the number of unused vertices of type b remaining at time t for $b = 1, \ldots, K$. Also, $y_{t+1}(b)$ for different b are independent. Note that $n_b \geq n_t(b) \geq n_b - w(n)$ for $b = 1, \ldots, K$. So, since, we have $|n_b/n - \pi_b| = O(n^{-1/2})$ for $b = 1, \ldots, K$, we get that,

$$|n_t(b) - \pi_b| < O\left(n^{-1/2} + w(n)/n\right) \quad \text{for } b = 1, \ldots, K$$

Now, we know that,

$$d_{TV}\left(\text{Bin}(m', \lambda/m), \text{Poi}(m'\lambda/m)\right) \leq \frac{\lambda}{m}, \qquad d_{TV}\left(\text{Poi}(\lambda), \text{Poi}(\lambda')\right) \leq |\lambda - \lambda'|$$

So, now, we have,

$$d_{TV}\left(P_{t+1}, Q_{t+1}\right) \leq O\left(n^{-1/2} \vee w(n)/n\right) = o(1)$$

where, P_{t+1} is the distribution of y_{t+1} under neighborhood exploration process and Q_{t+1} is the distribution of x_{t+1} under the branching process, and hence Lemma 1 follows.

Now, we restrict ourselves to the giant component of G_n. The size of the giant component of G_n, $\mathscr{C}_1(G_n)$, of a random graph generated from SBM(B, π) is related to the multi-type branching process through its survival probability as given in Definition 5. According to Theorem 3.1 of [8], we have,

$$\frac{1}{n}\mathscr{C}_1(G_n) \stackrel{P}{\rightarrow} \rho(B, \pi) \tag{15}$$

Under this additional condition of restricting to the giant component, the branching process can be coupled with another branching process with a different kernel. The kernel of that branching process is given in following lemma.

Lemma 2 *If v is in giant component of G_n, the new branching process has kernel* $\left(B_{ab}\left(2\rho(B, \pi)/K - \rho^2(B, \pi)/K^2\right)\right)_{a,b=1}^{K}$.

Proof The proof is given in Sect. 10 of [8].

Since, we will be restricting ourselves to the giant component of G_n, we shall be using the $B' \equiv \left(B_{ab}\left(2\rho(B, \pi)/K - \rho^2(B, \pi)/K^2\right)\right)_{a,b=1}^{K}$ matrix as the connectivity matrix in stead of B. We abuse notation by referencing to the matrix B' as B too.

We proceed to prove the limiting behavior of typical distance between vertices v and w of G_n, where, $v, w \in V(G_n)$. We first try to find a lower bound for distance between two vertices. We shall separately give an upper bound and lower bounds for the distance between two vertices of the same type and different types.

Lemma 3 *Under our model, for vertices $v, w \in V(G)$, if*

(a) type of v = type of w = a (say), then,

$$|\{\{v, w\} : d_G(v, w) \leq (1 - \varepsilon)\tau_1\}| \leq O(n^{2-\varepsilon}) \textit{ with high probability}$$

where, τ_1 is the minimum real positive t, which satisfies Eq. (6),

(b) type of $v = a \neq b =$ type of w (say), then,

$$|\{\{v, w\} : d_G(v, w) \leq (1 - \varepsilon)\tau_2\}| \leq O(n^{2-\varepsilon}) \textit{ with high probability}$$

where, τ_2 is the minimum real positive t, which satisfies Eq. (8).

Proof Let $\Gamma_d(v) \equiv \Gamma_d(v, G_n)$ denote the d-distance set of v in G_n, i.e., the set of vertices of G_n at graph distance exactly d from v, and let $\Gamma_{\leq d}(v) \equiv \Gamma_{\leq d}(v, G_n)$ denote the d-neighborhood $\cup_{d' \leq d} \Gamma_{d'}(v)$ of v. Let $\Gamma_{d,a}(v) \equiv \Gamma_{d,a}(v, G_n)$ denote the set of vertices of type a at d-distance in G_n and let $\Gamma_{\leq d,a}(v) \equiv \Gamma_{\leq d,a}(v, G_n)$ denote the d-neighborhood $\cup_{d' \leq d} \Gamma_{d',a}(v)$ of v consisting of vertices of type a. Let N_d^a be the number of particles at generation d of the branching process $\mathscr{B}_B(\delta_a)$ and $N_{d,c}^a$ be the number of particles at generation d of the branching process $\mathscr{B}_B(\delta_a)$ of type c. So, $N_d^a = \sum_{c=1}^K N_{d,c}^a$ and $Z_t(k) = \sum_{d=0}^t N_{d,k}^a$.

Lemma 1 involved first showing that, for n large enough, the neighborhood exploration process starting at a given vertex v of G_n with type a could be coupled with the branching process $\mathscr{B}_{B'}(\delta_a)$, where the B' is defined by Lemma 2. As noted we identify B' with B.

The neighborhood exploration process and multi-type branching process can be coupled so that for every d, $|\Gamma_d(v)|$ is at most the number $N_d + O\left(n^{-\frac{1}{2}} \vee w(n)/n\right)$, where, N_d is number of particles in generation d of $\mathscr{B}_B(\delta_a)$ and in d generations at most $w(n)$ vertices of G_n have been explored.

From Theorem 4, we get that with high probability

$$\left| \frac{\langle \phi_k, Z_t \rangle}{\lambda_k^t} - \langle \phi_k, Z_0 \rangle \right| \leq C(t+1)^2 (\log n)^{3/2}$$

Since, for any $x \in \mathbb{R}^K$, we get the unique representation, $x = \sum_{k=1}^K \langle x, \phi_k \rangle \phi_k$, for any basis $\{\phi_k\}_{k=1}^K$ of $\mathbb{R}^K$. If we take $x = e_b$, where, e_b is the unit vector with 1 at b-th co-ordinate and 0 elsewhere, $b = 1, \ldots, K$, we can get

$$Z_t(b) \leq \sum_{k=1}^K \phi_k(b) \lambda_k^t \phi_k(a) \left[Z_0(a) + C(t+1)^2 (\log n)^{3/2} \right]$$

Now, under our model one representation of the eigenvectors is $\phi_1 = \frac{1}{\sqrt{K}}(1, \ldots, 1)$, $\phi_2 = \frac{1}{\sqrt{2}}(-1, 1, 0, \ldots, 0)$, $\phi_3 = \frac{1}{\sqrt{6}}(-1, -1, 2, 0, \ldots, 0)$, $\cdots$, $\phi_{K-1} = \frac{1}{\sqrt{K(K-1)}}(-1, \ldots, -1, K-1)$. Now using the representation of eigenvectors for branching process starting from vertex of type a, $a \in [K]$, we get with high probability

$$\sum_{k=1}^K Z_t(k) \leq \lambda_1^t \left[Z_0(a) + C(t+1)^2 (\log n)^{3/2} \right]$$

$$Z_t(a) - Z_t(b) \geq \lambda_2^t \left[-Z_0(a) - C(t+1)^2 (\log n)^{3/2} \right], \quad b = 1, \ldots, K \text{ and } b \neq a.$$

So, we can simplify, for each $a \in [K]$ with $Z_0(a) = 1$, with high probability,

$$Z_t(a) \leq \frac{1}{K}\left(\lambda_1^t + (K-1)\lambda_2^t\right)\left[1 + C(t+1)^2(\log n)^{3/2}\right]$$
$$Z_t(b) \leq \frac{\lambda_1^t - \lambda_2^t}{K}\left[1 + C(t+1)^2(\log n)^{3/2}\right], \quad b \in [K] \text{ and } b \neq a.$$

Set $D_1 = (1-\varepsilon)\tau_1$, where, τ_1 is the solution to the equation

$$\left[\lambda_2^t + \frac{\lambda_1^t - \lambda_2^t}{K}\right] = n$$

and set $D_2 = (1-\varepsilon)\tau_2$, where, τ_2 is the solution to the equation

$$\left[\frac{\lambda_1^t - \lambda_2^t}{K}\right] = n$$

where, $\varepsilon > 0$ is fixed and small. Note that both τ_1 and τ_2 are of the order $O(\log n)$. Thus, with high probability, for v of type a and $w(n) = O(n^{1-\varepsilon})$,

$$|\Gamma_{\leq D_1,a}(v)| = \textstyle\sum_{d=0}^{D_1} N_{d,a}^a \leq Z_{D_1}(a) + O\left(D_1 n^{-\frac{1}{2}} \vee w(n)/n\right) = O(n^{1-\varepsilon})$$
$$|\Gamma_{\leq D_2,b}(v)| = \textstyle\sum_{d=0}^{D_2} N_{d,b}^a \leq Z_{D_2}(b) + O\left(D_2 n^{-\frac{1}{2}} \vee w(n)/n\right) = O(n^{1-\varepsilon})$$

So, summing over $v \in C_a$ and $v \in C_b$, where, $C_a = \{i \in V(G) | \boldsymbol{c}_i = a\}$ and $C_b = \{i \in V(G) | \boldsymbol{c}_i = b\}$, we have,

$$\sum_{v \in C_a} |\Gamma_{\leq D_1,a}(v)| = |\{\{v,w\} : d_G(v,w) \leq (1-\varepsilon)\tau_1, v, w \in C_a\}|$$
$$\sum_{v \in C_a} |\Gamma_{\leq D_2,b}(v)| = |\{\{v,w\} : d_G(v,w) \leq (1-\varepsilon)\tau_2, v \in C_a, w \in C_b\}|$$

and so with high probability

$$|\{\{v,w\} : d_G(v,w) \leq (1-\varepsilon)\tau_1, v, w \in C_a\}| = \sum_{v \in V(G_n)} |\Gamma_{\leq D,a}(v)| = O(n^{2-\varepsilon})$$
$$|\{\{v,w\} : d_G(v,w) \leq (1-\varepsilon)\tau_2, v \in C_a, w \in C_b\}| = \sum_{v \in V(G_n)} |\Gamma_{\leq D,b}(v)| = O(n^{2-\varepsilon})$$

The above statement is equivalent to

$$\mathrm{P}\left[|\{\{v,w\} : d_G(v,w) \leq (1-\varepsilon)\tau_1, v, w \in C_a\}| \leq O(n^{2-\varepsilon})\right] = 1 - o(1)$$
$$\mathrm{P}\left[|\{\{v,w\} : d_G(v,w) \leq (1-\varepsilon)\tau_2, v \in C_a, w \in C_b\}| \leq O(n^{2-\varepsilon})\right] = 1 - o(1)$$

for any fixed $\varepsilon > 0$.

Now, we upper bound the typical distance between two vertices of SBM graph G_n.

Lemma 4 *Under our model, for vertices $v, w \in V(G)$ and conditioned on the event that the exploration process starts from a vertex in the giant component of G, if,*

(a) type of v = type of $w = a$ (say), then,

$$P\left(d_G(v,w) < (1+\varepsilon)\tau_1\right) = 1 - exp(-\Omega(n^{2\eta}))$$

where, τ_1 is the minimum real positive t, which satisfies Eq. (6),

(b) type of $v = a \neq b$ = type of w (say), then,

$$P\left(d_G(v,w) < (1+\varepsilon)\tau_2\right) = 1 - exp(-\Omega(n^{2\eta}))$$

where, τ_2 is the minimum real positive t, which satisfies Eq. (8).

Proof We consider the multi-type branching process with probability kernel $P_{ab} = \frac{B_{ab}}{n}$ $\forall a, b = 1, \ldots, K$ and the corresponding random graph G_n generated from stochastic block model has in total n nodes. We condition that branching process $\mathscr{B}_K$ survives.

Note that an upper bound 1 is obvious, since we are bounding a probability, so it suffices to prove a corresponding lower bound. We may and shall assume that $B_{ab} > 0$ for some a, b.

Again, let $\Gamma_d(v) \equiv \Gamma_d(v, G_n)$ denote the d-distance set of v in G_n, i.e., the set of vertices of G_n at graph distance exactly d from v, and let $\Gamma_{\leq d}(v) \equiv \Gamma_{\leq d}(v, G_n)$ denote the d-neighborhood $\cup_{d' \leq d}\Gamma_{d'}(v)$ of v. Let $\Gamma_{d,a}(v) \equiv \Gamma_{d,a}(v, G_n)$ denote the set of vertices of type a at d-distance in G_n and let $\Gamma_{\leq d,a}(v) \equiv \Gamma_{\leq d,a}(v, G_n)$ denote the d-neighborhood $\cup_{d' \leq d}\Gamma_{d',a}(v)$ of v consisting of vertices of type a. Let N_d^a be the number of particles at generation d of branching process $\mathscr{B}_B(\delta_a)$ and $N_{d,c}^a$ be the number of particles at generation d of branching process $\mathscr{B}_B(\delta_a)$ of type c. So, $N_d^a = \sum_{c=1}^K N_{d,c}^a$ and $Z_t(k) = \sum_{d=0}^t N_{d,k}^a$.

By Lemma 1, for $w(n) = o(n)$,

$$|\Gamma_{d,c}(v)| \geq N_{d,c} - O\left(n^{-\frac{1}{2}} \vee w(n)/n\right), \; c = 1, \ldots, K. \tag{16}$$

for all d s.t. $|\Gamma_{\leq d}(v)| < \omega(n)$. This relation between the number of vertices at generation d of type c of branching process $\mathscr{B}_B(\delta_a)$, denoted by $N_{d,c}$ and the number of vertices of type c at distance d from v for the neighborhood exploration process of G_n, denoted by $|\Gamma_{d,c}(v)|$ becomes highly important later on in this proof, where, $c = 1, \ldots, K$. Note that the relation only holds when $|\Gamma_{\leq d}(v)| < \omega(n)$ for some $\omega(n)$ such that $\omega(n)/n \to 0$ as $n \to \infty$.

From Theorem 4 of the branching process, we get that with high probability

$$\left|\frac{\langle \phi_k, Z_t\rangle}{\lambda_k^t} - \langle \phi_k, Z_0\rangle\right| \leq C(\log n)^{3/2}$$

Now following the same line of argument as in proof of Lemma 3, for each $a \in [K]$ with $Z_0(a) = 1$, with high probability we get that,

$$Z_t(a) \leq \frac{1}{K}\left(\lambda_1^t + (K-1)\lambda_2^t\right)\left[1 + C(t+1)^2(\log n)^{3/2}\right]$$
$$Z_t(b) \leq \frac{\lambda_1^t - \lambda_2^t}{K}\left[1 + C(t+1)^2(\log n)^{3/2}\right], \quad b \in [K] \text{ and } b \neq a.$$

Let D_1 be the integer part of $(1+2\eta)\tau_1'$, where, τ_1' is the solution to the equation

$$\left[\lambda_2^t + \frac{\lambda_1^t - \lambda_2^t}{K}\right] = n^{1/2-\eta} \tag{17}$$

Thus conditioned on survival of the branching process $\mathscr{B}_B(\delta_a)$, $N^a_{D_1,a} \geq n^{1/2+\eta/2}$. Set $D_2 = (1+\eta)\tau_2'$, where, τ_2' is the solution to the equation

$$\lambda_1^t = n^{1/2+\eta} \tag{18}$$

Thus conditioned on survival of branching process $\mathscr{B}_B(\delta_a)$, $N^a_{D_2,b} \geq n^{1/2+\eta/2}$ for $b = 1,\ldots,K$. Furthermore $\lim_{d\to\infty} \mathrm{P}(N^a_d \neq 0) = \rho(B,a)$.

Now, we have conditioned that the branching process with kernel B is surviving. The right hand side tends to $\rho(B,a) = 1$ as $\eta \to 0$. Hence, given any fixed $\gamma > 0$, if we choose $\eta > 0$ small enough, and for large enough n, we have

$$\mathrm{P}\left(\forall b : N^a_{D_2,b} \geq n^{1/2+\eta/2}\right) = 1,$$
$$\mathrm{P}\left(N^a_{D_1,a} \geq n^{1/2+\eta/2}\right) = 1.$$

Now, the neighborhood exploration process and branching process can be coupled so that for every d, $|\Gamma_d(v)|$ is at most the number N_d of particles in generation d of $\mathscr{B}_B(a)$ from Lemma 1 and Eq. (16). So, we have for v of type a, with high probability,

$$|\Gamma_{\leq D_1,a}(v)| \leq \mathbb{E}\sum_{d=0}^{D_1} N_d = o(n^{2/3})$$

$$|\Gamma_{\leq D_2,b}(v)| \leq \mathbb{E}\sum_{d=0}^{D_2} N_d = o(n^{2/3})$$

if η is small enough, since D_1 is integer part of $(1+2\eta)\tau_1'$ and D_2 is the integer part of $(1+2\eta)\tau_2'$, where, τ_1' and τ_2' are solutions to Eqs. (17) and (18). Note that the power $2/3$ here is arbitrary, we could have any power in the range $(1/2, 1)$. So, now, we are in a position to apply Eq. (16), as we have $|\Gamma_{\leq D}(v)| \leq O(n_a^{2/3}) < \omega(n)$, with $\omega(n)/n \to 0$.

Now let v and w be two fixed vertices of $G(n,P)$, of types a and b respectively. We explore both their neighborhoods at the same time, stopping either when we reach distance D in both neighborhoods, or we find an edge from one to the other, in which case v and w are within graph distance $2D+1$. We consider two independent branching processes $\mathscr{B}_B(a)$, $\mathscr{B}_B'(b)$, with $N_{d,c}^a$ and $N_{d,c}^b$ vertices of type c in generation d respectively. By the previous argument, with high probability we encounter $o(n)$ vertices in the exploration so, by the argument leading to (16), whp either the explorations meet, or

$$|\Gamma_{d,c}^a(w)| \geq Z_d^{(a)}(c) - O\left(n^{-\frac{1}{2}} \vee n^{-\frac{1}{3}}\right),\ c = 1, \ldots, K, c \neq a$$

$$|\Gamma_{d,c}^b(w)| \geq Z_d^{(b)}(c) - O\left(n^{-\frac{1}{2}} \vee n^{-\frac{1}{3}}\right),\ c = 1, \ldots, K, c \neq b$$

with the explorations not meeting, where, $Z^{(a)}$ is the branching process starting from $Z_0 = \delta_a$, for $a = 1, \ldots, K$. Using bound on $N_{d,c}^a$ and the independence of the branching processes, it follows that for $a = b$,

$$\mathrm{P}\left(d(v,w) \leq 2D_1 + 1 \text{ or } |\Gamma_{D_1,c}^a(v)|, |\Gamma_{D_1,c}^a(w)| \geq n^{1/2+\eta}\right) \geq 1 - o(1).$$

and for $a \neq b$,

$$\mathrm{P}\left(d(v,w) \leq 2D_2 + 1 \text{ or } \forall c : |\Gamma_{D_2,c}^a(v)|, |\Gamma_{D_2,c}^b(w)| \geq n^{1/2+\eta}\right) \geq 1 - o(1).$$

Write these probabilities as $\mathrm{P}(A_j \cup B_j), j = 1, 2$. We now show that $\mathrm{P}(A_j^c \cap B_j) \to 0$ and since $\mathrm{P}(A_j \cup B_j) \to 1$, we will have $\mathrm{P}(A_j) \to 1$. We have not examined any edges from $\Gamma_D(v)$ to $\Gamma_D(w)$, so these edges are present independently with their original unconditioned probabilities. For any end vertex types c_1, c_2, the expected number of these edges is at least $|\Gamma_{D,c}^a(v)||\Gamma_{D,c}^a(w)|B_{c_1c_2}/n$ for first probability and $|\Gamma_{D,c_1}^a(v)||\Gamma_{D,c_2}^b(w)|B_{c_1c_2}/n$ for second probability. Choosing c_1, c_2 such that $B_{c_1c_2} > 0$, this expectation is $\Omega((n^{1/2+\eta/2})^2/n) = \Omega(n^\eta)$. It follows that at least one edge is present with probability $1 - \exp(-\Omega(n^\eta)) = 1 - o(1)$. If such an edge is present, then $d(v,w) \leq 2D_1 + 1$ for first probability and $d(v,w) \leq 2D_1 + 1$ for second probability. So, the probability that the second event in the above equation holds but not the first is $o(1)$. Thus, the last equation implies that

$$\mathrm{P}(d(v,w) \leq 2D_1 + 1) \geq (1-\gamma)^2 - o(1) \geq 1 - 2\gamma - o(1)$$
$$\mathrm{P}(d(v,w) \leq 2D_2 + 1) \geq (1-\gamma)^2 - o(1) \geq 1 - 2\gamma - o(1).$$

where, $\gamma > 0$ is arbitrary. Choosing η small enough, we have $2D + 1 \leq (1 + \varepsilon)\log(n)/\log\lambda$. As γ is arbitrary, we have

$$\mathrm{P}(d(v,w) \leq (1+\varepsilon)\tau_1) \geq 1 - \exp(-\Omega(n^{2\eta})),$$
$$\mathrm{P}(d(v,w) \leq (1+\varepsilon)\tau_2) \geq 1 - \exp(-\Omega(n^{2\eta})).$$

and the lemma follows.

Equations (6) and (8) control the asymptotic bounds for the graph distance $d_G(v,w)$ between two vertices v and w in $V(G_n)$. Under the condition (A3) it follows that $\lambda_2^2 > \lambda_1$. If we consider $\lambda_2^2 = c\lambda_1$, where, c is a constant, then Eqs. (6) and (8) can be written in the form of quadratic equations. So, the solutions τ_1 and τ_2 exist under the condition c^{τ_1} and c^{τ_2} are of the order $O(n)$ and the resulting solutions τ_1 and τ_2 are both of the order $O(\log n)$. Also, from the expression of the solutions τ_1 and τ_2, the limits $\frac{\tau_1}{\log n}$ and $\frac{\tau_2}{\log n}$ exist and we shall define the limit as σ_1 and σ_2 respectively.

4.3 *Proof of Theorems 2 and 3*

4.3.1 Proof of Theorem 2

We shall try to prove the limiting behavior of the typical graph distance in the giant component as $n \to \infty$. The Theorem essentially follows from Lemmas 3–4. Under the conditions mentioned in the Theorem, part (a) follows from Lemma 3(a) and 4(a) and part (b) follows from Lemma 3(b) and 4(b).

4.3.2 Proof of Theorem 3

From Definition 4, we have that $\mathbf{D}_{ij}$ = graph distance between vertices v_i and v_j, where, $v_i, v_j \in V(G_n)$. From Lemma 3, we get for any vertices v and w with high probability,

$$|\{\{v,w\} : d_G(v,w) \leq (1-\varepsilon)\tau_1\}| \leq O(n^{2-\varepsilon}), \text{ if type of } v = \text{ type of } w$$
$$|\{\{v,w\} : d_G(v,w) \leq (1-\varepsilon)\tau_2\}| \leq O(n^{2-\varepsilon}), \text{ if type of } v \neq \text{ type of } w.$$

Also, from Lemma 4, we get

$$\mathrm{P}\left(d_G(v,w) < (1+\varepsilon)\tau_1\right) = 1 - \exp(-\Omega(n^{2\eta})), \text{ if type of } v = \text{ type of } w,$$
$$\mathrm{P}\left(d_G(v,w) < (1+\varepsilon)\tau_2\right) = 1 - \exp(-\Omega(n^{2\eta})), \text{ if type of } v = \text{ type of } w.$$

Now, $\sigma_1 = \tau_1/\log n$ and $\sigma_2 = \tau_2/\log n$ are asymptotically constant as both τ_1 and τ_2 are of the order $\log n$ as follows from Eqs. (6) and (8). So, putting the two statements together, we get that with high probability,

$$\sum_{i,j=1:type(v_i)\neq type(v_j)}^{n} \left(\frac{\mathbf{D}_{ij}}{\log n} - \mathbb{D}_{ij}\right)^2 = O(n^{2-\varepsilon}) + O(n^2).\varepsilon^2$$

since, by Lemma 1, $\epsilon = o(1)$ and $(1 - \exp(-\Omega(n^{2\eta})))^{n^2} \to 1$ as $n \to \infty$. So, putting the two cases together, we get that with high probability, for some $\varepsilon > 0$,

$$\sum_{i,j=1}^{n} \left(\frac{\mathbf{D}_{ij}}{\log n} - \mathbb{D}_{ij}\right)^2 = O(n^{2-\varepsilon}) + O(n^2).\varepsilon^2 = o(n^2).$$

Hence, for some $\varepsilon > 0$,

$$\left\|\frac{\mathbf{D}}{\log n} - \mathbb{D}\right\|_F \leq o(n).$$

We have completed proofs of Theorems 2 and 3.

4.4 Perturbation Theory of Linear Operators

We now establish part II of our program. D can be considered as a perturbation of the operator $\mathbb{D}$.

The Davis-Kahan Theorem [12] gives a bound on perturbation of eigenspace instead of eigenvector, as discussed previously.

Theorem 6 (Davis-Kahan [12]) *Let $\mathbf{H}, \mathbf{H}' \in \mathbb{R}^{n\times n}$ be symmetric, suppose $\mathcal{V} \subset \mathbb{R}$ is an interval, and suppose for some positive integer d that $\mathbf{W}, \mathbf{W}' \in \mathbb{R}^{n\times d}$ are such that the columns of $\mathbf{W}$ form an orthonormal basis for the sum of the eigenspaces of $\mathbf{H}$ associated with the eigenvalues of $\mathbf{H}$ in $\mathcal{V}$ and that the columns of $\mathbf{W}'$ form an orthonormal basis for the sum of the eigenspaces of $\mathbf{H}'$ associated with the eigenvalues of $\mathbf{H}'$ in $\mathcal{V}$. Let δ be the minimum distance between any eigenvalue of $\mathbf{H}$ in $\mathcal{V}$ and any eigenvalue of $\mathbf{H}$ not in $\mathcal{V}$. Then there exists an orthogonal matrix $\mathbf{R} \in \mathbb{R}^{d\times d}$ such that $||\mathbf{WR} - \mathbf{W}'||_F \leq \sqrt{2}\frac{||\mathbf{H}-\mathbf{H}'||_F}{\delta}$.*

4.5 Proof of Theorem 1

The behavior of the eigenvalues of the limiting operator $\mathbb{D}$ can be stated as follows:

Lemma 5 *Under our model, the eigenvalues of* $\mathbb{D}$ - $|\mu_1(\mathbb{D})| \geq |\mu_2(\mathbb{D})| \geq \cdots \geq |\mu_n(\mathbb{D})|$, *can be bounded as follows:*

$$\mu_1(\mathbb{D}) = O(n\sigma_1),\ |\mu_K(\mathbb{D})| = O(n(\sigma_1 - \sigma_2)),\ \mu_{K+1}(\mathbb{D}) = \cdots = \mu_n(\mathbb{D}) = -\sigma_1 \tag{19}$$

Also, With high probability it holds that $|\mu_K(\mathbf{D}/\log n)| = O(n(\sigma_1 - \sigma_2))$ *and* $\mu_{K+1}(\mathbf{D}/\log n) \leq o(n)$.

Proof The matrix $\mathbb{D} + \sigma_1 \mathrm{I}_{n\times n}$ is a block matrix with blocks of sizes $\{n_a\}_{a=1}^K$, with $\sum_{a=1}^K n_a = n$. The elements of (a, b)th block are all same and equal to σ_1, if $a = b$ and equal to σ_2, if $a \neq b$. Note, diagonal of $\mathbb{D}$ is zero, as diagonal of $\mathbf{D}$ is also zero. Now, we have the eigenvalues of the $K \times K$ matrix of the values in $\mathbb{D}$ to be $(\sigma_1+(K-1)\sigma_2, \sigma_1-\sigma_2, \ldots, \sigma_1-\sigma_2)$. If we consider, $\lambda_{\frac{1}{2}}^2 = c\lambda_1$, then, if $c > 1$, we will have $\sigma_1 > \sigma_2$. So, under our model, we have that $\sigma_1 > \sigma_2$. So, because of repetitions in the block matrix $\mu_1(\mathbb{D}) = O(n\sigma_1) = O(n)$ and $\mu_K(\mathbb{D}) = O(n(\sigma_1 - \sigma_2)) = O(n)$, since, by assumption (A3), $n_a = O(n)$, for all $a = 1, \ldots, K$. Now, the rest of the eigenvalues of $\mathbb{D} + \sigma_1 \mathrm{Id}_{n\times n}$ is zero, so the rest of eigenvalues of $\mathbb{D}$ is $-\sigma_1$.

Now, about the second part of Lemma, By Weyl's Inequality, for all $i = 1, \ldots, n$,

$$||\mu_i(\mathbf{D}/\log n)| - |\lambda_i(\mathbb{D})|| \leq ||\mathbf{D}/\log n - \mathbb{D}||_F \leq o(n)$$

Since, from (A1)–(A3), it follows that $\sigma_1 - \sigma_2 > c > 0$, for some constant c, so, $|\lambda_K(\mathbf{D}/\log n)| = O(n(\sigma_1 - \sigma_2)) - o(n) = O(n(\sigma_1 - \sigma_2))$ for large n and $|\lambda_{K+1}(\mathbf{D}/\log n)| \leq -\sigma_1 + o(n) = o(n)$.

Now, let $\mathbf{W}$ be the eigenspace corresponding to the top K absolute eigenvalues of $\mathbb{D}$ and $\tilde{\mathbf{W}}$ be the eigenspace corresponding to the top K absolute eigenvalues of $\mathbf{D}$. Using Davis-Kahan

Lemma 6 *With high probability, there exists an orthogonal matrix* $\mathbf{R} \in \mathbb{R}^{K\times K}$ *such that* $||\mathbf{W}\mathbf{R} - \tilde{\mathbf{W}}||_F \leq o\left((\sigma_1 - \sigma_2)^{-1}\right)$

Proof The top K eigenvalues of both $\mathbb{D}$ and $\mathbf{D}/\log n$ lies in (Cn, ∞) for some $C > 0$. Also, the gap $\delta = O(n(\sigma_1 - \sigma_2))$ between top K and $K + 1$th eigenvalues of matrix $\mathbb{D}$. So, now, we can apply Davis-Kahan Theorem 6 and Theorem 3, to get that,

$$||\mathbf{W}\mathbf{R} - \tilde{\mathbf{W}}||_F \leq \sqrt{2}\frac{||\mathbf{D}/\log n - \mathbb{D}||_F}{\delta} \leq \frac{o(n)}{O(n(\sigma_1 - \sigma_2))} = o\left((\sigma_1 - \sigma_2)^{-1}\right)$$

Now, the relationship between the rows of W can be specified as follows:

Lemma 7 *For any two rows* i, j *of* $\mathbf{W}_{n\times K}$ *matrix,* $||u_i - u_j||_2 \geq O(1/\sqrt{n})$, *if type of* $v_i \neq$ *type of* v_j.

Proof The matrix $\mathbb{D} + \sigma_1 \mathrm{Id}_{n\times n}$ is a block matrix with blocks of sizes $\{n_a\}_{a=1}^K$, with $\sum_{a=1}^K n_a = n$. The elements of (a, b)th block are all same and equal to σ_1, if $a = b$ and equal to σ_2, if $a \neq b$. Note, diagonal of $\mathbb{D}$ is zero, as diagonal of $\mathbf{D}$ is also zero.

Now, we have the rows of eigenvectors of the $K \times K$ matrix of the values in $\mathbb{D}$ that have a constant difference. Under our model, we have that $\sigma_1 > \sigma_2$. So, because of repetitions in the block matrix, rows of $\mathbb{D}$ as well as the projection of $\mathbb{D}$ into its top K eigenspace has difference of order $O(n^{-1/2})$ between rows of matrix.

Now, if we consider K-means criterion as the clustering criterion on $\tilde{\mathbf{W}}$, then, for the K-means minimizer centroid matrix $\mathbf{C}$ is an $n \times K$ matrix with K distinct rows corresponding to the K centroids of K-means algorithm. By property of K-means objective function and Lemma 6, with high probability,

$$\begin{aligned} ||\mathbf{C} - \tilde{\mathbf{W}}||_F &\leq ||\mathbf{WR} - \tilde{\mathbf{W}}||_F \\ ||\mathbf{C} - \mathbf{WR}||_F &\leq ||\mathbf{C} - \tilde{\mathbf{W}}||_F + ||\mathbf{WR} - \tilde{\mathbf{W}}||_F \\ ||\mathbf{C} - \mathbf{WR}||_F^2 &\leq 4||\mathbf{WR} - \tilde{\mathbf{W}}||_F^2 \\ &\leq o\left((\sigma_1 - \sigma_2)^{-2}\right) \end{aligned}$$

By Lemma 7, for large n, we can get constant C, such that, K balls, $B_1, \ldots, B_K$, of radius $r = Cn^{-1/2}$ around K distinct rows of $\mathbf{W}$ are disjoint.

Now note that with high probability the number of rows i such that $||\mathbf{C}_i - (\mathbf{WR})_i|| > r$ is at most $\frac{cn}{(\sigma_1 - \sigma_2)^2}$, with arbitrarily small constant $c > 0$. If the statement does not hold then,

$$\begin{aligned} ||\mathbf{C} - \mathbf{WR}||_F^2 &> r^2.\left(\frac{cn}{(\sigma_1 - \sigma_2)^2}\right) \\ &\geq Cn^{-1}.\left(\frac{cn}{(\sigma_1 - \sigma_2)^2}\right) = O\left((\sigma_1 - \sigma_2)^{-2}\right) \end{aligned}$$

So, we get a contradiction, since $||\mathbf{C} - \mathbf{WR}||_F^2 \leq o\left((\sigma_1 - \sigma_2)^{-2}\right)$. Thus, the number of mistakes should be at most $\left(\frac{cn}{(\sigma_1 - \sigma_2)^2}\right)$, with arbitrarily small constant $c > 0$.

So, for each $v_i \in V(G_n)$, if $\boldsymbol{c}(v_i)$ is the type of v_i and $\hat{\boldsymbol{c}}(v_i)$ is the type of v_i as estimated from applying K-means on top K eigenspace of geodesic matrix $\mathbf{D}$, we get that for arbitrarily small constant, $c > 0$,

$$\left[\frac{1}{n}\sum_{i=1}^{n} \mathbf{1}\left(\boldsymbol{c}(v_i) \neq \hat{\boldsymbol{c}}(v_i)\right) < \frac{c}{(\sigma_1 - \sigma_2)^2}\right] \to 1$$

So, for constant σ_1 and σ_2, we get $c > 0$ such that,

$$\left[\frac{1}{n}\sum_{i=1}^{n} \mathbf{1}\left(\boldsymbol{c}(v_i) \neq \hat{\boldsymbol{c}}(v_i)\right) < \frac{1}{2}\right] \to 1$$

5 Conclusion

We have given an overview of spectral clustering in the context of community detection of networks and clustering. We have also introduced a new method of community detection in the paper and we have shown bounds on theoretical performance of the method.

References

1. Abbe, E., Bandeira, A.S., Hall, G.: Exact recovery in the stochastic block model (2014). arXiv preprint arXiv:1405.3267
2. Amini, A.A., Levina, E.: On semidefinite relaxations for the block model (2014). arXiv preprint arXiv:1406.5647
3. Amini, A.A., Chen, A., Bickel, P.J., Levina, E.: Pseudo-likelihood methods for community detection in large sparse networks. Ann. Stat. **41**(4), 2097–2122 (2013). doi:10.1214/13-AOS1138. http://dx.doi.org/10.1214/13-AOS1138
4. Bhamidi, S., Van der Hofstad, R., Hooghiemstra, G.: First passage percolation on the Erds-Renyi random graph. Comb. Probab. Comput. **20**(5), 683–707 (2011)
5. Bhattacharyya, S., Bickel, P.J.: Community detection in networks using graph distance (2014). arXiv preprint arXiv:1401.3915
6. Bickel, P.J., Chen, A.: A nonparametric view of network models and Newman–Girvan and other modularities. Proc. Natl. Acad. Sci. **106**(50), 21068–21073 (2009)
7. Bickel, P., Choi, D., Chang, X., Zhang, H.: Asymptotic normality of maximum likelihood and its variational approximation for stochastic blockmodels. Ann. Stat. **41**(4), 1922–1943 (2013). doi:10.1214/13-AOS1124. http://dx.doi.org/10.1214/13-AOS1124
8. Bollobás, B., Janson, S., Riordan, O.: The phase transition in inhomogeneous random graphs. Random Struct. Algorithm. **31**(1), 3–122 (2007)
9. Bordenave, C., Lelarge, M., Massoulié, L.: Non-backtracking spectrum of random graphs: community detection and non-regular Ramanujan graphs (2015). arXiv preprint arXiv:1501.06087
10. Celisse, A., Daudin, J.J., Pierre, L.: Consistency of maximum-likelihood and variational estimators in the stochastic block model. Electron. J. Stat. **6**, 1847–1899 (2012). doi:10.1214/12-EJS729. http://dx.doi.org/10.1214/12-EJS729
11. Chatelin, F.: Spectral Approximation of Linear Operators. SIAM, Philadelphia (1983)
12. Davis, C., Kahan, W.M.: The rotation of eigenvectors by a perturbation. III. SIAM J. Numer. Anal. **7**(1), 1–46 (1970)
13. Decelle, A., Krzakala, F., Moore, C., Zdeborová, L.: Asymptotic analysis of the stochastic block model for modular networks and its algorithmic applications. Phys. Rev. E **84**(6), 066106 (2011)
14. Fiedler, M.: Algebraic connectivity of graphs. Czechoslov. Math. J. **23**(98), 298–305 (1973)
15. Floyd, R.W.: Algorithm 97: shortest path. Commun. ACM **5**(6), 345 (1962)
16. Gao, C., Ma, Z., Zhang, A.Y., Zhou, H.H.: Achieving optimal misclassification proportion in stochastic block model (2015). arXiv preprint arXiv:1505.03772
17. Girvan, M., Newman, M.E.: Community structure in social and biological networks. Proc. Natl. Acad. Sci. **99**(12), 7821–7826 (2002)
18. Hartigan, J.A.: Clustering Algorithms. Wiley Series in Probability and Mathematical Statistics. Wiley, New York/London/Sydney (1975)
19. Holland, P.W., Laskey, K.B., Leinhardt, S.: Stochastic blockmodels: first steps. Soc. Netw. **5**(2), 109–137 (1983)

20. Johnson, D.B.: Efficient algorithms for shortest paths in sparse networks. J. ACM **24**(1), 1–13 (1977)
21. Katō, T.: Perturbation Theory for Linear Operators, vol. 132. Springer, Berlin (1995)
22. Massoulié, L.: Community detection thresholds and the weak Ramanujan property. In: Proceedings of the 46th Annual ACM Symposium on Theory of Computing, pp. 694–703. ACM, New York (2014)
23. Mode, C.J.: Multitype Branching Processes: Theory and Applications, vol. 34. American Elsevier Pub. Co., New York (1971)
24. Mossel, E., Neeman, J., Sly, A.: Stochastic block models and reconstruction (2012). arXiv preprint arXiv:1202.1499
25. Mossel, E., Neeman, J., Sly, A.: A proof of the block model threshold conjecture (2013). arXiv preprint arXiv:1311.4115
26. Ng, A.Y., Jordan, M.I., Weiss, Y., et al.: On spectral clustering: analysis and an algorithm. Adv. Neural Inf. Process. Syst. **2**, 849–856 (2002)
27. Rohe, K., Chatterjee, S., Yu, B.: Spectral clustering and the high-dimensional stochastic blockmodel. Ann. Stat. **39**(4), 1878–1915 (2011). doi:10.1214/11-AOS887. http://dx.doi.org/10.1214/11-AOS887
28. Rousseeuw, P.J., Leroy, A.M.: Robust Regression and Outlier Detection. Wiley Series in Probability and Mathematical Statistics: Applied Probability and Statistics. Wiley, New York (1987). doi:10.1002/0471725382. http://dx.doi.org/10.1002/0471725382
29. Shi, J., Malik, J.: Normalized cuts and image segmentation. IEEE Trans. Pattern Anal. Mach. Intell. **22**(8), 888–905 (2000)
30. Sussman, D.L., Tang, M., Fishkind, D.E., Priebe, C.E.: A consistent adjacency spectral embedding for stochastic blockmodel graphs. J. Am. Stat. Assoc. **107**(499), 1119–1128 (2012). doi:10.1080/01621459.2012.699795. http://dx.doi.org/10.1080/01621459.2012.699795
31. von Luxburg, U.: A tutorial on spectral clustering. Stat. Comput. **17**(4), 395–416 (2007)
32. von Luxburg, U., Belkin, M., Bousquet, O.: Consistency of spectral clustering. Ann. Stat. **36**(2), 555–586 (2008). doi:10.1214/009053607000000640. http://dx.doi.org/10.1214/009053607000000640
33. Warshall, S.: A theorem on boolean matrices. J. ACM **9**(1), 11–12 (1962)

Bayesian Hierarchical Mixture Models

Leonardo Bottolo and Petros Dellaportas

Abstract When massive streams of data are collected, it is usually the case that different information sources contribute to different levels of knowledge, or inferences about subgroups may suffer from small or inadequate sample size. In these cases, Bayesian hierarchical models have been proven to be valuable, or even necessary, modelling tools that provide the required multi-level modelling structure to deal with the statistical inferential procedure. We investigate the need to generalize the inherent assumption of exchangeability which routinely accompanies these models. By modelling the second-stage parameters of a Bayesian hierarchical model as a finite mixture of normals with unknown number of components, we allow for parameter partitions so that exchangeability is assumed within each partition. This more general model formulation allows better understanding of the data generating mechanism and provides better parameter estimates and forecasts. We discuss choices of prior densities and MCMC implementation in problems in actuarial science, finance and genetics.

1 Introduction

The simplest form of the standard Bayesian hierarchical model can be described as follows. Suppose that an exchangeable sequence of observations $x_1, x_2, \ldots, x_I$ are available from I different, but related sources. The first stage of the hierarchy specifies a parametric model $f(x_i|\psi_i)$ for each of the I sequences, where ψ_i are unknown parameter vectors of dimension J. In the second stage, prior beliefs about the structural relationship of ψ_i's, specified through the premise that they are judged to be exchangeable, provide a prior that is expressed through the assumption that each ψ_i is distributed from a density $p(\psi_i|\gamma)$. γ is a vector of parameters usually called hyper-parameters, which has typically an interpretation in terms of

L. Bottolo (✉)
Department of Mathematics, Imperial College London, London, UK
e-mail: l.bottolo@imperial.ac.uk

P. Dellaportas
Department of Statistics, Athens University of Economics and Business, Athens, Greece
e-mail: petros@aueb.gr

A. Frigessi et al. (eds.), *Statistical Analysis for High-Dimensional Data*,
Abel Symposia 11, DOI 10.1007/978-3-319-27099-9_5

the characteristics of $p(\psi_i|\gamma)$, usually mean and variance. Finally, it is often the case that no reliable prior information is available on γ so a non-informative prior density $p(\gamma)$ is assigned to the unknown set of hyper-parameters.

Bayesian hierarchical models have turned out to be an essential modeling tool for applied statisticians because their structure allows combining information, or borrowing strength, from different experiments. This means that the second stage prior affects the posterior means of ψ_i by shrinking them towards a central value. The importance of such an inferential procedure has been documented and studied in detail in frequentist, empirical Bayes and Bayesian literature in the case of inference for a multivariate normal mean problem from both expected risk and predictive performance perspective; see, for example, the recent review by George et al. [11]. Moreover, the enormous advances of computational techniques during the last twenty years facilitated the implementation of Bayesian paradigm and have made possible the widespread use of hierarchical models in nearly all areas of applied statistics. A recent general discussion can be found in [10].

Adoption of Bayesian hierarchical models is natural in many practical applications with massive streams of data. For example, it is usually the case that different information sources contribute to different levels of knowledge or inferences about subgroups may suffer from small or inadequate sample size. Then, the issue of borrowing strength or sharing information is essential when posterior summaries of interest are required for specific experimental units. In these cases, Bayesian hierarchical models have been proven to be valuable, or even necessary, modelling tools that provide the required multilevel modelling structure to deal with the statistical inferential procedure.

One important part of model criticism in the Bayesian hierarchical models refers exactly to the second stage density $p(\psi_i|\gamma)$. Albert and Chib [1] discuss various departures from the second stage implicit assumptions. In particular they point out that the density of $p(\psi_i|\gamma)$ should capture departures such as outliers or two-group clustering of ψ_i's, and they provide Bayesian model choice methodologies that can test these models through Bayes factors. The exchangeability principle assumes that the ψ_i's are similar enough to be modelled by a common density, but clearly testing the above violations requires prior knowledge of some structure that implies non-exchangeability. Note that in most practical scenarios this prior evidence is usually not available and the structural departures from exchangeability are obtained by inspecting the residuals in the basic exchangeable model.

In this article we claim not only that the assumption of exchangeability is usually very strong, but that it also has some undesirable consequences in the Bayesian inference and prediction processes. The hierarchical smoothing achieved by the standard hierarchical model shrinks the estimates for each unit towards the average of ψ_i's, with the shrinkage being greater for those ψ_i that correspond to sources based on smaller sample sizes. Although bias is increased, inferences are typically improved when the exchangeability assumption is valid, but it is questionable whether this holds in the presence on non-exchangeability. For example, it is often desirable to avoid oversmoothing when some kind of heterogeneity produced by clustering or outliers is present. We call these models "Bayesian hierarchical mixture models" (BHMM).

Given the flexibility allowed by the current computational power, we discuss and propose a general parametric modelling framework that is more general than the standard Bayesian hierarchical model in the following sense. Instead of testing for possible departures from the assumption of exchangeability, it seems natural to adopt a general parametric family at the second stage of the hierarchy that is based on a belief of partial exchangeability. This can be expressed by assuming that the ψ_i's follow a discrete mixture of normal distributions with unknown means, variances and number of components; or, one may view it as partitioning ψ_i's into an (unknown) number of groups such that within each group exchangeability holds. An inferential consequence of this model is that the parameters are shrunk towards the within group mean value. Another way to view it is that it is a compromise between the fully exchangeable model and a pure independence model in which the second stage density $p(\psi_i \mid \gamma)$ does not depend on a common parameter γ but it is just a prior density that expresses prior beliefs about ψ_i and shrinkage does not take place. We note here that another way to express similar modelling assumptions is achieved via Dirichlet process models that we believe are less intuitive and more restrictive (see, for example, [12]).

In the past, there have been three papers that proposed the modelling framework above. Nobile and Green [18] presented an analysis for factorial experiments in which main effects and interactions are modelled as finite mixtures of normals with unknown number of components. Bottolo et al. [5] modelled insurance claims extreme data by proposing mixture models similar to [18] to all parameters that specify the intensity of a Poisson process. Bottolo and Consonni [3] used the same procedure developed in [5] to cluster the probability of under-over-expression across genes in a microarray experiment. We review these papers and extend the discussion and applicability of BHMM by presenting one further applications in time series. The examples serve as illustration of the kind of difficulties one is faced with when trying to fit such complex models, but they also demonstrate the power and flexibility of BHMM. In particular, we will discuss issues of choice of prior densities and MCMC implementation.

The rest of the paper proceeds as follows. Section 2 introduces the general notation and formulation. Section 3 introduces the four examples. Section 4 discusses issues of prior specification, whereas Sect. 5 deals with key ideas in MCMC implementation. We conclude with a brief discussion in Sect. 6.

2 Bayesian Hierarchical Mixture Models

Typically, application of BHMM's require first a transformation of each element of the parameter vector ψ_i so that a resulting vector λ_i has elements $\lambda_{ij}, j = 1, \dots, J$ that take values in the whole real line. We can then proceed by assuming that for each j

$$\lambda_{ij} \sim \sum_{h_j=1}^{k_j} \omega_{h_j} \, \mathrm{N}(\theta_{h_j}, \xi_{h_j}), \; i = 1, \dots, I, \tag{1}$$

where $\sum_{h_j} \omega_{h_j} = 1$ and the number of components k_j is unknown. In the third stage of the model we assign a discrete uniform prior on the number of components, $k_j \sim \text{Unif}(0, K_j)$ with $K_j \leq I$. Moreover, let z_{ij} be an allocation parameter that indicates to which mixture component λ_{ij} belongs, so the mixture model (1), can be interpreted as follows: conditionally on the mixture weights $\omega_j = (\omega_{1_j}, \ldots, \omega_{k_j})'$, each z_{ij} is independently drawn from a multinomial distribution with $\Pr(z_{ij} = h_j) = \omega_{h_j}$. The hierarchical structure is further specified by assigning a symmetric prior density on the mixture weights $\omega_j \sim \text{Dir}(d_1, \ldots, d_{k_j})$. It is completed by specifying a prior density for the prior mean and precision component $\theta_{h_j} \sim \text{N}(m_j, 1/\tau_j)$ and $\xi_{h_j}^{-1} \sim \text{Ga}(a_{\xi j}, b_{\xi j})$, respectively, with $\tau_j \sim \text{Ga}(a_{\tau j}, b_{\tau j})$.

The above formulation has been introduced by Nobile and Green [18] and, as the authors pointed out, it follows the modern Bayesian trend to adopt priors not solely for testing and inference, but as modelling instruments for inferences that take into account model uncertainty. Moreover, there is some resemblance with the priors suggested by Consonni and Veronese [6] who propose, for each j, placing priors on partitions of λ_{ij} and then assuming exchangeability within the partitions.

3 Applications

We describe here four different applications in which BHMM's turned out to be useful modelling tool for inference or predictions.

3.1 *Factorial Experiments*

Assume that conditionally on parameter vectors ψ, the data vectors are normally distributed replicate observations from a two-way layout model. Under the general assumption of exchangeability across data units, rows and columns, we obtain the usual random effects, or "fully random model" (see, for example, [7]). Thus, the vectors ψ correspond to the parameters contributing to the systematic mean component and the error variance. In particular, the mean vector has dimension equal to the product of rows and columns produced by the experimental layout and can be conveniently parameterized as an overall mean, mean effects λ_{i1} and λ_{i2}, and interaction effects λ_{i3}. Here, i takes values that correspond to the respected parameters obtained from the number of rows and columns and the usual sum to zero constraints imposed to the model. Nobile and Green [18] considered this model and placed priors of the form (1) to the three groups of parameters λ_{ij}, for $j = 1, 2, 3$.

Apart for testing the indistinguishability of factor levels or whether contrasts are zero, the BHMM formulation provides a Bayesian model average posterior predictive density of next observations conditioned on factor level combinations. Moreover, in unreplicated experiments where typically a model without interactions is appropriate, the BHMM provides the extra flexibility to an incorporate interaction term which can explain the variability which cannot be accounted for by the main effects.

3.2 Extreme Values

Bottolo et al. [5] improved upon the Bayesian hierarchical model of [23] by applying a BHMM to extreme data from different types of insurance claims. For every claim type i, $i = 1, \ldots, I$, a threshold u_i is associated so that exceedances over these thresholds are recorded in the form of data vectors x_i. Then, conditional on parameters ψ_i, a model [22] for the observed exceedances over thresholds assumes that x_i are generated by a Poisson process of intensity

$$\Lambda_{y_i} = \left(1 + \xi_i \frac{y_i - \mu_i}{\sigma_i}\right)_+^{-1/\xi_i}, \tag{2}$$

where $y_+ = \max(0, y)$. Let $\psi_i = (\mu_i, \sigma_i, \xi_i)'$ be the parameter vector of the ith insurance claim type and with $\lambda_i = (\lambda_{i1}, \lambda_{i2}, \lambda_{i3})'$ the transformed parameter vector which takes values in the real line. Bottolo et al. [5] argued that heterogeneity between claim types should be taken into account by applying priors of the form (1) to λ_{ij}.

Prediction of future exceedances for a specific claim-type is of primary importance in actuarial science. The BHMM provides remarkable discrepancies when compared to MLE-based estimates (see Fig. 1) and appreciable difference with the standard hierarchical model. By borrowing strength only between similar claim types more sensible and general predictions are available (see [5]).

3.3 Gene Profiling

A crucial objective of studies based on microarray for gene expression is gene clustering based on the similarity of their level of expression. A related clustering task is molecular profiling it and aims at identifying similarities across samples based on a few genes identified from the gene clustering stage of the analysis. Bottolo and Consonni [3] considered a subset, a 460 × 203 matrix, of expression measurements data of human lung carcinomas [2]. Of the 203 samples, 17 were normal lung specimens ("NL"); the 186 lung cancer specimens include histologically defined lung adenocarcinomas (127) ("adeno"), squamous cell lung carcinomas (21) ("SQ"), pulmonary carcinoids (20) ("PC"), small-cell lung carcinoma (6) ("SCLC"), while the remaining 12 adenocarcinomas were suspected to be extrapulmonary metastases based on clinical history ("adenoEM"). They extended the model of

[19] using a two-level mixtures in a very distinct fashion. First of all, each of the I expression measurements are assumed to originate from a three-component mixture distribution, see [9, 19], representing the underlying population classes (baseline, under-expression and over-expression) of samples relative to gene-expression. For each gene i, they specify a specific (random) probability of belonging to any of the three classes. In the second stage, they assume that each gene specific probability arises from a mixture of prior distributions with an unknown number of components. Denoting by ψ_{i1} and ψ_{i2} the probability for gene i to be under- over-expressed, [3] applied a BHMM by focusing on these parameters. Specifically, after a logit transformation, ψ_{i1} and ψ_{i2} are denoted as λ_{i1} and λ_{i2} and priors of the form (1) were placed.

Except from the partial exchangeability assumption which allows to borrow strength within groups of tumors with similar probabilities of abnormal expression, another important empirical advantage of BHHM is evident from the analysis of [3]. Since partitions that correspond to probabilities of abnormal low/high expressions z_{λ_1} and z_{λ_2} are readily available, joint partitions can be obtained by taking their intersection $z_{\lambda_1,\lambda_2} = z_{\lambda_1} \cap z_{\lambda_2}$. The mode of the posterior number of components k_{λ_1,λ_2} (obtained in a post-processing analysis by intersecting $z^{(t)}_{\lambda_1,\lambda_2} = z^{(t)}_{\lambda_1} \cap z^{(t)}_{\lambda_2}$ at each MCMC iteration and counting the number of distinctive groups) specifies a unique partition of the genes. As a final step, a bivariate normal kernel density estimate was fitted to $\{\mathrm{E}(\lambda_{1i}|\text{data}), \mathrm{E}(\lambda_{2i}|\text{data})\}$ separately for each joint partition. Then a "representative gene" for each cluster is identified as that with values closest to the modal value of the bivariate normal density. Similar ideas about discriminatory variables in clustering or small subsets of variables that characterize clusters can be found also in [14, 15]. Using all the "representative genes", the joint posterior probability of the three expression states can be calculated and their differences across tumors can be utilized to derive profiling of patients. The same procedure can be used to identify the genetic signature of tumor and refine the subgroup classification of cancer specimens going beyond the histological definition of tumor.

3.4 Volatility Prediction

Bottolo and Dellaportas [4] consider financial time series where prediction of volatility of each series is of interest. Perhaps the most popular model to deal with this problem is the AR(1)-GARCH(1,1) model with Student-t errors. In particular, suppose that for each stock i, $i = 1, \ldots, I$, a times series or returns $(x_{t,i})_{t=1}^{T}$ is observed and assume that, for each of them,

$$x_{t,i} = \mu_i + \rho_i x_{t-1,i} + \epsilon_{t,i} \tag{3}$$

with the innovation $\epsilon_{t,i} \sim \sigma_{t,i}t(\nu_i)$, where $t(d)$ is the density function of a standard Student-t distribution with d degrees of freedom and

$$\sigma_{t,i}^2 = \eta_i + \alpha_i \epsilon_{t-1}^2 + \beta_i \sigma_{t-1,i}^2. \tag{4}$$

We denote with $\psi_i = (\mu_i, \rho_i, \eta_i, \alpha_i, \beta_i)'$ the parameter vector of the ith stock and with $\lambda_i = (\lambda_{i1}, \lambda_{i2}, \lambda_{i3}, \lambda_{i4}, \lambda_{i5})'$ the transformed parameter vector which takes values in the real line.

The standard Bayesian hierarchical setup assumes exchangeability across units in a population, allowing borrowing strength and shrinkage towards a central overall mean. Bottolo and Dellaportas [4] suggest the use of (1) so that parameters within each normal component are shrunk towards a group-dependent central value. The results in a large empirical study that involves 100 stocks of the FTSE UK Index indicate that the BHMM has better predictive ability than both the standard Bayesian hierarchical model as well as the model in which each stock is treated entirely independently from the other stocks. This exercise is indicative that BHMM may play an important role in a series of financial econometric studies in which predictions of multivariate returns are considered.

4 Priors

Assume that we deal with the standard model of the form (1) where λ_{ij} are observable. Even in this case, this model requires prior specifications for the parameters θ_{h_j} and ξ_{h_j} that are far from non-informative. This issue has been dealt with in detail by Richardson and Green [20] and it is now well established that such models are non-identifiable without some, at least vague, prior information. Clearly, for the BHHM's where λ_{ij} are unobservable, the choice of informative priors is both necessary and important. We will describe here a series of ideas on how to choose these priors based on the four models of Sect. 3.

Nobile and Green [18] argue that in the case of the full random model, prior densities should incorporate the experimenter's subjective judgement about what differences, Δ, in factor levels are considered negligible. Although some minimal use of data is used in the prior specification, their primary message is that the choice of the prior hyperparameters is an important part of this model and informative prior information should be incorporated. Bottolo et al. [5] adopted the idea of specifying "negligible differences" between parameters but they replaced the genuine prior information which is extremely hard to be specified for the parameters of the model presented in Sect. 3.2 with an empirical Bayes estimate as follows. For each j in (1), they constructed an empirical random variable Δ based on all the $I(I-1)/2$ pairwise absolute differences of the MLE, $|\hat{\lambda}_{ij} - \hat{\lambda}_{lj}|$, $i, l = 1, \ldots, I$ with $i > l$. Then, they based their prior choice to the belief that two parameters do not differ substantially if their pairwise difference is less than a selected percentile of this empirical distribution. For example, when the median is chosen, two parameters

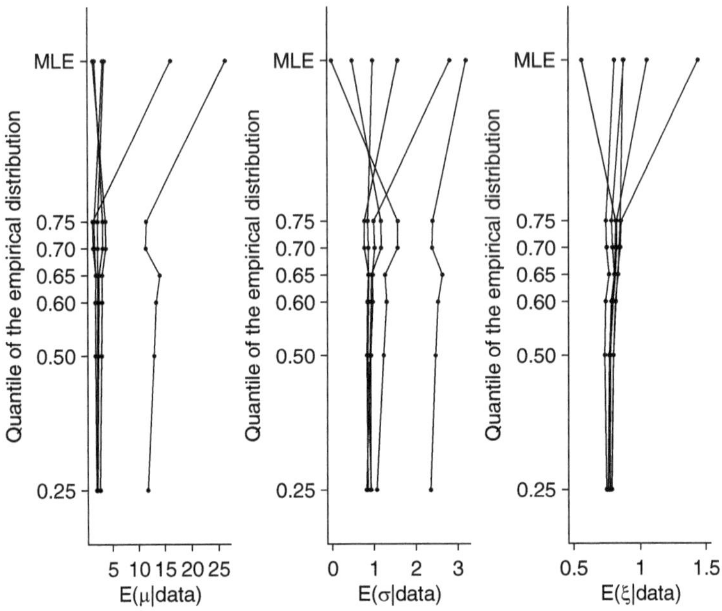

Fig. 1 Crossover diagram for location parameter μ, for scale parameter σ and for shape parameter ξ for six different types of insurance claims. MLE and posterior means marked as *dots* for various choices of the quantiles of empirical distribution of Δ

are considered coming from distinct components if their distance is larger than the majority of the pairwise distances. Finally, they derive the within/between variance hyper-parameters for a fixed percentile of Δ. As expected and illustrated in [5], different percentiles lead to a posteriori to different partitions. Figure 1 shows the varying degree of shrinkage that takes place as Δ is allowed to vary between the first and third quartile and the striking discrepancies when compared to MLE.

If we are interested in constructing a default, non-informative prior without prior information, natural extension is to use the Δ parameter of [18] but instead of fixing it [4] suggest placing a prior density based on the data. For ease of notation, in the following we bypass the subscripts j and h_j in the prior (1). Bottolo and Dellaportas [4] build a data-based empirical distribution of the random variable Δ by assuming that Δ has a right truncated gamma density, $\Delta \sim \text{Ga}(a_\Delta, b_\Delta, \Delta_B)$, with a_Δ, b_Δ parameters that fit the sample of the MLEs of the parameters λ_i conditionally on Δ_B, the maximum absolute difference observed. This resemblances the specification of an hyper-prior for the precision parameter of a Dirichlet process, where the total mass of the base-line measure is used to tune the distribution of the number of distinct components, see, for example, [8]. Thus, the smoothed random proximity variable Δ has support in $[0, \Delta_B]$ and for each value of Δ different b_ξ and b_τ are derived. However, the derivation of the two hyper-parameters is computational expensive since a time consuming root-finding algorithm must be applied. For implementation purposes, a crucial element in [4], prior construction is the discretization of the right truncated gamma density based on B evenly spaced points, $b = 1, \dots, B$. Thus, for each point Δ_b, b_ξ and b_τ are calculated and stored.

Since two parameters are considered coming from the same mixture component if $p_0 = \Pr(|\lambda_i - \lambda_l| \leq \Delta_b)$, once the generic within-component variance ξ is integrated out, $\lambda_i - \lambda_l \sim \{a_\xi/(2b_\xi)\}^{1/2} t(2a_\xi)$, the numerical value of the hyper-parameter is obtained by solving the equation with respect to b_ξ

$$b_\xi = \frac{a_\xi}{2} \Delta_b^2 \left\{ F^{-1} \left(\frac{1 + p_0}{2}; 2a_\xi \right) \right\}^{-2}, \tag{5}$$

where p_0 is close to 1 and $F(d)$ is the distribution function of a standard Student-t distribution with d degrees of freedom.

Fixing the hyper-parameter b_τ that controls the spread between the components is slightly more elaborated. Bottolo and Dellaportas [4] naturally require that the component means are well separated and in fact their spread should be larger than the within-component variance. To this aim, they impose that for any two components r and s, the density of $(\lambda_i - \lambda_l)$ is higher than the density of $(\theta_r - \theta_s)$ in the interval $(-\Delta_b, \Delta_b)$, where θ_r, θ_r are the components' mean, see Eq. (1). Since $\tau \sim (2b_\tau)^{-1} \chi^2(2a_\tau)$, where $\chi^2(d)$ is the chi-square distribution with d degrees of freedom, once the generic between-components variance τ is integrated out, $(\theta_r - \theta_s) \sim \{a_\tau/(2b_\tau)\}^{1/2} t(2a_\tau)$, the above requirement implies that hyper-parameter b_τ should satisfy the condition

$$t \left\{ \Delta_b \left(\frac{a_\xi}{2b_\xi} \right)^{\frac{1}{2}}; 2a_\xi \right\} \left(\frac{a_\xi}{2b_\xi} \right)^{\frac{1}{2}} = t \left\{ \Delta_b \left(\frac{a_\tau}{2b_\tau} \right)^{\frac{1}{2}}; 2a_\tau \right\} \left(\frac{a_\tau}{2b_\tau} \right)^{\frac{1}{2}}. \tag{6}$$

The the non-trivial solution of b_τ that can obtained by applying a bisection algorithm on (6). Finally, setting $B = 200$ and using (5) and (6), for each value of Δ_b, Bottolo and Dellaportas [4] construct a $B \times 1$ look-up tables for b_ξ and b_τ, respectively. Finally, they set both $a_\xi = 3$ and $a_\tau = 3$ to ensure the existence of the second moment of ξ and τ.

5 MCMC Implementation

The complex model specification of BHHM can only be dealt with an MCMC algorithm. The design of such an algorithm borrows from numerous papers that adopt MCMC in Bayesian hierarchical models, so we only note here the following key ingredients in the required Gibbs steps. Conditional on λ_{ij}, sampling from the parameters of the J finite mixtures of normals with unknown number of components requires simultaneous parallel implementation of J reversible jump algorithms proposed and studied in detail by Richardson and Green [20]. Conditional on all the parameters in RHS of (1) used in the finite mixtures specification, the full conditional density of λ_{ij} is derived by just multiplying a normal density obtained by (1) and the density coming from the likelihood contribution from the top level of the hierarchy. If the top level is modelled with a normal density, and $\psi_{ij} = \lambda_{ij}$ as in the example of Sect. 3.1, this density is normal and a Gibbs sampling step is required; otherwise we need to adopt a Metropolis step for λ_{ij}. Given the large number I of first-stage parameter to be sampled, see for instance the example of Sect. 3.3, an automatic tuning of the Metropolis proposal density for each first-stage parameter is sought. Both adaptive Metropolis [21] or multiple try Metropolis [17] can be used to make the MCMC algorithm fully automatic.

6 An Application Based on FTSE UK Index

We demonstrate the power of BHMM's by analysing 100 stocks from the FTSE UK Index using the model of Sect. 3.4. We used 240 working days to fit the AR(1)-GARCH(1,1) model with t-errors and we applied the BHMM (1) with the default prior specification suggested in Sect. 4. In fact, since we deal here with times series data, instead of using the MLE estimates of the AR(1)-GARCH(1,1) model for the actual data we analyse, we performed the same procedure described in Sect. 4 employing historical data observed *before* the first day of the data we used for inference. Specifically, we used 480 days to create the look-up tables for b_ξ and b_τ. Therefore, our prior is not data-based but expresses genuine prior information based on historical data [13].

There are two competing Bayesian hierarchical models with which one would compare the inference of BHMM. The first is the simple Bayesian independent model in which the data from each stock are treated separately and non-informative priors, independent from the priors of other stocks, are placed in each parameter of the model. No shrinkage is achieved and when the priors are diffuse enough the posterior densities coincide with the normalised likelihood functions. At the other extreme, one may adopt the fully exchangeable model which is a special case of the BHMM when there is only one normal component. Here the shrinkage of all 100 corresponding parameters to a central value takes place and the effect of borrowing strength between stocks is maximized.

Figures 2 and 3 present how the posterior means of the AR(1) and GARCH(1,1) specification vary in the three models. Notice that the shrinkage in BHMM is weaker than the one achieved in the fully exchangeable model, especially for the auto-regressive parameter ρ, but the well-known phenomenon of order reversal effect is still being observed.

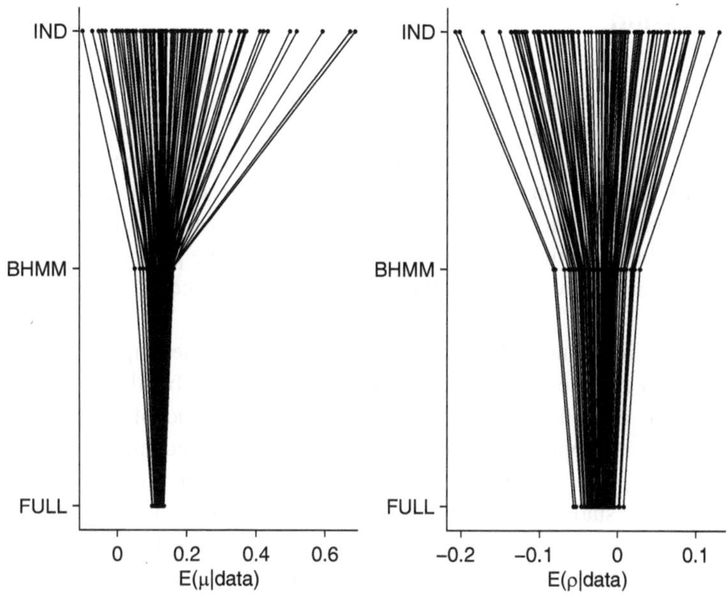

Fig. 2 Posterior means of the parameter η and ρ in model described in Sect. 3.4 for 100 stocks of FTSE UK Index under the independence (IND), partial exchangeability (BHMM) and full exchangeability (FULL) model

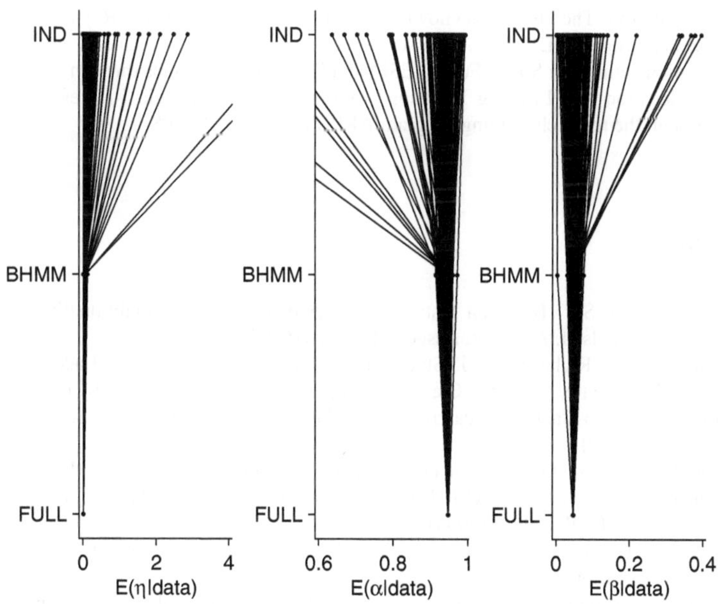

Fig. 3 Posterior means of the parameter η, α and β in model described in Sect. 3.4 for 100 stocks of FTSE UK Index under the independence (IND), partial exchangeability (BHMM) and full exchangeability (FULL) model

7 Discussion

We have reviewed a generalisation of Bayesian hierarchical models [16] which specifies a more general modelling structure based on partial exchangeability assumption in the second stage of the hierarchy. Careful prior specifications and intensive MCMC implementation are essential in constructing the proposed models. We believe that when these issues are taken care of, the resulting modelling freedom that exploits the modern Bayesian viewpoint of specifying priors that lead to model averaging inferences will be a valuable tool for inference in complex statistical models.

Modelling simultaneously first-stage parameters is one important area which in our opinion requires further work. In Sect. 3.3 the probability of under- over-expression are modelled separately, merely on the ground of simplicity. Indeed it would be more appropriate to analyse them jointly, because of the constraint $\psi_{i3} = 1 - \psi_{i1} - \psi_{i2}$, where ψ_{i3} is the probability of normal expression. In Sect. 3.4, strong stationarity of the GARCH process is attained by imposing the constraint $\alpha_i + \beta_i \leq 1$. Also in this case the two first-stage parameters are treated independently for simplicity. Nonetheless extending BHMM to the multivariate case is not straightforward, mainly because it will be difficult to specify "joint negligible differences" between parameters. Alternative models that go beyond this definition are therefore required.

Acknowledgements The authors acknowledge financial support from the Royal Society (International Exchanges grant IE110977). The second author acknowledges financial support from the European Union (European Social Fund—ESF) and Greek national funds through the Operational Program "Education and Lifelong Learning" of the National Strategic Reference Framework (NSRF) through the research funding program ARISTEIA-LIKEJUMPS.

References

1. Albert, J., Chib, S.: Bayesian tests and model diagnostics in conditionally independent hierarchical models. J. Am. Stat. Assoc. **92**(439), 916–925 (1997)
2. Bhattacharjee, A., Richards, W.G., Staunton, J., Li, C., Monti, S., Vasa, P., Ladd, C., Beheshti, J., Bueno, R., Gillette, M., et al.: Classification of human lung carcinomas by mrna expression profiling reveals distinct adenocarcinoma subclasses. Proc. Natl. Acad. Sci. USA **98**(24), 13790–13795 (2001)
3. Bottolo, L., Consonni, G.: Bayesian clustering of gene expression microarray data for subgroup identification. In: Atti della XLII Riunione Scientifica della Societa' Italiana di Statistica, pp. 187–198. CLEUP, Padova (2004)
4. Bottolo, L., Dellaportas, P.: Bayesian hierarchical mixture models for financial time series (2015, in preparation)
5. Bottolo, L., Consonni, G., Dellaportas, P., Lijoi, A.: Bayesian analysis of extreme values by mixture modeling. Extremes **6**(1), 25–47 (2003)
6. Consonni, G., Veronese, P.: A Bayesian method for combining results from several binomial experiments. J. Am. Stat. Assoc. **90**(431), 935–944 (1995)

7. Dawid, A.P.: Exchangeability and its ramifications. In: Damien, P., Dellaportas, P., Polson, N.G., Stephens, D.A. (eds.) Bayesian Theory and Applications, pp. 19–30. Oxford University Press, Oxford (2013)
8. Escobar, M.D., West, M.: Bayesian density estimation and inference using mixtures. J. Am. Stat. Assoc. **90**(430), 577–588 (1995)
9. Garrett, E.S., Parmigiani, G.: POE: statistical methods for qualitative analysis of gene expression. In: The Analysis of Gene Expression Data, pp. 362–387. Springer, Berlin (2003)
10. Gelfand, A.E., Ghosh, S.: Hierarchical modelling. In: Damien, P., Dellaportas, P., Polson, N.G., Stephens, D.A. (eds.) Bayesian Theory and Applications, pp. 33–49. Oxford University Press, Oxford (2013)
11. George, E.I., Liang, F., Xu, X.: From minimax shrinkage estimation to minimax shrinkage prediction. Stat. Sci. **27**(1), 82–94 (2012)
12. Green, P.J., Richardson, S.: Modelling heterogeneity with and without the Dirichlet process. Scand. J. Stat. **28**(2), 355–375 (2001)
13. Ibrahim, J.G., Chen, M.-H.: Power prior distributions for regression models. Stat. Sci. **15**(1), 46–60 (2000)
14. Lee, H., Li, J.: Variable selection for clustering by separability based on ridgelines. J. Comput. Graph. Stat. **21**(2), 315–337 (2012)
15. Lin, L., Chan, C., West, M.: Discriminative variable subsets in bayesian classification with mixture models, with application in flow cytometry studies. Biostatistics (2015, in press)
16. Lindley, D.V., Smith, A.F.: Bayes estimates for the linear model. J. R. Stat. Soc. B **34**(1), 1–41 (1972)
17. Martino, L., Read, J.: On the flexibility of the design of multiple try Metropolis schemes. Comput. Stat. **28**(6), 2797–2823 (2013)
18. Nobile, A., Green, P.J.: Bayesian analysis of factorial experiments by mixture modelling. Biometrika **87**(1), 15–35 (2000)
19. Parmigiani, G., Garrett, E.S., Anbazhagan, R., Gabrielson, E.: A statistical framework for expression-based molecular classification in cancer. J. R. Stat. Soc. B **64**(4), 717–736 (2002)
20. Richardson, S., Green, P.J.: On Bayesian analysis of mixtures with an unknown number of components (with discussion). J. R. Stat. Soc. B **59**(4), 731–792 (1997)
21. Roberts, G.O., Rosenthal, J.S.: Examples of adaptive MCMC. J. Comput. Graph. Stat. **18**(2), 349–367 (2009)
22. Smith, R.L.: Extreme value analysis of environmental time series: an application to trend detection in ground-level ozone. Stat. Sci. **4**(4), 367–377 (1989)
23. Smith, R.L., Goodman, D.: Bayesian risk analysis. In: Embrechts, P. (ed.) Extremes and Integrated Risk Management, pp. 235–251. Risk Books, London (2000)

iBATCGH: Integrative Bayesian Analysis of Transcriptomic and CGH Data

Alberto Cassese, Michele Guindani, and Marina Vannucci

Abstract We describe a method for the integration of high-throughput data from different sources. More specifically, `iBATCGH` is a package for the integrative analysis of transcriptomic and genomic data, based on a hierarchical Bayesian model. Through the specification of a measurement error model we relate the gene expression levels to latent copy number states which, in turn, are related to the observed surrogate CGH measurement via a hidden Markov model. Selection of relevant associations is performed employing variable selection priors that explicitly incorporate dependence information across adjacent copy number states. Posterior inference is carried out through Markov chain Monte Carlo techniques that efficiently explores the space of all possible associations. In this chapter we review the model and present the functions provided in `iBATCGH`, an R package based on a C implementation of the inferential algorithm. Lastly, we illustrate the method via a case study on ovarian cancer.

1 Introduction

In recent years, the field of genomics has seen the development of modern profiling high-throughput techniques that have resulted in the generation of large-scale data sets. The development of these modern techniques has made available several platforms to profile DNA, RNA and proteins, at different levels of accuracy. Integrating data from those different sources has emerged as a challenging problem in genomics, and a fundamental step in the understanding of many diseases. For example, it is now well known that cancer is the consequence of a dynamic interplay

A. Cassese
Maastricht University, Maastricht, The Netherlands
e-mail: alberto.cassese@maastrichtuniversity.nl

M. Guindani
UT MD Anderson Cancer Center, Houston, TX, USA
e-mail: mguindani@mdanderson.org

M. Vannucci (✉)
Department of Statistics, Rice University, Houston, TX, USA
e-mail: marina@rice.edu

A. Frigessi et al. (eds.), *Statistical Analysis for High-Dimensional Data*,
Abel Symposia 11, DOI 10.1007/978-3-319-27099-9_6

at different levels (DNA, mRNA and protein). Multilevel studies that try to integrate different types of data have therefore become of great interest.

Here we focus on the combined analysis of gene expression data and DNA copy number aberrations. Gene expression data are measurements of the abundance of a set of transcripted genes in a specific tissue. At the DNA level, many different kinds of aberration can occur and, for this reason, many different methods have been developed to detect them. Here we focus on Comparative Genomic Hybridization (CGH), a method able to detect copy number changes. This technique has a relatively high resolution and can span a large part of the genome in a single experiment. CGH data are well suited for cancer studies, since cancer is the result of a number of complex biological events and as such it cannot be attributed to a single mutation. Thus, discovering amplification of oncogenes or deletion of tumor suppressors is an important step for elucidating tumorigenesis.

Some methods that rely on regression models as a way to integrate gene expression data with copy number variants have been developed [21, 28]. These methods do not infer the underlying copy number information, but rather use their surrogate CGH measurements as regressors. Alternatively, methods have been proposed that first estimate copy number latent states using available methodology, and, as a second step, use these estimates as regressors [3, 33]. Here we describe a novel method we have proposed for the joint estimation of copy number aberrations and their association with copy number variants [7, 8]. More specifically, we have developed a model that regresses gene expression on copy number states, while simultaneously estimating the latent copy number states of the observed surrogate CGH data. This modeling strategy is able to take into account the uncertainty on the latent unobserved copy number states typical of CGH data, while simultaneously assessing their association with gene expression. The model employs selection priors to detect significant associations, incorporating information on the physical distance between neighboring DNA probes and their latent copy number and association status. The latent copy number states are estimated via a hidden Markov model, which is able to capture the peculiar stickiness of CGH data.

In this chapter, after reviewing the proposed methodology, we describe in details the implementation of the methods via the package `iBATGH`, released under the GNU General Public License within the R project, and freely available on the CRAN website. The package is mainly based on an algorithm using C-code and the interface with the R environment is handled using the packages `Rcpp` and `RcppArmadillo` [13]. This choice achieves a good performance in terms of computational speed, with the advantage of a user friendly interface as provided by the R environment.

The rest of this chapter is organized as follows. In Sect. 2 we describe the model, the priors and the posterior inferential algorithm. In Sect. 3 we describe the R package `iBATCGH`. In Sect. 4 we illustrate the method via a case study.

2 Model

Let us first introduce the notation that will be used throughout the following sections. Let $\boldsymbol{Y} = [Y_{ig}]_{n \times G}$ be the $n \times G$ matrix of gene expression measurements on G genes in n subjects. Let $\boldsymbol{X} = [X_{im}]_{n \times M}$ denote the matrix of CGH measurements on M DNA probes, on the same samples ($i = 1, \ldots, n$). We assume the CGH probes ordered according to their chromosomal location and refer to two consecutive probes as adjacent. Lastly, let $\boldsymbol{Z} = [\boldsymbol{Y}, \boldsymbol{X}]_{n \times (G+M)}$ denote the $(n \times (G + M))$ matrix containing all data measurements.

In our modeling approach we treat the observed CGH intensities $\boldsymbol{X}$ as surrogates for the unobserved copy number states. In particular, we introduce $\boldsymbol{\xi} = [\xi_{im}]_{n \times M}$, a latent matrix of copy number states, and consider a four copy number states classification [15]:

$$
\begin{aligned}
\xi_{im} &= 1 \quad \text{for copy number loss (less than two copies of the fragment)} \\
\xi_{im} &= 2 \quad \text{for copy-neutral state (exactly two copies of the fragment)} \\
\xi_{im} &= 3 \quad \text{for a single copy gain (exactly three copies of the fragment)} \\
\xi_{im} &= 4 \quad \text{for multiple copy gains (more than three copies of the fragment).}
\end{aligned}
$$

We assume that, conditional on the latent state $\boldsymbol{\xi}$, the corresponding observed surrogate $\boldsymbol{X}$ does not contain additional information on the outcome $\boldsymbol{Y}$, that is, $f(\boldsymbol{Y}|\boldsymbol{\xi}, \boldsymbol{X}) = f(\boldsymbol{Y}|\boldsymbol{\xi})$. In the statistical literature this modeling framework is commonly referred to as a *non-differential measurement error model* [27], and allows the factorization of the joint distribution of $\boldsymbol{Z}$ as the product of two conditionally independent sub models: an outcome model, that in our modeling context relates the gene expressions with the latent copy number states, and a measurement model, that relates the latent states to the observed surrogate CGH measurements, $f(\boldsymbol{Z}|\boldsymbol{\xi}) = f(\boldsymbol{Y}|\boldsymbol{\xi})f(\boldsymbol{X}|\boldsymbol{\xi})$. As commonly done in the literature on integrative genomics, we assume conditional independence of the gene expression measurements, $\boldsymbol{Y}_i \perp \boldsymbol{Y}_j|\xi_1, \ldots, \boldsymbol{\xi}_M$. We also assume independence of the CGH measurements, conditional on their latent states, $\boldsymbol{X}_i \perp \boldsymbol{X}_j|\boldsymbol{\xi}_1, \ldots, \boldsymbol{\xi}_M$. Given those assumptions, we can write our proposed model as

$$
f(\mathbf{Z}|\boldsymbol{\xi}) = \prod_{i=1}^{n} \left\{ \prod_{g=1}^{G} f(Y_{ig}|\boldsymbol{\xi}_i) \prod_{m=1}^{M} f(X_{im}|\xi_{im}) \right\}. \tag{1}
$$

Below we provide detailed specification of the outcome and the marginal models.

2.1 Outcome Model with Measurement Error

We follow current literature on models that integrate gene expression levels with genetic data and specify the outcome model as a linear regression of the gene expression measurements on the latent copy number states [21, 28]. For each gene $g = 1, \ldots, G$ the regression is defined as follows,

$$Y_{ig} = \mu_g + \boldsymbol{\xi}_i \boldsymbol{\beta}_g + \epsilon_{ig}, \qquad i = 1, \ldots, n, \tag{2}$$

where μ_g is a gene specific intercept and $\epsilon_{ig} \sim \mathcal{N}(0, \sigma_g^2)$ are independent normally distributed errors, with σ_g^2 a gene specific variance. We further assume conjugate prior distributions for the intercept, $\mu_g | \sigma_g^2 \sim \mathcal{N}(0, c_\mu^{-1} \sigma_g^2)$, and gene specific precisions, $\sigma_g^{-2} \sim \text{Ga}(\frac{\delta}{2}, \frac{d}{2})$, with c_μ, δ and d hyperparameters to be chosen.

We look at the identification of copy number variations associated with gene expression levels as a variable selection problem. We therefore introduce a latent binary matrix $\boldsymbol{R} = [r_{gm}]_{G \times M}$, where the generic element r_{gm} is set to one if the corresponding regression coefficient β_{gm} is different from zero, and $r_{gm} = 0$ otherwise. As commonly done in the Bayesian variable selection literature, we adopt spike and slab priors on the conditional distribution of the regression coefficients,

$$\beta_{gm} | r_{gm}, \sigma_g^2 \sim r_{gm} \mathcal{N}(0, c_\beta^{-1} \sigma_g^2) + (1 - r_{gm}) \delta_0(\beta_{gm}), \tag{3}$$

with $\delta_0(\cdot)$ a point mass at zero, σ_g^2 is a gene specific variance, and c_β an hyperparameter to be chosen [5, 14]. Equation (3) is completed with a prior on r_{gm}. The simplest choice is to assume an independent Bernoulli prior, $r_{gm} \sim \text{Bern}(p)$ with p a fixed hyperparameter. However, in Sect. 2.3 below, we describe two alternative priors that accounts for spatial information [7, 8], borrowing strength across genes.

2.2 Marginal Model

We now describe the marginal model that relates the latent copy number states with the surrogate CGH measurements. In the literature this problem has been tackled by using modeling strategies that employ either circular binary segmentation, a method that infers change points [35], or clustering based methods [6, 25]. In addition, Bayesian nonparametric methods have been applied to CGH modeling [1, 12, 38], as well as methods that rely on hidden Markov models [9, 15, 36]. Here we extend the latter approaches, in particular the one proposed by Guha et al. [15], to handle multiple samples in a single modeling framework.

A hidden Markov model is a state space model with discrete hidden states. It comprises of a Markov chain with stochastic measurements on the hidden states and, conditionally on the states, of an independent emission distribution. In the context of our specific application, conditional on the latent copy number states, the observed CGH measurements are assumed independent and normally distributed, and the emission distribution is defined as

$$X_{im}|(\xi_{im} = j) \overset{iid}{\sim} \mathcal{N}(\eta_j, \sigma_j^2), \tag{4}$$

with η_j and σ_j^2 denoting respectively the expected $\log_2$ ratio and variance of all CGH probes in state j ($j = 1, \ldots, 4$). As for the latent copy number states, we choose a first order HMM, which assumes that the probability of being in a particular copy number state for a given probe m depends only on the state of the previous probe $(m - 1)$,

$$P(\xi_{im}|\xi_{i1}, \ldots, \xi_{i(m-1)}) = P(\xi_{im}|\xi_{i(m-1)}) = a_{\xi_{i(m-1)}\xi_{im}}, \tag{5}$$

with $\boldsymbol{A} = [a_{hj}]_{4\times 4}$ a matrix of transition probabilities with strictly positive elements. We also assume that the distribution of the first probe is given by the unique stationary distribution of $\boldsymbol{A}$, denoted by π_A. We further assume the samples to be independent, and that they share the same transition matrix. In summary, the proposed HMM can be factorized as

$$\begin{aligned} P(\boldsymbol{X}_1, \ldots, \boldsymbol{X}_M, \boldsymbol{\xi}_1, \ldots, \boldsymbol{\xi}_M) = &\prod_{i=1}^{n} P(X_{i1}|\xi_{i1})P(\xi_{i1}) \\ &\prod_{m=2}^{M} P(X_{im}|\xi_{im})P(\xi_{im}|\xi_{i(m-1)}). \end{aligned} \tag{6}$$

To complete our prior specification of the HMM, we choose conjugate priors. In particular, we assume each row of the transition matrix $\boldsymbol{A}$ as a draw from independent Dirichlet distributions, $\boldsymbol{a}_h = [a_{h1}, a_{h2}, a_{h3}, a_{h4}] \sim \text{Dir}(\phi_1, \phi_2, \phi_3, \phi_4)$, for $h = 1, \ldots, 4$, with $\boldsymbol{\phi} = [\phi_1, \phi_2, \phi_3, \phi_4]$ a vector of hyperparameters to be chosen. As for the state specific mean η_j and variance σ_j^2, we assume $\eta_j \sim N(\delta_j, \tau_j^2)\boldsymbol{I}\{low_{\eta_j} < \eta_j < upp_{\eta_j}\}$ and $\sigma_j^{-2} \sim \text{Gamma}(b_j, l_j)\boldsymbol{I}\{\sigma_j^{-2} > upp_{\sigma_j}\}$, for $j = 1, \ldots, 4$. Lastly, we set $low_{\eta_1} = -\infty$, $upp_{\eta_4} = \infty$, while all other hyperparameters are defined by the user on the base of the platform [15].

2.3 Spatially Informed Variable Selection Priors

Our choice of the selection prior relies on the consideration that two contiguous regions of copy number variants might correspond to the same aberration. As a consequence, they are more likely to jointly affect gene expression. We therefore define a prior that accounts for the selection status of the adjacent probes. In other words, the prior probability $p(r_{gm})$ of an association between gene g and probe m depends on the values of $r_{g(m-1)}$ and $r_{g(m+1)}$. As a first step of the prior construction, we define a probe specific quantity that incorporates, in a multiplicative fashion, information on the physical distance among probes and on the frequency of copy number change points across samples as

$$s_{(m-1)m} = \left\{ \frac{\exp\{1 - \frac{d_m}{D}\} - 1}{\exp\{1\} - 1} \right\} \left\{ \frac{1}{n} \sum_{i=1}^{n} \boldsymbol{I}\{\xi_{im} = \xi_{i(m-1)}\} \right\}, \tag{7}$$

where d_m denotes the distance between adjacent probes $[m-1, m]$ and where D is the total length of the DNA fragment, for example the length of the chromosome under study. We then explore two different ways of employing these quantities in the definition of the selection prior [7, 8]. More specifically, we have investigated a mixture prior and a Probit prior.

(a) **Mixture prior**: We start defining the quantities,

$$\gamma_m = \frac{\alpha}{\alpha + s_{(m-1)m} + s_{m(m+1)}},$$
$$\omega_m^{(1)} = \frac{s_{(m-1)m}}{\alpha + s_{(m-1)m} + s_{m(m+1)}}, \quad \omega_m^{(2)} = \frac{s_{m(m+1)}}{\alpha + s_{(m-1)m} + s_{m(m+1)}}, \tag{8}$$

with α set to a positive real value, and then define a mixture prior with two components

$$\pi(r_{gm}|r_{g(m-1)}, r_{g(m+1)}, \boldsymbol{\xi}, \pi_1) = \gamma_m[\pi_1^{r_{gm}}(1-\pi_1)^{(1-r_{gm})}] + \sum_{j=1}^{2} \omega_m^{(j)} \boldsymbol{I}\{r_{gm} = r_{g(m+(-1)^j)}\}. \tag{9}$$

According to Eq. (9), with probability γ_m, the r_{gm}'s are distributed Bern(π_1), independently of the neighboring values. Otherwise, r_{gm} assumes the same value as in $r_{g(m-1)}$ or $r_{g(m+1)}$, with probability $\omega_m^{(1)}$ or $\omega_m^{(2)}$, respectively. We note that the weights in Eq. (8) sum up to one, i.e. $\gamma_m + \omega_m^{(1)} + \omega_m^{(2)} = 1$, and that the case $\gamma_m = 1$ reduces to an independent Bernoulli prior. We further note that $\alpha \to \infty$ implies $\gamma_m \to 1$, that is the independent prior, while when $\alpha = 0$, r_{gm} depends only on the values $r_{g(m-1)}$ and $r_{g(m+1)}$, with weights proportional to $s_{(m-1)m}$ and $s_{m(m+1)}$, respectively. As a consequence, lower values of α implies a stronger dependence on the selection status of the adjacent probes. In addition, larger values of $s_{(m-1)m}$ imply a stronger dependence of probe m on probe $(m-1)$, and viceversa. This reflects the assumption that two probes physically close and that share a similar copy number status are more likely to have the same association pattern. In [7] we suggest to chose α in the range $\alpha = [20, 50]$, for a good balance in terms of false positives and false negatives. We complete our prior specification by imposing a Beta hyperprior on $\pi_1 \sim$ Beta(e,f), and integrating it out. This results in the following equation

$$\pi(r_{gm}|r_{g(m-1)},r_{g(m+1)},\boldsymbol{\xi}) = \gamma_m \frac{\Gamma(e+f)\Gamma(e+r_{gm})\Gamma(f+1-r_{gm})}{\Gamma(e+f+1)\Gamma(e)\Gamma(f)} + \sum_{j=1}^{2} \omega_m^{(j)} \boldsymbol{I}_{\{r_{gm}=r_{g(m+(-1)^j)}\}}. \tag{10}$$

(b) **Probit prior**: Let us first define the quantity Q_m as

$$Q_m = (-1)^{r_{g(m-1)}} s_{(m-1)m} + (-1)^{r_{g(m+1)}} s_{m(m+1)}. \tag{11}$$

Note that Q_m can either increase or decrease based on the selection status of the adjacent probes, and that the amount of increase or decrease depends on $s_{(m-1)m}$ and $s_{m(m+1)}$. We define the probability of inclusion for r_{gm} as

$$\pi(r_{gm}=1|r_{g(m-1)},r_{g(m+1)},\boldsymbol{\xi}) = 1-\Phi(\alpha_0+\alpha_1 Q_m), \tag{12}$$

where Φ indicates the c.d.f. of a standard normal distribution, and α_0 and $\alpha_1 > 0$ are hyperparameters to be set. In particular, α_0 represents a baseline intercept that can be set according to an a priori specified "level of significance", in absence of other covariates. Similarly, α_1 can be interpreted as a coefficient that captures the strength of the association between adjacent probes. We note that $\pi(r_{gm})$ is a monotonic function of Q_m, therefore it increases or decreases, based on the selection status of the adjacent probes, by an amount determined by $s_{(m-1)m}$ and $s_{m(m+1)}$. This reflects the assumption that two probes physically close and that share a similar copy number status are more likely to have the same association pattern. Even though the prior specifications (9) and (12) share the same assumptions and employ similar quantities, prior (12) is of more easy interpretation and has produced better results on simulated data [8].

2.4 Posterior Inference

In this section we describe the approach employed to perform posterior inference. In particular, the methodology aims at estimating the association matrix $\boldsymbol{R}$ and the matrix of copy number states $\boldsymbol{\xi}$. We rely on a Markov chain Monte Carlo algorithm that employs stochastic search variable selection techniques [5, 7, 8, 14, 28, 29, 31]. In order to simplify the algorithm and to improve the mixing of the chain, we integrate out the regression coefficients μ_g, β_g and σ_g^2 [5, 29, 32]. The marginal likelihood reduces to

$$f(\boldsymbol{Y}_g|\boldsymbol{\xi},\boldsymbol{R}) = \frac{(2\pi)^{-\frac{n}{2}}(\frac{c_\mu}{c_\mu+n})^{\frac{1}{2}}(c_\beta)^{\frac{k_g}{2}}\Gamma(\frac{n+\delta}{2})(\frac{d}{2})^{\frac{\delta}{2}}}{|\boldsymbol{U}_g|^{\frac{1}{2}}\Gamma(\frac{\delta}{2})(\frac{d+q_g}{2})^{(\frac{n+\delta}{2})}}, \tag{13}$$

Algorithm 1 Selection of the subsets of rows of $\boldsymbol{R}$ and $\boldsymbol{\xi}$ to be updated at every MCMC iteration

set *cumsum* $= 0$
repeat
  Generate ζ from Geom(p)
  Sum ζ to *cumsum*
  Add *cumsum* to the set of selected features
until *cumsum* $> F$

with $q_g = \boldsymbol{Y}_g^T \boldsymbol{H}_s \boldsymbol{Y}_g - \boldsymbol{Y}_g^T \boldsymbol{H}_s \boldsymbol{\xi}_R \boldsymbol{U}_g^{-1} \boldsymbol{\xi}_R^T \boldsymbol{H}_s \boldsymbol{Y}_g$, $\boldsymbol{U}_g = c_\beta \boldsymbol{I}_{k_g} + \boldsymbol{\xi}_R^T \boldsymbol{H}_s \boldsymbol{\xi}_R$ and $\boldsymbol{H}_s = \boldsymbol{I}_n - \frac{\boldsymbol{1}_n \boldsymbol{1}_n^T}{n+c_\mu}$, where k_g indicates the number of selected regressors for the gth regression. Aiming at more efficient MCMC steps, we perform multiple updates of $\boldsymbol{R}$ and $\boldsymbol{\xi}$. This is accomplished relying on Algorithm 1 for the selection of a subset of rows to be updated at every MCMC iteration. The MCMC consists of four steps and is described below.

- Update $\boldsymbol{R}$ using a Metropolis step. First use Algorithm 1 with parameters $p = p_R$ and $F = G$ to select at random a set of genes. Then, for each gene in the set, choose between an Add/Delete or Swap moves, with probability ρ and $(1 - \rho)$ respectively. For the Add/Delete move, choose at random one element of the row and change its selection status. For the Swap move, select at random two elements of the row with different inclusion status and swap their values. In order to efficiently explore the space of all possible associations, we do not consider some CGH probes as possible regressors. In particular, we exclude those CGH probes that have been called in neutral state in a fraction of samples larger than p_{MC}, at the current MCMC iteration. Note that p_{MC} is a parameter set by the user, for example 10 % is the default argument in the package. We accept the proposed move with probability

$$\min\left[\frac{f(\boldsymbol{Y}|\boldsymbol{\xi}, \boldsymbol{R}^{new})\pi(\boldsymbol{R}^{new}|\boldsymbol{\xi})}{f(\boldsymbol{Y}|\boldsymbol{\xi}, \boldsymbol{R}^{old})\pi(\boldsymbol{R}^{old}|\boldsymbol{\xi})}, 1\right].$$

- Update $\boldsymbol{\xi}$ using a Metropolis-Hastings step. First select a column of $\boldsymbol{\xi}$ and then use Algorithm 1 with parameters $p = p_\xi$ and $F = N$ to select at random a subset of samples. For each selected element sample a candidate state using the current transition matrix $\boldsymbol{A}$. In other words, we propose ξ_{im}^{new} conditional on ξ_{im}^{old}. Accept the proposed move with probability

$$\min\left[\frac{f(\boldsymbol{Y}|\boldsymbol{\xi}^{new}, \boldsymbol{R})f(\boldsymbol{X}|\boldsymbol{\xi}^{new})\pi(\boldsymbol{R}|\boldsymbol{\xi}^{new})\pi(\boldsymbol{\xi}^{new}|\boldsymbol{\xi}^{old}, \boldsymbol{A})q(\boldsymbol{\xi}^{old}|\boldsymbol{\xi}^{new})}{f(\boldsymbol{Y}|\boldsymbol{\xi}^{old}, \boldsymbol{R})f(\boldsymbol{X}|\boldsymbol{\xi}^{old})\pi(\boldsymbol{R}|\boldsymbol{\xi}^{old})\pi(\boldsymbol{\xi}^{old}|\boldsymbol{\xi}^{old}, \boldsymbol{A})q(\boldsymbol{\xi}^{new}|\boldsymbol{\xi}^{old})}, 1\right].$$

- Update η_j, for $j = 1, \ldots, 4$ using a Gibbs step. Sample $\eta_j|\boldsymbol{X}, \boldsymbol{\xi}, \sigma_j \sim \mathcal{N}(\nu_j, \theta_j^{-2})\mathbf{I}_{\{low_{\eta_j} < \eta_j < upp_{\eta_j}\}}$, with precision $\theta_j = \tau_j^{-2} + n_j\sigma_j^{-2}$ and weighted mean $\nu_j = \theta_j^{-2}(\delta_j\tau_j^{-2} + \bar{X}_j n_j \sigma_j^{-2})$, where $n_j = \sum_{m=1}^{M}\sum_{i=1}^{n} \boldsymbol{I}\{\xi_{im} = j\}$ and $\bar{X}_j = \frac{1}{n_j}\sum_{m=1}^{M}\sum_{i=1}^{n} X_{im}\boldsymbol{I}\{\xi_{im} = j\}$.

- Update σ_j, for $j = 1, \ldots, 4$ using a Gibbs step. Sample $\sigma_j|\boldsymbol{X}, \boldsymbol{\xi}, \eta_j \sim \text{IG}(b_j + \frac{n_j}{2}, l_j + \frac{V_j}{2})\boldsymbol{I}_{\{\sigma_j^{-2} > upp_{\sigma_j}\}}$, where $n_j = \sum_{m=1}^{M}\sum_{i=1}^{n} \boldsymbol{I}_{\{\xi_{im}=j\}}$ and $V_j = (X_{im} - \eta_j)^2 \boldsymbol{I}_{\{\xi_{im}=j\}}$.
- Update $\boldsymbol{A}$ using a Metropolis step. Generate for each row of $\boldsymbol{A}$ a new vector as $\boldsymbol{A}_{.j}^{new}|\boldsymbol{\xi} \sim Dir(\phi_1 + o_{h1}, \phi_2 + o_{h2}, \phi_3 + o_{h3}, \phi_4 + o_{h4})$, where $o_{hj} = \sum_{i=1}^{n}\sum_{m=1}^{M-1} \boldsymbol{I}_{\{\xi_{im}=h, \xi_{i(m+1)}=j\}}$, and accept it with probability

$$\min\left[1, \prod_{i=1}^{n} \frac{\pi_{A^{new}}(\xi_{i1})}{\pi_{A^{old}}(\xi_{i1})}\right].$$

We summarize the output of the MCMC as follows. Inference on $\boldsymbol{R}$ is performed computing the marginal probability of inclusion (PPI) for each of its elements. More specifically, PPIs are obtained by counting for each element of the matrix the number of iterations it was set to one after burn-in, and dividing by the total number of iteration after burn-in. A selection of the most relevant associations can be made by thresholding the PPIs based on some decision theoretic criterion, see for example [2, 23]. As for the inference on $\boldsymbol{\xi}$ we select for every position of the matrix the modal state after burn-in, i.e. the state that shows the highest count. Inference on the HMM parameters $\boldsymbol{A}$, $\boldsymbol{\mu}$ and $\boldsymbol{\sigma}$ is performed by averaging their values across the MCMC iterations, after burn-in.

3 The iBATCGH Package

The package `iBATCGH` is released under the GNU General Public License within the R project, and is freely available on the CRAN website. It uses the libraries `Rcpp` and `RcppArmadillo`, and it is based on a backbone C implementation [13]. The package comprises of nine functions and two data sets. The first data set, `NCI_60`, consists of the processed and filtered NCI-60 cancer cell lines data, as used in [7]. The second one, `TCGA_lung`, is the processed and filtered TCGA lung squamous cell carcinoma data set, as used in [8]. In the rest of the section, we describe the main R functions and provide an example on how to run them. A summary of the functions with their arguments, output and a brief description can be found in Table 1. Throughout this Section, the variables in the code will be written using `teletypefont`, while the corresponding notation used in Sect. 2 will be reported in parenthesis.

The functions `Scenario1` and `Scenario2` generate two types of simulated data sets, with `Scenario2` explicitly assuming dependence among the regression coefficients [7]. Their only argument is the error variance of the regression model `sigmak` (σ_ϵ), set to 0.1 by default. Those functions return a list composed by the

Table 1 Available functions of the package `iBATCG`, their arguments, output and brief description

Function	Arguments	Output	Description
`Center`	Y	$\bar{Y}$	*Preprocessing*, center each column of the gene expression matrix
`iBAT`	$\boldsymbol{Y}, \boldsymbol{X}, \boldsymbol{d}, D$, *intercept*, $\boldsymbol{\xi}$, $\boldsymbol{R}, \boldsymbol{A}, \eta, \boldsymbol{\sigma}, c_{\mu}, c_{\beta}, \delta, d$, $e, f, \alpha, \boldsymbol{\delta}$, ***tau***, $\boldsymbol{upp}_{\eta}$, $\boldsymbol{low}_{\eta}, \boldsymbol{b}, \boldsymbol{l}, \boldsymbol{upp}_{\sigma}, \boldsymbol{\phi}$, *niter*, *burnin*, *Cout*, ϕ, p_R, p_{MC}, p_{ξ}	**MCMC output**	*Main*, function for the model that employs the mixture prior
`iBATProbit`	$\boldsymbol{Y}, \boldsymbol{X}, \boldsymbol{d}, D$, *intercept*, $\boldsymbol{\xi}$, $\boldsymbol{R}, \boldsymbol{A}, \eta, \boldsymbol{\sigma}, c_{\mu}, c_{\beta}, \delta, d$, $\alpha_0, \alpha_1, \boldsymbol{\delta}$, ***tau***, $\boldsymbol{upp}_{\eta}$, $\boldsymbol{low}_{\eta}, \boldsymbol{b}, \boldsymbol{l}, \boldsymbol{upp}_{\sigma}, \boldsymbol{\phi}$, *niter*, *burnin*, *Cout*, ϕ, p_R, p_{MC}, p_{ξ}, *indep*	**MCMC output**	*Main*, function for the model that employs the Probit prior
`Inference`	**MCMC output**, G, M, *niter*, *burnin*, *threshold*	$\hat{\boldsymbol{R}}, \hat{\boldsymbol{\xi}}, \hat{\boldsymbol{A}}, \hat{\boldsymbol{\mu}}, \hat{\boldsymbol{\sigma}}$	*Postprocessing*, perform posterior inference on the output of the main function
`InitMu`	$\boldsymbol{\delta}, \boldsymbol{\tau}, \boldsymbol{low}_{\eta}, \boldsymbol{upp}_{\eta}$	$\boldsymbol{\mu}$	*Initialization*, initialize $\boldsymbol{\mu}$, sampling from the prior distribution
`InitXi`	$\boldsymbol{X}$	$\boldsymbol{\xi}$	*Initialization*, initialize $\boldsymbol{\xi}$, using a crude estimator on $\boldsymbol{X}$
`Scenario1`	σ_{ϵ}	$\boldsymbol{Y}, \boldsymbol{X}, \boldsymbol{\xi}, \boldsymbol{A}, \boldsymbol{\mu}, \boldsymbol{\sigma}, \boldsymbol{B}, \boldsymbol{d}, D$	*Simulated data*, simulate the data as described in [7, 8]
`Scenario2`	σ_{ϵ}	$\boldsymbol{Y}, \boldsymbol{X}, \boldsymbol{\xi}, \boldsymbol{A}, \boldsymbol{\mu}, \boldsymbol{\sigma}, \boldsymbol{B}, \boldsymbol{d}, D$	*Simulated data*, simulate the data as described in [7, 8]
`Tran`	$\boldsymbol{\xi}$	$\boldsymbol{A}$	*Preprocessing*, compute the transition matrix corresponding to a specific $\boldsymbol{\xi}$

A **bold** variable in the arguments/output represents a vector, matrix or list

two data matrices `Y` ($\boldsymbol{Y}$) and `X` ($\boldsymbol{X}$), and the empirical parameters of the HMM, `Xi` ($\boldsymbol{\xi}$), `A` ($\boldsymbol{A}$), `mu` ($\boldsymbol{\mu}$) and `Sd` ($\boldsymbol{\sigma}$). Also, they return a matrix of regression coefficients `coeff` ($\boldsymbol{B}$), a vector of distances between probes `distance` ($\boldsymbol{d}$) and the total length of the DNA fragment `disfix` (D).

The function `Center` takes as argument a matrix of gene expression measurements `Y` ($\boldsymbol{Y}$) and returns the matrix obtained after centering each column with respect to its mean. As for the initialization of the parameters, `InitMu` initializes the state specific mean vector, by sampling each element independently from its prior, i.e.

Algorithm 2 Crude estimator employed to initialize $\boldsymbol{\xi}$

for i=1 **to** i=N **do**

  for m=1 **to** m=M **do**

    if $X_{im} < bounds_1$ **then**
      set $\xi_{im} = 1$
    else if $X_{im} < bounds_2$ **then**
      set $\xi_{im} = 2$
    else if $X_{im} < bounds_3$ **then**
      set $\xi_{im} = 3$
    else
      set $\xi_{im} = 4$
    end if
  end for
end for

truncated normal distribution. This function has default arguments and can be run simply as `> mu = InitMu()`. However the user can change the arguments of the vector of state specific means `deltak` ($\boldsymbol{\delta}$), standard deviations `tauk` ($\boldsymbol{\tau}$), lower bound `low_bounds` ($\boldsymbol{low}_\eta$) and upper bound `upp_bounds` ($\boldsymbol{upp}_\eta$). The function `InitXi` takes a matrix of CGH data as the only argument and returns a crude estimate of the corresponding latent copy number states. More specifically, given a vector of threshold `bounds`, set by default to $[-0.5, 0.29, 0.79]$, the function simply applies the thresholding to the data and groups them into four subsets. Each subset is associated to a specific latent state as described in Algorithm 2. Given a matrix of latent states $\boldsymbol{\xi}$, an empirical transition matrix can be computed. In order to initialize $\boldsymbol{A}$, we use this empirical transition matrix computed on the initialized value of $\boldsymbol{\xi}$. The function implemented for this purpose is `Tran` and takes `xi` as only argument.

We now focus on the two main functions implemented for the integrative Bayesian analysis of gene expression and CGH data. More specifically, `iBAT` employs the mixture prior and `iBATProbit` employs the Probit prior. Tables 2 and 3 show a description of their arguments. In particular, the first column reports the arguments used in the code, the second column recalls the corresponding math notation as introduced in Sect. 2, and the third column adds a brief description. Note that the case of spatially independent variable selection priors can be obtained by setting the option `indep` to one or `alpha1` to zero, respectively in `iBAT` and `iBATProbit`. The output consists of an R list composed by `4*niter+3` objects, where `niter` is the number of MCMC iterations. The first `niter` objects of the list are vectors, each containing the positions of the association matrix set to one, at the corresponding MCMC iteration. Each of the following `niter` objects of the list are the transition matrices at the corresponding MCMC iteration, while the third and the fourth set of `niter` objects are the vectors of state specific mean and state specific variance, respectively. The last three objects of the list consist of three matrices counting the number of times the corresponding latent state has been set to 1, 3 and 4, respectively.

Table 2 Arguments of `iBAT`: name in the code, corresponding math notation, and brief description

Argument	Math	Description
`Y`	$\boldsymbol{Y}$	Matrix of gene expression data
`X`	$\boldsymbol{X}$	Matrix of CGH data
`distance`	$\boldsymbol{d}$	Vector of distance between CGH probes
`disfix`	D	Length of the chromosome under investigation
`intercept`	NA	If set to one an intercept is included in the regression model
`xi`	$\boldsymbol{\xi}$	Initialized matrix of latent states
`R`	$\boldsymbol{R}$	Initialized association matrix in a vector form. Default set to -1, that automatically creates a vector with all the positions set to zero
`tran`	$\boldsymbol{A}$	Initialized transition matrix
`mu`	$\boldsymbol{\mu}$	Initialized state specific mean vector
`sigma`	$\boldsymbol{\sigma}$	Initialized state specific standard deviation vector
`cmu`	c_{μ}	Parameter that controls the variance of the prior on the intercept
`c`	c_{β}	Parameter that determines the shrinkage in the model
`delta`	δ	Parameter of the Inverse-Gamma prior on the error variance
`d`	d	Parameter of the Inverse-Gamma prior on the error variance
`e`	e	Parameter of the Beta prior on the inclusion probability
`f`	f	Parameter of the Beta prior on the inclusion probability
`alpha`	α	Parameter that regulates the strength of the independent part of the mixture
`deltak`	$\boldsymbol{\delta}$	Vector of mean of the prior on the state specific mean
`tauk`	$\boldsymbol{\tau}$	Vector of standard deviation parameters of the prior on the state specific mean
`upp_bounds`	$\boldsymbol{upp}_{\eta}$	Vector of upper bounds of the prior on the state specific mean
`low_bounds`	$\boldsymbol{low}_{\eta}$	Vector of lower bounds of the prior on the state specific mean
`alpha_IG`	$\boldsymbol{b}$	Vector of parameters of the prior on the state specific standard deviation
`beta_IG`	$\boldsymbol{l}$	Vector of parameters of the prior on the state specific standard deviation
`low_IG`	$\boldsymbol{upp}_{\sigma}$	Truncation of the prior on the state specific standard deviation
`a`	$\boldsymbol{\phi}$	Vector of parameters of the prior on the transition matrix
`niter`	NA	Number of Markov Chain Monte Carlo iterations
`burnin`	NA	Burn-in
`Cout`	NA	Print the number of iterations ran every `Cout` iterations
`phi`	ϕ	Probability of an A/D step
`pR`	p_R	Parameter of the distribution used to select the rows to be updated at every MCMC iteration
`selectioncgh`	p_{MC}	Number of samples not in neutral state in order to consider a CGH as a potential candidate for association with gene expression. Default set to -1 that automatically set it to 10 % of the samples
`pXI`	p_{ξ}	Parameter of the distribution used to select the rows to be updated at every MCMC iteration
`indep`	NA	If set to an integer different from zero, run the analysis with an independent prior, i.e. setting $\alpha \to \infty$

Table 3 Arguments of `iBATProbit`: name in the code, corresponding math notation, and brief description

Argument	Math	Description
`Y`	$\boldsymbol{Y}$	Matrix of gene expression data
`X`	$\boldsymbol{X}$	Matrix of CGH data
`distance`	$\boldsymbol{d}$	Vector of distance between CGH probes
`disfix`	D	Length of the chromosome under investigation
`intercept`	NA	If set to one an intercept is included in the regression model
`xi`	$\boldsymbol{\xi}$	Initialized matrix of latent states
`R`	$\boldsymbol{R}$	Initialized association matrix in a vector form. Default set to -1, that automatically creates a vector with all the positions set to zero
`tran`	$\boldsymbol{A}$	Initialized transition matrix
`mu`	$\boldsymbol{\mu}$	Initialized state specific mean vector
`sigma`	$\boldsymbol{\sigma}$	Initialized state specific standard deviation vector
`cmu`	c_μ	Parameter that controls the variance of the prior on the intercept
`c`	c_β	Parameter that determines the shrinkage in the model
`delta`	δ	Parameter of the Inverse-Gamma prior on the error variance
`d`	d	Parameter of the Inverse-Gamma prior on the error variance
`alpha0`	α_0	Baseline intercept of the selection prior
`alpha1`	α	Parameter that regulates the strength of the spatially informed dependence
`deltak`	$\boldsymbol{\delta}$	Vector of mean of the prior on the state specific mean
`tauk`	$\boldsymbol{\tau}$	Vector of standard deviation parameters of the prior on the state specific mean
`upp_bounds`	$\boldsymbol{upp}_\eta$	Vector of upper bounds of the prior on the state specific mean
`low_bounds`	$\boldsymbol{low}_\eta$	Vector of lower bounds of the prior on the state specific mean
`alpha_IG`	$\boldsymbol{b}$	Vector of parameters of the prior on the state specific standard deviation
`beta_IG`	$\boldsymbol{l}$	Vector of parameters of the prior on the state specific standard deviation
`low_IG`	$\boldsymbol{upp}_\sigma$	Truncation of the prior on the state specific standard deviation
`a`	$\boldsymbol{\phi}$	Vector of parameters of the prior on the transition matrix
`niter`	NA	Number of Markov Chain Monte Carlo iterations
`burnin`	NA	Burn-in
`Cout`	NA	Print the number of iterations ran every `Cout` iterations
`phi`	ϕ	Probability of an A/D step
`pR`	p_R	Parameter of the distribution used to select the rows to be updated at every MCMC iteration
`selectioncgh`	p_{MC}	Number of samples not in neutral state in order to consider a CGH as a potential candidate for association with gene expression Default set to -1, that automatically set it to 10 % of the samples
`pXI`	p_ξ	Parameter of the distribution used to select the rows to be updated at every MCMC iteration

The last function that we discuss summarizes the output of the MCMC chains and, therefore, allows to perform posterior inference. More specifically, the arguments of the function `Inference` are the output of the MCMC `listComplete`, the number of gene expression probes `G`, the number of CGH probes `M`, the number of MCMC iteration `niter`, the number of iterations to be discarded as burn-in `burnin`, and the threshold on the PPIs `threshold`, set by default to 0.5. The output of the function is a list made by five elements: `R`, the binary matrix of estimated association, `Xi`, the matrix of estimated copy number states, `A`, the estimated transition matrix, `Mu`, the estimated vector of state specific means, and `Sd`, the estimated vector of state specific standard deviations.

We now give an example of the use of the code. First get the data,

```
> data(NCI_60)
> Y = NCI_60$Affy
> X = NCI_60$aCGH
> distance = NCI_60$distance
```

then initialize ξ, $\boldsymbol{A}$ and η and center the measurements of each gene in the gene expression matrix,

```
> xi = InitXi(X)
> tran = Tran(xi)
> mu = InitMu()
> Y = Center(Y)
```

finally run the main function and summarize the results.

```
> res = iBAT(Y=Y,X=X,distance=distance,
disfix=146274826,xi=xi,tran=tran,
mu=mu,d=0.2587288)
> summRes = Inference(res,G=dim(Y)[[2]],
M=dim(X)[[2]],niter=niter,bi=bi,threshold=0.5)
```

The example above takes approximately 5 min to run 1000 iterations, using a double core ® Intel ® Xeon processor with 16 GB of memory, 2.2 GHz.

4 Case Study

In order to illustrate the performance of the model and the type of inference it allows, we further used the function `iBATProbit` to analyze data from a study of ovarian cancer obtained from The Cancer Genome Atlas (TCGA) data portal, currently not included in the package. We used the level 3 Affymetrix HG-U133A array data as gene expression levels, and the normalized 415K array as CGH data. We selected a total of 350 samples, as those for which both data types were available. We further focused our attention on a subset of genes with highest variation across the samples (coefficient of variation). As for the CGH probes, we focused on the probes belonging to chromosome 17, which is highly involved in ovarian cancer [24]. We further reduced the complexity of the CGH data by smoothing the original signal via replacing each value with the median in a window of three elements, using the R function `runmed`. We then selected one probe every 5. After reduction, the data set consisted of $G = 119$ genes and $M = 2265$ probes.

We ran our analysis using the default parameters of the function `iBATProbit`, except for $\boldsymbol{upp}_\eta = [-0.3, 0.3, 0.73, \infty]$, $\boldsymbol{low}_\eta = [-Inf, -0.3, 0.3, 0.73]$ and $p_{MC} = 5$. The default choice for $\alpha_1 = 1$ and $\alpha_0 = 2.32$ were used. We ran our MCMC for 500,000 iterations and we discarded the first 300,000 as burn-in. We report here the results by selecting associations with $PPI > 0.5$, that is the modal model selected by our method [2]. The selected set of associations contained 16 unique target genes and 22 unique CGH probes. As an example of the output of our analysis, Fig. 1 shows the marginal posterior probability of inclusion for each element of the matrix $\boldsymbol{R}$. The horizontal red line corresponds to the threshold used for our analysis. As for the inference on $\boldsymbol{\xi}$, Fig. 2 shows the frequency of copy number gains (states 3 and 4) and loss (state 1) across the samples for every CGH probe considered in our analysis. Note that there are a large number of CGH probes with high frequency of copy number loss, in line with what reported in the literature [34].

We assessed the biological relevance of our findings by using the database for annotation visualization and integrated discovery (DAVID) tool [11]. In particular, we performed a gene ontology (GO) analysis on the list of selected gene expressions and CGHs separately. We first focused on the enrichment analysis for the gene expressions, see Fig. 3 for a schematic representation of our findings. We found enrichment for six different GO terms. More specifically, we found enrichment

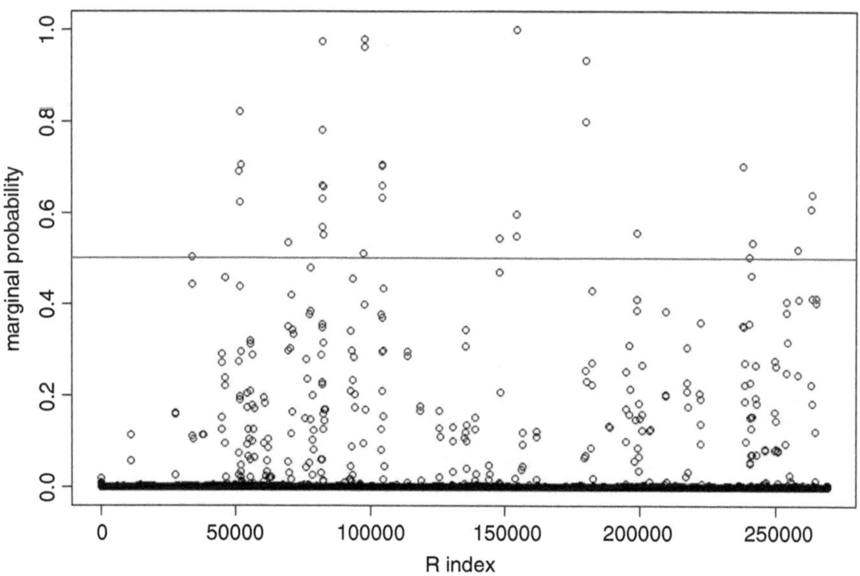

Fig. 1 Marginal posterior probabilities of inclusion of the single elements of the matrix $\boldsymbol{R}$, with the *horizontal red line* corresponding to the threshold used in our analysis

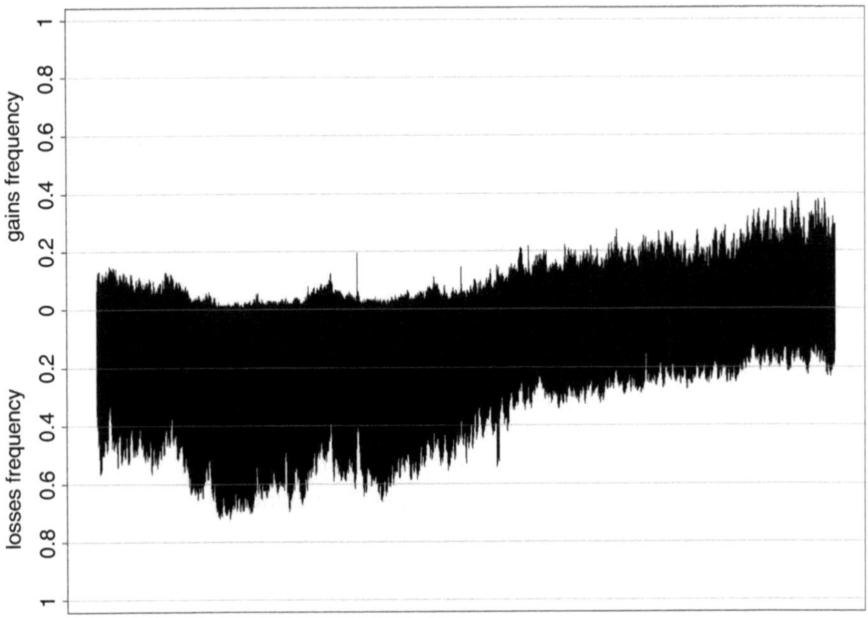

Fig. 2 Frequency of copy number gains (states 3 and 4) and loss (state 1) across the samples for every CGH probe considered in our analysis

for genes that code for skeletal system development, acute phase response, proteolysis, response to wounding, acute inflammatory response and regulation of lipid metabolic process. In particular, genes IGF2 and SERPINA3 are members of the acute phase response, response to wounding, acute inflammatory response and regulation of lipid metabolic process terms, and IGF2 is also a member of the skeletal system development. IGF2 is an insulin-like growth factor and has been previously found inhibited after treatment of responsive RMS-13 cells with 5-fluorouracil and betulinic acid in a study on the effect of the combination of these two acids on ovarian carcinoma cells [37]. SERPINA3, a serpin peptidase inhibitor, has been found over expressed in recurrent ovarian tumors, when compared to the expression in the primary tumor [17]. Focusing on the single genes identified by our analysis a large number of them have been found as associated with tumors in general (HOXB6, FAP, MMP1, GSTA, TAX3, FABP6, SERPINB2, HGMA2) and with ovarian cancer in particular (POSTN). In addition HGMA2 is a promising target for ovarian cancer silencing therapy [20]. Also, although it has not been confirmed yet, MAGEA4 may play a role in embrional development and tumor transformation or aspects of tumor progression [4, 16, 26]. Lastly, we also found enrichment for PPAR signaling KEGG pathway. This pathway inhibits proliferation in PC3 prostate carcinoma cells [30].

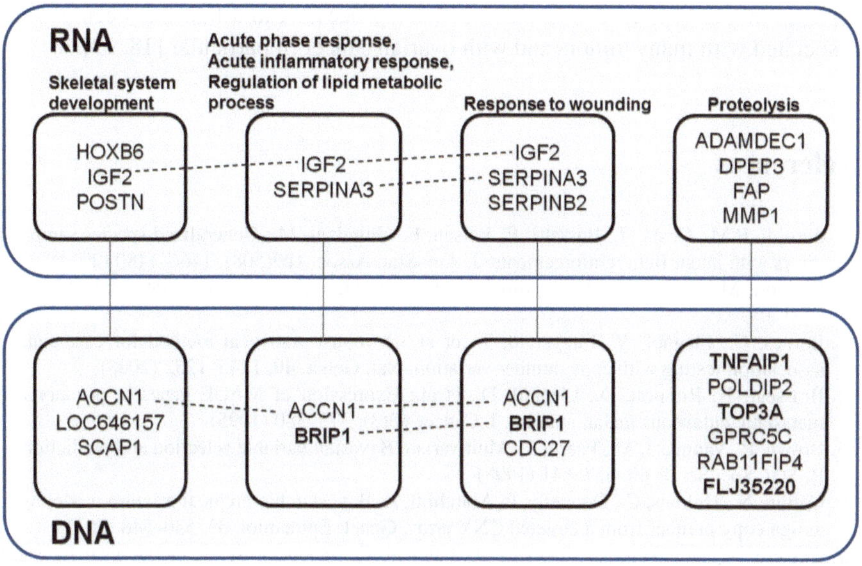

Fig. 3 Schematic representation of a GO analysis of the gene expressions identified by our model, via thresholding the posterior probabilities of inclusion. The *upper box* (labeled RNA) shows the enriched molecular functions together with the corresponding lists of target genes. The *lower box* (labeled DNA) reports the lists of CGH probes that our model found to be associated with the gene expressions. Bold CGH probes highlight those elements found enriched for molecular functions in the GO analysis on the CGH probes. The *solid connecting lines* indicate estimated associations between target genes and CNVs; *dashed lines* indicate genes that appear in multiple lists

As for the enrichment analysis of the CGH probes identified by our method, we found enrichment for six GO terms. More specifically, we found enrichment for the DNA metabolic process, cellular response to stress, DNA repair, cell projection organization, cellular response to DNA damage stimulus and cell projection assembly. A very interesting result is that we found enrichment for three terms that are linked to cellular response to DNA damage (DNA repair and DNA damage stimulus) and external stimulus (cellular response to stress). The DNA repair mechanism is often altered in ovarian cancer. Indeed mutations on the genes BRCA1 and BRCA2 are genes involved in DNA repair, and are very well know for their association with increased breast and ovarian cancer risks [19]. We also found enrichment for two terms related to cell movement and migration, cell projection organization and cell projection assembly. Cellular reorganization is often involved in acquisition of motility ability by cancer cells. This is a key process for the cell invasion and metastasis, two important stages of tumor progression. Further confirmation of our results comes from inspecting the single genes. As an example we identified BRIP1, the official symbol of BRCA1, and MAP2K4, the mitogen-activated protein kinase kinase 4, both well known tumor suppressor genes in ovarian cancer [10, 19]. Also, we identified TNFAIP1, a tumor necrosis factor, SFRS1, a proto oncogene upregulated in various tumors and SUMO2, a gene that play a role in DNA replication and repair, among other cellular processes, and that has been already associated with many tumors and with ovarian cancer in particular [18, 22].

References

1. Airoldi, E.M., Costa, T., Bassetti, F., Leisen, F., Guindani, M.: Generalized species sampling priors with latent Beta reinforcements. J. Am. Stat. Assoc. **109**(508), 1466–1480 (2014)
2. Barbieri, M.M., Berger, J.O.: Optimal predictive model selection. Ann. Stat. **32**(3), 870–897 (2004)
3. Barnes, C., Plagnol, V., Fitzgerald, T., et al.: A robust statistical method for case-control association testing with copy number variation. Nat. Genet. **40**, 1245–1252 (2008)
4. Brasseur, F., Rimoldi, D., Liénard, D., et al.: Expression of MAGE genes in primary and metastatic cutaneous melanoma. Int. J. Cancer **63**(3), 375–380 (1995)
5. Brown, P., Vannucci, M., Fearn, T.: Multivariate Bayesian variable selection and prediction. J. R. Stat. Soc. Ser. B **60**, 627–641 (1998)
6. Cardin, N., Holmes, C., Donnelly, P., Marchini, J.: Bayesian hierarchical mixture modeling to assign copy number from a targeted CNV array. Genet. Epidemiol. **35**, 536–548 (2011)
7. Cassese, A., Guindani, M., Tadesse, M., Falciani, F., Vannucci, M.: A hierarchical Bayesian model for inference of copy number variants and their association to gene expression. Ann. Appl. Stat. **8**(1), 148–175 (2014)
8. Cassese, A., Guindani, M., Vannucci, M.: A bayesian integrative model for genetical genomics with spatially informed variable selection. Cancer Informat. **13**(S2), 29–37 (2014)
9. Colella, S., Yau, C., Taylor, J., et al.: QuantiSNP: an objective Bayes hidden-Markov model to detect and accurately map copy number variation using SNP genotyping data. Nucleic Acids Res. **35**(6), 2013–2025 (2007)
10. Davis, S.J., Choong, D.Y., Ramakrishna, M., Ryland, G.L., Campbell, I.G., Gorringe, K.L.: Analysis of the mitogen-activated protein kinase kinase 4 (MAP2K4) tumor suppressor gene in ovarian cancer. BMC Cancer **1**(11), 173 (2011)
11. Dennis, G., Sherman, B.T., Hosack, D.A., Yang, J., Gao, W., Lane, H.C., Lempicki, R.A.: DAVID: database for annotation, visualization, and integrated discovery. Genome Biol. **4**(5), P3 (2003)
12. Du, L., Chen, M., Lucas, J., Carlin, L.: Sticky hidden Markov modeling of comparative genomic hybridization. IEEE Trans. Signal Process **58**(10), 5353–5368 (2010)
13. Eddelbuettel, D., Francois, R.: Rcpp: seamless R and C++ integration. J. Stat. Softw. **40**(8), 1–18 (2011)
14. George, E., McCulloch, R.: Approaches for Bayesian variable selection. Stat. Sin. **7**, 339–373 (1997)
15. Guha, S., Li, Y., Neuberg, D.: Bayesian hidden Markov modelling of array cgh data. J. Am. Stat. Assoc. **103**(482), 485–497 (2008)
16. Imaia, Y., Shichijo, S., Yamada, A., Katayama, T., Yano, H., Itoh, K.: Sequence analysis of the MAGE gene family encoding human tumor-rejection antigens. Gene **160**(2), 287–290 (1995)
17. Jinawath, N., Vasoontara, C., Jinawath, A., et al.: Oncoproteomic analysis reveals co-upregulation of RELA and STAT5 in carboplatin resistant ovarian carcinoma. PLoS One **5**(6), e11198 (2010)
18. Karni, R., de Stanchina, E., Lowe, S.W., Sinha, R., Mu, D., Krainer, A.R.: The gene encoding the splicing factor SF2/ASF is a proto-oncogene. Nat. Struct. Mol. Biol. **14**(3), 185–193 (2007)
19. King, M.C., Marks, J.H., Mandell., J.B.: Breast and ovarian cancer risks due to inherited mutations in BRCA1 and BRCA2. Science **302**(5645), 643–646 (2003)
20. Malek, A., Bakhidze, E., Noske, A., et al.: HMGA2 gene is a promising target for ovarian cancer silencing therapy. Int. J. Cancer **132**(2), 348–356 (2008)

21. Monni, S., Tadesse, M.: A stochastic partitioning method to associate high-dimensional responses and covariates. Bayesian Anal. **4**(3), 413–436 (2009)
22. Morris, J.R., Boutell, C., Keppler, M., et al.: The SUMO modification pathway is involved in the BRCA1 response to genotoxic stress. Nature **462**(7275), 886–890 (2009)
23. Newton, M.A., Noueiry, A., Sarkar, D., Ahlquist, P.: Detecting differential gene expression with a semiparametric hierarchical mixture method. Biostatistics **5**(2), 155–176 (2004)
24. Pharoah, P.D., Tsai, Y.Y., Ramus, S.J., et al.: GWAS meta-analysis and replication identifies three new susceptibility loci for ovarian cancer. Nat. Genet. **45**(4), 362–370 (2013)
25. Picard, F., Robin, S., Lebarbier, E., Daudin, J.: A segmentation-clustering model for the analysis of array CGH data. Biometrics **63**(3), 758–766 (2007)
26. Resnick, M.B., Sabo, E., Kondratev, S., Kerner, H., Spagnoli, G.C., Yakirevich, E.: Cancer-testis antigen expression in uterine malignancies with an emphasis on carcinosarcomas and papillary serous carcinomas. Int. J. Cancer **101**(2), 190–195 (2002)
27. Rihardson, S., Gilks, W.R.: Conditional independence models for epidemiological studies with covariate measurement error model. Stat. Med. **12**, 1703–1722 (1993)
28. Richardson, S., Bottolo, L., Rosenthal, J.: Bayesian models for sparse regression analysis of high dimensional data. Bayesian Stat. **9**, 539–569 (2010)
29. Sha, N., Vannucci, M., Tadesse, M., et al.: Bayesian variable selection in multinomial probit models to identify molecular signatures of disease stage. Biometrics **60**(3), 812–819 (2004)
30. Shappell, S.B., Gupta, R.A., Manning, S., et al.: 15S-Hydroxyeicosatetraenoic acid activates peroxisome proliferator-activated receptor gamma and inhibits proliferation in PC3 prostate carcinoma cells. Cancer Res. **61**(2), 497–503 (2001)
31. Stingo, F., Chen, Y., Vannucci, M., Barrier, M., Mirkes, P.A.: Bayesian graphical modelling approach to microRNA regulatory network inference. Ann. Appl. Stat. **4**(4), 2024–2048 (2010)
32. Stingo, F., Chen, Y., Tadesse, M., Vannucci, M.: Incorporating biological information into linear models: a Bayesian approach to the selection of pathways and genes. Ann. Appl. Stat. **5**(3), 1978–2002 (2011)
33. Subirana, I., Diaz-Uriarte, R., Lucas, G., Gonzalez, J.: CNVassoc: association analysis of CNV data using R. BMC Med. Genomics **4**, 47 (2011)
34. Tavassoli, M., Ruhrberg, C., Beaumont, V., Reynolds, K., Kirkham, N., Collins, W.P., Farzaneh F.: Whole chromosome 17 loss in ovarian cancer. Genes Chromosom. Cancer **8**(3), 195–198 (1993)
35. Venkatraman, E., Olshen, A.: A faster circular binary segmentation algorithm for the analysis of array CGH data. Bioinformatics **23**(6), 657–663 (2007)
36. Wang, K., Li, M., Hadley, D., et al.: PennCNV: an integrated hidden Markov model designed for high-resolution copy number variation detection in whole-genome SNP genotyping data. Genome Res. **17**(11), 1665–1674 (2007)
37. Wang, Y.J., Liu, J.B., Dou, Y.C.: Sequential treatment with betulinic acid followed by 5-fluorouracil shows synergistic cytotoxic activity in ovarian cancer cells. Int. J. Clin. Exp. Pathol. **8**(1), 252–259 (2015)
38. Yau, C., Papaspiliopoulos, O., Roberts, G.O., Holmes, C.: Bayesian nonparametric hidden Markov models with application to the analysis of copy-number-variation in mammalian genomes. J. R. Stat. Soc. Ser. B **73**(1), 37–57 (2011)

Models of Random Sparse Eigenmatrices and Bayesian Analysis of Multivariate Structure

Andrew Cron and Mike West

Abstract We discuss probabilistic models of random covariance structures defined by distributions over sparse eigenmatrices. The decomposition of orthogonal matrices in terms of Givens rotations defines a natural, interpretable framework for defining distributions on sparsity structure of random eigenmatrices. We explore theoretical aspects and implications for conditional independence structures arising in multivariate Gaussian models, and discuss connections with sparse PCA, factor analysis and Gaussian graphical models. Methodology includes model-based exploratory data analysis and Bayesian analysis via reversible jump Markov chain Monte Carlo. A simulation study examines the ability to identify sparse multivariate structures compared to the benchmark graphical modelling approach. Extensions to multivariate normal mixture models with additional measurement errors move into the framework of latent structure analysis of broad practical interest. We explore the implications and utility of the new models with summaries of a detailed applied study of a 20-dimensional breast cancer genomics data set.

1 Introduction

We are interested in Bayesian modelling approaches to sparsity in variance and precision matrices in multivariate normal distributions. With interests in parsimony and scalability of analyses of multivariate data in models such as Gaussian mixtures for classification, priors that encourage sparse component covariance patterns are increasingly key as dimension increases. New modelling frameworks also need to enable efficient computational methods for model fitting, which can otherwise be a barrier to application.

A. Cron
84.51°, 100 W. 5th St., Cincinnati, OH 45202, USA
e-mail: andrew.j.cron@gmail.com

M. West (✉)
Department of Statistical Science, Duke University, Durham, NC 27708-0251, USA
e-mail: mw@stat.duke.edu

A. Frigessi et al. (eds.), *Statistical Analysis for High-Dimensional Data*,
Abel Symposia 11, DOI 10.1007/978-3-319-27099-9_7

Among recent related developments, traditional sparsity priors from model selection in regression have been exploited in sparse extensions of Bayesian factor analysis [3, 36, 39], and in complementary approaches using Gaussian graphical models [8, 19, 30]. The developments in the current work represent natural extensions of the thinking behind these models—building sparsity into variance or precision matrices—while naturally linking and bridging between factor models and graphical models.

The new "sparse Givens" models introduced and developed here arise from new theory of random sparse eigenmatrices; these define eigenstructure of variance and precision matrices, and so induce new classes of priors over Gaussian graphical models. Compared to factor analysis, we avoid the assumption of a reduced dimensional latent factor structure, and the choices it involves. Our new models arise from an inherent theoretical feature of eigenmatrices, rather than hypothesized model structures. We also face fewer challenges in hyper-parameter specification and tuning to fit models. Our models can in fact be viewed as full-rank factor models with sparse, square factor loadings matrices. Additional related work has explored new classes of priors over variance matrices through varying parametrizations, such as partial correlations or Cholesky decompositions [6, 23], that could be extended with sparsity priors. Some such extensions to time series contexts [13, 29] show the utility of various Cholesky-style approaches. Our approach relates to this general literature in that it uses an inherent theoretical property of eigenmatrices that naturally defines the reparametrization as well as an underlying set of parameters that, when set to zero, define parsimonious models.

Section 2 introduces the theoretical and modelling ideas; the approach is based on the Givens rotation representation of full-rank eigenmatrices [1]. We describe how this can be exploited to define new classes of random sparse eigenmatrices, and relate these to decomposable graphical models. Section 3 considers prior specification over variance matrices using this new parametrization, in the context of normal random samples. Section 4 discusses properties of the likelihood and aspects of exploratory data analysis that give insights into sparsity structure of eigenmatrices in our framework, with an example using a 20-dimensional gene expression data set. Section 5 discusses full Bayesian model fitting using a customized reversible jump Markov Chain Monte Carlo approach. We make a detailed, simulation-based comparison with traditional Gaussian graphical modelling (GGM) in Sect. 6. Section 7 discusses embedding the basic model into more practicable contexts involving measurement errors and normal mixture models. That section concludes with a detailed example using breast cancer gene expression data, where underlying components relate to known, broad and intersecting cancer subtypes with expected sparsity in dependence, and conditional dependence patterns of subsets of the genes. Section 8 concludes with additional comments and potential extensions.

2 Structure and Sparsity in Eigenmatrices

We discuss Givens representations of variance matrices, introduce the general idea of sparsity modelling in this context, and explore aspects of the theoretical structures that emerge under priors over the resulting models.

2.1 Givens Rotator Product Representation

Consider a random q-vector $\boldsymbol{x}$ with variance matrix $\boldsymbol{V} = Var(\boldsymbol{x})$. The spectral representation (principal component decomposition) is $\boldsymbol{V} = \boldsymbol{RDR}'$ where $\boldsymbol{R}$ is the $q \times q$ orthogonal matrix of eigenvectors—the eigenmatrix—and $\boldsymbol{D} = \mathrm{diag}(d_1, \ldots, d_q)$ is the matrix of non-negative eigenvalues. The corresponding precision matrix is $\boldsymbol{K} = \boldsymbol{RAR}'$ with $\boldsymbol{A} = \boldsymbol{D}^{-1} = \mathrm{diag}(a_1, \ldots, a_q)$. The general Givens rotator product representation of $\boldsymbol{R}$ [1, 38] is

$$\begin{aligned} \boldsymbol{R} = \boldsymbol{O}_{1,2}(\omega_{1,2})\ \boldsymbol{O}_{1,3}(\omega_{1,3}) \ldots \boldsymbol{O}_{1,q}(\omega_{1,q}) \times& \\ \boldsymbol{O}_{2,3}(\omega_{2,3}) \ldots \boldsymbol{O}_{2,q}(\omega_{2,q}) \times& \\ \vdots\quad& \\ \boldsymbol{O}_{q-1,q}(\omega_{q-1,q}) \times \boldsymbol{Q}& \end{aligned} \tag{1}$$

where $\boldsymbol{Q}$ is diagonal with elements ± 1, and each $\boldsymbol{O}_{i,j}(\omega_{i,j})$ is a Givens rotation matrix

$$\boldsymbol{O}_{i,j}(\omega_{i,j}) = \begin{array}{cc} & \begin{array}{ccccc} & i & & j & \end{array} \\ \begin{array}{c} \\ i \\ \\ j \\ \\ \end{array} & \begin{pmatrix} I & 0 & 0 & 0 & 0 \\ 0 & \cos(\omega_{i,j}) & 0 & \sin(\omega_{i,j}) & 0 \\ 0 & 0 & I & 0 & 0 \\ 0 & -\sin(\omega_{i,j}) & 0 & \cos(\omega_{i,j}) & 0 \\ 0 & 0 & 0 & 0 & I \end{pmatrix} \end{array} \tag{2}$$

for some rotator angles $\omega_{i,j}$, $(i = 1 : q, j = i + 1 : q)$. Some comments and notation follow.

- The angles $\omega_{i,j}$ lie in $(-\pi/2, \pi/2]$. Write $\boldsymbol{\omega}$ for the set of these $m = q(q-1)/2$ angles.
- This decomposition of $\boldsymbol{R}$ into m angles is unique and linked to the specific order of the variables in $\boldsymbol{x}$.
- For our goal of covariance modelling, note that $\boldsymbol{Q}$ cancels in $\boldsymbol{RDR}'$; hence, $\boldsymbol{Q}$ plays no role and we set $\boldsymbol{Q} = \boldsymbol{I}_q$ with no loss when focused on modelling variance matrices via this decomposition.
- Covariance patterns in $\boldsymbol{V}$ can be viewed as successively built-up by pairwise rotations of initial uncorrelated random variables. Take a q-vector $\boldsymbol{e}$ with $Var(\boldsymbol{e}) = \boldsymbol{D}$; then dependencies are defined by successive left multiplication of

$\boldsymbol{e}$ by the rotator matrices: first by $\boldsymbol{O}_{q-1,q}(\omega_{i,j})$, then $\boldsymbol{O}_{q-2,q}(\omega_{i,j})$, and so on up to $\boldsymbol{O}_{1,2}(\omega_{i,j})$ to define $\boldsymbol{x} = \boldsymbol{Re}$ (assuming $\boldsymbol{Q} = \boldsymbol{I}_q$ as noted).

- If $\omega_{i,j} = 0$ for any (i,j), then $\boldsymbol{O}_{i,j}(0) = \boldsymbol{I}_q$ and that rotation has no contribution to the build-up of dependencies and is effectively removed from the representation of Eq. (1).
- If $\omega_{i,j} = \pi/2$ for any (i,j), then $\boldsymbol{O}_{i,j}(\pi/2)\boldsymbol{M}\boldsymbol{O}'_{i,j}(\pi/2)$ permutes rows i and j, and columns i and j, of any square matrix $\boldsymbol{M}$ and hence does not affect the sparsity of $\boldsymbol{M}$.
- The spectral representations of $\boldsymbol{V}$ and $\boldsymbol{K}$ are unique only up to permutations of the columns $\boldsymbol{R}$, i.e., reordering of the eigenvalues. Any reordering of the eigenvalues will generate a decomposition as in Eq. (1) but with different values of the rotator angles. For identification, therefore, we will constrain to $d_1 > d_2 > \cdots d_q$. For variance matrices in models of data distributions, the d_i will be distinct so a strict ordering can be assumed.

2.2 Sparse Givens Models

The general representation above reparametrizes $\boldsymbol{V}$ to the $m = q(q-1)/2$ angles in $\boldsymbol{\omega}$ and the q eigenvalues in $\boldsymbol{D}$. We note above the role of zero angles, and this opens the path to defining sparse Givens models, i.e., products of fewer than the full set of rotators defining a resulting sparse eigenmatrix: if a large number of the angles are zero, then $\boldsymbol{R}$ will become sparse. This can induce a sparse variance matrix $\boldsymbol{V}$ and, equivalently, a sparse precision matrix $\boldsymbol{K}$ as a result.

Let $\mathscr{M} = \{(i,j);\ i = 1:(q-1), j = (i+1):q\}$ with $|\mathscr{M}| = q(q-1)/2 := m$. Then Eq. (1) is compactly written as $\boldsymbol{R} = \prod_{k=1}^{m} \boldsymbol{O}_{m_k}(\omega_{m_k})$ where m_k is the kth pair of dimensions in $\mathscr{M}$. Now allow exact zeros in $\boldsymbol{\omega}$. Define a sparsity defining index sequence $\mathscr{S} = \{(i,j) \in \mathscr{M} : \omega_{i,j} = 0\}$ with cardinality $|\mathscr{S}| = s$, and set $\mathscr{Z} = \mathscr{M} \setminus \mathscr{S}$ with size $z = m - s$. In words, $\mathscr{Z}$ is a sequence of $z \leq m$ ordered pairs (i_k, j_k) denoting the relevant, non-identity Givens rotation matrices in Eq. (1) and

$$\boldsymbol{R} = \prod_{k=1}^{z} \boldsymbol{O}_{Z_k}(\omega_{i_k j_k}). \tag{3}$$

Assuming that priors support exact zeros in $\boldsymbol{\omega}$, a primary modelling goal is then to learn $\mathscr{Z}$ and the corresponding non-zero angles.

Among the features of this approach is that we are able to model full-rank, orthogonal matrices with a parsimonious set of angles, and we maintain the computational convenience of the full-rank spectral parametrization when inverting $\boldsymbol{V}$ and $\boldsymbol{K}$. This is especially useful in evaluating density functions in Metropolis Hastings acceptance ratios and, later, in computing normal mixture classification probabilities.

2.3 Conditional Independence Graphs

The process of successively building dependencies by adding rotators (from right to left) in Eq. (3) induces ties between the variables whose variance matrix is the resulting $\boldsymbol{V}$. The resulting structure of $\boldsymbol{K} = \boldsymbol{V}^{-1}$ connects to Gaussian graphical modelling [2, 7, 8, 19, 21, 30].

View the q variables in $\boldsymbol{x}$ as nodes of a graph in which conditional independencies are represented by lack of edges between node pairs. Specifically, this is the undirected graph $\mathscr{G} = (\mathscr{V}, \mathscr{E})$ with the q nodes, or vertices, in the vertex set $\mathscr{V} = \{1 : q\}$; two vertices (i, j) are connected by an edge in the graph if, and only if, $K_{i,j} \neq 0$ where $K_{i,j}$ is the (i, j)-element of $\boldsymbol{K}$. The edge set is $\mathscr{E} = \{(i, j) : K_{i,j} \neq 0\}$.

Any precision matrix $\boldsymbol{K}_0$ having some off-diagonal zero elements has an implied graph $\mathscr{G}_0$. Now take $\boldsymbol{K}_1 = \boldsymbol{O}_{i,j}\boldsymbol{K}_0\boldsymbol{O}'_{i,j}$ where $\omega_{i,j} \neq 0$ and $\omega_{i,j} \neq \pi/2$, with implied graph $\mathscr{G}_1$. Notice that left multiplication of $\boldsymbol{R}_0$ by $\boldsymbol{O}_{i,j}$ simply replaces the ith and jth rows of with a linear combination of the two. Therefore, the indices of the non-zero elements of the ith and jth rows of $\boldsymbol{R}_1$ are the union of the indices of the ith and jth rows of $\boldsymbol{R}_0$. Similar comments apply to right multiplication. As a result, the sparsity pattern of $\boldsymbol{K}_1$ is the same as that of $\boldsymbol{K}_0$ except in rows and columns i and j. Specifically, those rows and columns have sparsity indices that are the unions of the those in $\boldsymbol{K}_0$. This shows that the additional rotator $\boldsymbol{O}_{i,j}$ maps the graph $\mathscr{G}_0 = (\mathscr{V}, \mathscr{E}_0)$ to $\mathscr{G}_1 = (\mathscr{V}, \mathscr{E}_1)$ as follows. With $\mathscr{N}_j(i) = \{(j, k) : (i, k) \in \mathscr{E}_0\}$, then $\mathscr{E}_1 = \mathscr{E}_0 \cup (i, j) \cup \mathscr{N}_i(j) \cup \mathscr{N}_j(i)$. In words, $\mathscr{G}_1$ takes $\mathscr{G}_0$, connects i and j, and unions their neighborhoods.

This structure also generates constructive insights into the nature of the graphical models so defined. It shows that adding a new rotator to an existing sparse Givens model merges the complete subgraphs (cliques) in which the rotators pair (i, j) reside into one larger clique. Starting at an empty graph, this leads to graphs that are decomposable, formally shown as follows.

Theorem 1 *The conditional independence graph $\mathscr{G}$ implied by a sparse $\boldsymbol{K} = \boldsymbol{RAR}'$ under $\mathscr{Z}$ is a decomposable graph.*

Proof It is enough to show that $\mathscr{G}$ has a perfect elimination ordering; that is, an ordering of the vertices of the graph such that, for each vertex $v \in \mathscr{V}$, the neighbors of v that occur after v in the order form a clique [11]. We do this by induction, beginning with no rotations: $\boldsymbol{R}_0 = \boldsymbol{I}_q$ and $\boldsymbol{K}_0 = \boldsymbol{A}$. This implies that $\mathscr{G}_0$ is the empty graph and the perfect elimination ordering is trivial. For the inductive step, assume that an ordering exists for the graph implied by a current set of Givens rotations defining $\boldsymbol{R}_0$ and $\mathscr{G}_0$. Now take $\boldsymbol{K}_1 = \boldsymbol{O}_{i,j}\boldsymbol{K}_0\boldsymbol{O}'_{i,j}$ where $\omega_{i,j} \neq 0$ and $\omega_{i,j} \neq \pi/2$, with implied graph $\mathscr{G}_1$. Note that there is no loss of generality here; $\omega_{i,j} = \pi/2$ would imply simply swapping the i and j rows and columns of $\boldsymbol{K}_0$ to make $\boldsymbol{K}_1$, and so always yields another decomposable graph. It is now enough to show that $\mathscr{G}_1$ has a perfect elimination ordering.

Start with the ordering of $\mathscr{G}$ given by $\mathscr{U} = \{v_1, v_2, \ldots, v_q\} \equiv \{1, 2, \ldots, q\}$. Now take the ordering for $\mathscr{G}_1$ to be $\tilde{\mathscr{U}} = \{v_1, \ldots, v_{i-1}, \ldots, v_{i+1}, \ldots, v_{j-1}, v_{j+1}, \ldots, v_q, v_i, v_j\}$. It is enough to show that $\tilde{\mathscr{U}}$ is a perfect elimination ordering for $\mathscr{G}_1$. Take $v^\star \in \tilde{\mathscr{U}}$ and let η be $v^\star$ and its neighbors that occur after $v^\star$ in $\tilde{\mathscr{U}}$. We need to show that η forms a clique in $\mathscr{G}_1$. If $v^\star = v_1, v_i$, or v_j, this is trivial. If $v^\star$ is not a neighbor of either v_i or v_j in $\mathscr{G}_0$, the rotation has no effect on the neighborhood of $v^\star$ and η is a clique. Now suppose that $v^\star$ is a neighbor of v_i in $\mathscr{G}_0$. Due to our construction of $\mathscr{G}_1$, the neighbors of $v^\star$ in $\mathscr{G}_0$ become neighbors of v_i in $\mathscr{G}_1$. Since $\eta \backslash v_i$ is a clique in $\mathscr{G}_0$, then η will remain a clique in $\mathscr{G}_1$. Since v_i and v_j were moved to the end of the ordering and $\eta \backslash v_i$ comes after $v^\star$ in $\tilde{\mathscr{U}}$ by the inductive hypothesis, then $\tilde{\mathscr{U}}$ is a perfect elimination ordering of $\mathscr{G}_1$.

Note that the above concerns general, unrestricted values of the non-zero angles. Furthermore, this applies to any ordering of the rotators where Eq. (1) is a special case. There are sparse precision matrices whose graphs are decomposable but that do not have a sparse Givens representations for their eigenmatrices. These arise, in particular, in parametric models where the variance and precision matrix are initially defined as functions of lower dimensional parameters to begin; in such cases, the resulting eigenmatrices are inherently structured and typically not sparse, even though the precision matrices are sparse. The simplest example is that of the dependence structure for a set of q consecutive values of a stationary, linear, Gaussian first-order autoregressive process. There $\boldsymbol{K}$ is tri-diagonal, and neither $\boldsymbol{R}$ nor $\boldsymbol{V}$ is sparse. While $\boldsymbol{R}$ has the Givens representation, all m angles are required and they are deterministically related.

In the next section we define priors for the rotator angles $\boldsymbol{\omega}$. This includes conditional priors for the effective angles—excluding values of 0 and $\pi/2$—under which these angle are a random sample from a continuous distribution. In such cases, which can be regarded as all practicable cases for applied data analysis, we find a surprising connection between sparse graphical models and sparse factor models; that is, they coincide in this new sparse Givens approach.

Theorem 2 *If the angles $\omega_{i,j} \in \mathscr{X}$ defining a sparse eigenmatrix are a random sample from a continuous distribution, then the resulting patterns of zeros in* $\mathbf{V}$ *and* $\boldsymbol{K} = \mathbf{V}^{-1}$ *are the same with probability one.*

Proof For any (i,j) pair,

$$V_{i,j} = \sum_{k=1}^{q} d_k R_{i,k} R_{j,k} \text{ and } K_{i,j} = \sum_{k=1}^{q} a_k R_{i,k} R_{j,k}.$$

Therefore, zero values of $V_{i,j}$ and $K_{i,j}$ follow when

$$\forall k \in \{1, \ldots, q\}\ R_{i,k} = 0 \text{ or } R_{j,k} = 0.$$

However, any other case giving $V_{i,j} = 0$ requires specific values of $\boldsymbol{D}$, and/or specific relationships among elements of $\boldsymbol{V}$ and $\boldsymbol{D}$ defining the deterministic constraint that the above sum be zero. Such a constraint will not yield $K_{i,j} = 0$ under a continuous prior over the angles.

3 Sparsity Priors on Eigenstructures

We overlay the theoretical framework above with priors that define interesting theoretical models of random variance matrices as well as the specifications necessary for Bayesian analysis.

3.1 Class of Priors

We specify priors that give positive probability to zero values among the angles, allowing row and column flips via angles of $\pi/2$, and that otherwise draw angles independently from a continuous distribution. Specifically, the m angles $\omega_{i,j}$ are a random sample from a distribution with density

$$p(\omega) = \beta_{\frac{\pi}{2}} I(\omega = \pi/2) + (1 - \beta_{\frac{\pi}{2}})\beta_0 I(\omega = 0) + (1 - \beta_{\frac{\pi}{2}})(1 - \beta_0) p_c(\omega) \qquad (4)$$

where $I(\cdot)$ is the indicator function and $p_c(\omega)$ a continuous density on $(-\pi/2, \pi/2)$.

Since $\omega_{i,j} = \pi/2$ does not effect the sparsity of R and is needed for permuting the effects of the eigenvalues as discussed earlier, we do not want to penalize permutations in the same way as other non-zero angles. We specify the prior in three stages. First with probability $\beta_{\frac{\pi}{2}}$, $\omega_{i,j} = \pi/2$ to complement the constraint on eigenvalues d_i being ordered. Then, for angles that do not induce a permutation, we allow zero values with a non-zero conditional probability β_0. Finally, conditional on $\omega_{i,j} \neq 0$ or $\pi/2$, it follows a continuous prior $p_c(\cdot)$.

There are various choices of the continuous prior component $p_c(\cdot)$. Our examples here use a specific form that seems relevant for use as a routine, namely

$$p_c(\omega) = c(\kappa) \exp\left\{\kappa \cos^2(\omega)\right\} I(|\omega| < \pi/2) \qquad (5)$$

where $\kappa > 0$ and $c(\kappa)$ is a normalizing constant. In Bayesian analyses via reversible jump MCMC methods we need the value of $c(\kappa)$ and it can be easily evaluated using any standard numerical integration technique. This prior is unimodal and symmetric about zero, so represents appropriate centering relative to the "null hypothesis" value at zero. The prior concentrates more around zero for larger values of κ, while $\kappa \to 0$ leads to the limiting uniform distribution on $(-\pi/2, \pi/2)$. The specific mathematical form is also suggested by the forms of conditional likelihood functions for angles in normal models, as noted below in Sect. 4.

The prior is completed by specifying a distribution for the eigenvalues $\boldsymbol{D} = \text{diag}(d_1, d_2, \ldots, d_q)$ of $\boldsymbol{V}$. As discussed above, we take them ordered as $d_1 > d_2 > \cdots > d_q$. The natural, conditionally conjugate class of priors takes the d_j as ordered values of q independent draws from an inverse gamma distribution: given some chosen hyperparameters (η_1, η_2), draw $d_i^{-1} \sim Ga(\eta_1/2, \eta_2/2)$ independently then impose the ordering.

A specified prior over $(\boldsymbol{\omega}, \boldsymbol{D})$ leads to the implied prior over $\boldsymbol{V}$ and $\boldsymbol{K}$, and within that a prior over the sparsity structure that relates to the random graphical model induced. Simulation of $p(\boldsymbol{\omega}, \boldsymbol{D})$ yields simulations from the latter. One aspect of interest is to understand how sparsity in $\boldsymbol{R}$ is related to the number of rotators. A follow-on question is how these then relate to sparsity in $\boldsymbol{K}$ and hence the sparsity of the implied graph. This is trivially explored by simulation and then simply counting the number of zeros in $\boldsymbol{R}$ and $\boldsymbol{K}$. For a given set of rotator pairs $\mathscr{Z}$ with $z = |\mathscr{Z}|$, randomly pick which rotations will be non-zero then sample their angles uniformly and generate $\boldsymbol{R}$ and $\boldsymbol{K}$. We repeat this process 10,000 times for each $0 < z < m$. For each dimension $q = 20, 30$, Fig. 1 shows the median proportion of zeros in $\boldsymbol{R}$ and $\boldsymbol{K}$ as the proportion of non-zero rotators increases. Note how quickly the sparsity of $\boldsymbol{K}$, defining the sparsity of the underlying graph, decreases relative to $\boldsymbol{R}$. This gives some insights into how the choice of the prior sparsity probability β_0 plays a role in generating sparse graphs.

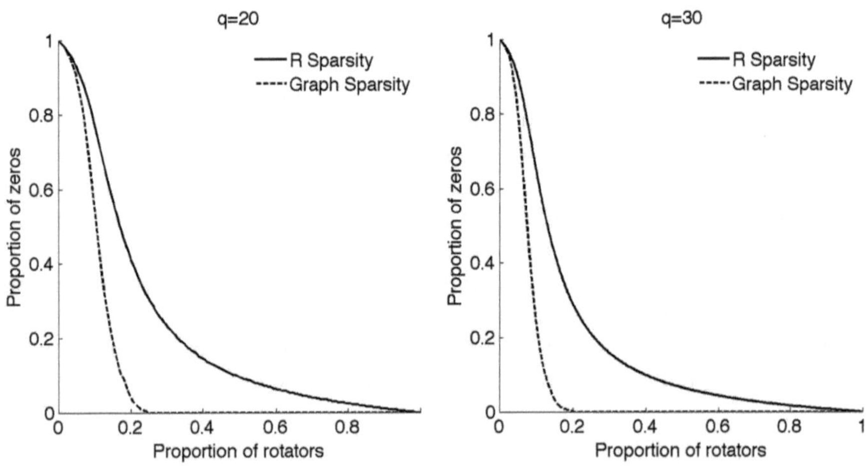

Fig. 1 Sparsity of $\boldsymbol{R}$ and the graphical model represented by $\boldsymbol{K}$ conditional on the number of random rotators in the model. For $q = 20$ and 30, this displays the prior median percent sparsity, i.e., proportion of zeros in $\boldsymbol{R}$ and $\boldsymbol{K}$ out of the possible $q(q-1)$ and $q(q-1)/2$ respectively. The prior for location of rotator pairs and values of the non-zero angles are each uniform, conditional on a given number of rotators selected

4 Likelihood and Exploratory Analyses

We discuss aspects of the likelihood function for the new parametrization $(\boldsymbol{\omega}, \boldsymbol{A})$ without considering sparsity, and then link that to an easily implemented forward selection algorithm that we have found of use in defining starting values for full MCMC analysis under our sparsity priors.

4.1 Likelihood

Consider a random sample $\boldsymbol{X} = \{\boldsymbol{x}_1, \ldots, \boldsymbol{x}_n\}$ where $\boldsymbol{x}_i \sim N_q(\boldsymbol{0}, \boldsymbol{V})$. With sum-of-squares matrix $\boldsymbol{S}$, the log likelihood function has a form in $\boldsymbol{R}$ that is a constant minus $\mathrm{tr}(\boldsymbol{RAR}'\boldsymbol{S})/2$. Note that $\boldsymbol{O}_{i,j}(\omega_{i,j})$ can be mapped onto an underlying 2×2 rotation matrix $\boldsymbol{G}(\omega)$ where, for any ω,

$$\boldsymbol{O}_{i,j}(\omega) = \boldsymbol{I}_q + \boldsymbol{H}'_{i,j}(\boldsymbol{G}(\omega) - \boldsymbol{I}_2)\boldsymbol{H}_{i,j} \quad \text{with} \quad \boldsymbol{G}(\omega) = \begin{pmatrix} \cos(\omega) & \sin(\omega) \\ -\sin(\omega) & \cos(\omega) \end{pmatrix} \tag{6}$$

and

$$\boldsymbol{H}_{i,j} = \begin{pmatrix} 0 & \cdots & 0 & \overset{i}{1} & 0 & \cdots & 0 & \overset{j}{0} & 0 & \cdots & 0 \\ 0 & \cdots & 0 & 0 & 0 & \cdots & 0 & 1 & 0 & \cdots & 0 \end{pmatrix}. \tag{7}$$

Write $\boldsymbol{R} = \boldsymbol{R}_{i,j,0}\boldsymbol{O}_{i,j}(\omega_{i,j})\boldsymbol{R}_{i,j,1}$; that is, $\boldsymbol{R}_{i,j,0}$ is the product of ordered rotators preceding $\boldsymbol{O}_{i,j}(\omega_{i,j})$, and $\boldsymbol{R}_{i,j,1}$ that following. Also, define $\boldsymbol{S}_{i,j} = \boldsymbol{R}'_{i,j,0}\boldsymbol{S}\boldsymbol{R}_{i,j,0}$ and $\boldsymbol{A}_{i,j} = \boldsymbol{R}_{i,j,1}\boldsymbol{A}\boldsymbol{R}'_{i,j,1}$. Note that $\boldsymbol{S}_{i,j}$ has the interpretation of a decorrelated version of $\boldsymbol{S}$ based on the subset of rotators represented in $\boldsymbol{R}_{i,j,0}$, i.e., all those preceding (i,j) in the product making up $\boldsymbol{R}$. Then, as a function of $\omega_{i,j}$ conditional on all other parameters, the log likelihood reduces to

$$\log p(\boldsymbol{X}|\omega_{i,j}, -) = \mathrm{c} - \mathrm{tr}[\boldsymbol{\Psi}_{i,j}\boldsymbol{G}(\omega_{i,j})'\boldsymbol{\Phi}_{i,j}\boldsymbol{G}(\omega_{i,j}) + \boldsymbol{G}(\omega_{i,j})'\boldsymbol{\Gamma}_{i,j}]/2 \tag{8}$$

where $\boldsymbol{\Phi}_{i,j} = \boldsymbol{H}_{i,j}\boldsymbol{S}_{i,j}\boldsymbol{H}'_{i,j}$, $\boldsymbol{\Psi}_{i,j} = \boldsymbol{H}_{i,j}\boldsymbol{A}_{i,j}\boldsymbol{H}_{i,j}$ and $\boldsymbol{\Gamma}_{i,j} = \boldsymbol{H}_{i,j}\boldsymbol{A}_{i,j}\boldsymbol{S}_{i,j}\boldsymbol{H}'_{i,j} - \boldsymbol{\Psi}_{i,j}\boldsymbol{\Phi}_{i,j}$. Some specific points to note are as follows:

- The form of the conditional likelihood is the kernel of a matrix Bingham von-Mises Fisher distribution for $\boldsymbol{G}(\omega_{i,j})$ [17], which suggests such distributions as conditionally conjugate priors.
- As a function of the scalar angle $\omega_{i,j}$, it is trivially shown that the log likelihood is a quadratic form in $(\sin(\omega_{i,j}), \cos(\omega_{i,j}))$. It is easy to numerically maximize this conditional log likelihood. As a result, iterative maximum likelihood estimates can be derived by sequentially maximizing the above conditional likelihood

functions as we iterate over rotators (i,j), coupled with conditional maximization over the eigenvalues.

- In the special case of $\boldsymbol{R}_{i,j,1} = \boldsymbol{I}_q$, i.e., when (i,j) is the right-most rotator pair and $\boldsymbol{A}_{i,j} = \boldsymbol{A}$, the conditional likelihood can be maximized analytically if the diagonal of $\boldsymbol{A}$ is not constrained to be ordered. The maximizing $\omega_{i,j}$ value satisfies $\tan(2\hat{\omega}_{i,j}) = 2s_{i,j}/(s_{j,j} - s_{i,i})$ where $s_{a,b}$ are the scalar entries of the "decorrelated" sample variance matrix $\boldsymbol{S}_{i,j}$. Given this value, including $\boldsymbol{A}$ in the conditional log likelihood maximization gives the following:

$$\begin{aligned}
\hat{\omega}_{i,j} &= \frac{1}{2}\arctan\left(\frac{2s_{i,j}}{s_{j,j} - s_{i,i}}\right), \\
n\hat{a}_i^{-1} &= s_{i,i}\cos^2(\hat{\omega}_{i,j}) + s_{j,j}\sin^2(\hat{\omega}_{i,j}) + 2s_{i,j}\cos(\hat{\omega}_{i,j})\sin(\hat{\omega}_{i,j}), \\
n\hat{a}_j^{-1} &= s_{j,j}\cos^2(\hat{\omega}_{i,j}) + s_{i,i}\sin^2(\hat{\omega}_{i,j}) - 2s_{i,j}\cos(\hat{\omega}_{i,j})\sin(\hat{\omega}_{i,j}), \\
n\hat{a}_k^{-1} &= s_{k,k} \text{ for } k \neq i,j.
\end{aligned} \tag{9}$$

- Continuing in the above case, if all correlation between variables i and j has been rotated away by the application of the preceding rotators so that $s_{i,j} = 0$, then the conditional MLE of $\omega_{i,j}$ is zero. In this case, it can also be shown that the conditional likelihood function in $\omega_{i,j}$ is proportional to $\cos^2(\omega_{i,j})$.
- The above confirms the role of a continuous prior $p_c(\cdot)$, as in Eq. (5), as a conditionally conjugate prior centered around the region of no residual correlation between the two variables.

4.2 An Exploratory Analysis Algorithm

The investigations of likelihood structure above suggests a simple exploratory analysis that can be of use in generating insights into potential sparsity structure as well as, particularly, defining starting values for a full Bayesian MCMC-based analysis of the sparse eigenmatrix model. This is discussed here in the case of $\kappa = 0$ in the prior, for simplicity, although could be trivially modified.

Begin with $\boldsymbol{S}_* = \boldsymbol{S}$ and $\boldsymbol{R}_* = \boldsymbol{I}_q$ defining the "current" versions of the decorrelated sample variance matrix and corresponding candidate eigenmatrix, respectively.

1. Set variable index $i = 1$ and $j = 2$.
2. Compute the sample correlation $r_{i,j}$ from $\boldsymbol{S}_*$.
3. If $|r_{i,j}|$ is large enough based on some pre-specified threshold which can be linked to the log likelihood difference it implies, add a rotator on pair (i,j) with angle $\hat{\omega}_{i,j}$ from Eq. (9).
4. If the choice is to include a new rotator, update $\boldsymbol{R}_*$ to $\boldsymbol{R}_*\boldsymbol{O}(\hat{\omega}_{i,j})$ and further decorrelate the sample variance matrix by updating $\boldsymbol{S}_*$ to $\boldsymbol{O}(\hat{\omega}_{i,j})'\boldsymbol{S}_*\boldsymbol{O}(\hat{\omega}_{i,j})$.

5. Sequence through the remaining (i,j) in the order of the rotations in Eq. (1). Finally, set $\boldsymbol{A}_*$ to be the MLE based on the decorrelated $\boldsymbol{S}_*$.

This forward selection process successively adds optimized rotators via right multiplication, building up the corresponding sequence of pairs of variable indices (i,j) to define an empirical set $\mathscr{L}$ of included rotators. It delivers this empirical estimate of $\mathscr{L}$ and the corresponding, optimized estimate of $\boldsymbol{R}$, and hence of $\boldsymbol{V}$ and $\boldsymbol{K}$ based on a final re-maximization of the likelihood for $\boldsymbol{A}$ given the optimized $\boldsymbol{R}$. There are many rules that can be used for the thresholding in step 3. For instance, we could use the absolute value of the conditional MLE, $\hat{\omega}_{i,j}$. However, the effect of the rotation on the likelihood is unclear as it depends on the eigenvalues which makes a particular threshold hard to interpret. Simple thresholding on the current, "residual" sample correlation $|r_{i,j}|$ is natural and interpretable; the squared correlation is the degree of residual structure in S_* that will be removed in that iteration of the exploratory algorithm. Hence a natural approach is to add a new rotator so long as $|r_{i,j}| > \rho$ for some specified threshold ρ.

We note that this fast exploratory algorithm cannot constrain the diagonal of our estimate $\boldsymbol{A}_*$ to be ordered. For exploration purposes, this is not an issue as the resulting estimate of $\boldsymbol{V}$ and $\boldsymbol{K}$ will not be affected. Furthermore if we denote by $\boldsymbol{A}_*$ an exploratory estimate, and let $\boldsymbol{P}$ be the permutation matrix such that $\boldsymbol{A} = \boldsymbol{P}\boldsymbol{A}_*\boldsymbol{P}'$ where the diagonal of $\boldsymbol{A}$ is ordered, then $\boldsymbol{V} = \boldsymbol{R}\boldsymbol{A}\boldsymbol{R}'$ where $\boldsymbol{R} = \boldsymbol{R}_*\boldsymbol{P}$. In words, we are simply finding a sparse spectral decomposition that has the interpretation of a forward selection process based on residual correlation. We then order the eigenvalues and their corresponding eigenvectors. Generating MCMC starting values for $\boldsymbol{\omega}$ is now simply a matter of finding the unique $\boldsymbol{\omega}$ that represents $\boldsymbol{R}$ in the general Givens rotator product representation. Anderson et al. [1] recursively derive $\boldsymbol{\omega}$ exactly from $\boldsymbol{R}$. Just as many zero elements in $\boldsymbol{\omega}$ induce zeros in $\boldsymbol{R}$, the starting value for $\boldsymbol{\omega}$ based on the decomposition of the sparse $\boldsymbol{R}$ will have many elements set to zero making this a very fast and effective method for finding sparse starting values.

In supporting material, we provide code implementing this overall algorithm for interested readers.

4.3 A Breast Cancer Genomics Example

We consider a subset of the microarray-based gene expression data that is analyzed in more detail in Sect. 7 below. The subset of size $n = 66$ represents tumors that would be regarded as aggressive in term of their expression profiles, based on higher levels of expression of genes related to the two key hormonal pathway: the ER (estrogen receptor) and Her2 growth factor pathways [18, 37]. Activity of genes in these two primary, distinct pathways, and their interactions with multiple other biological pathways in cell growth and development, play into our understanding of the heterogeneity of breast cancer, and critically into advances in understanding

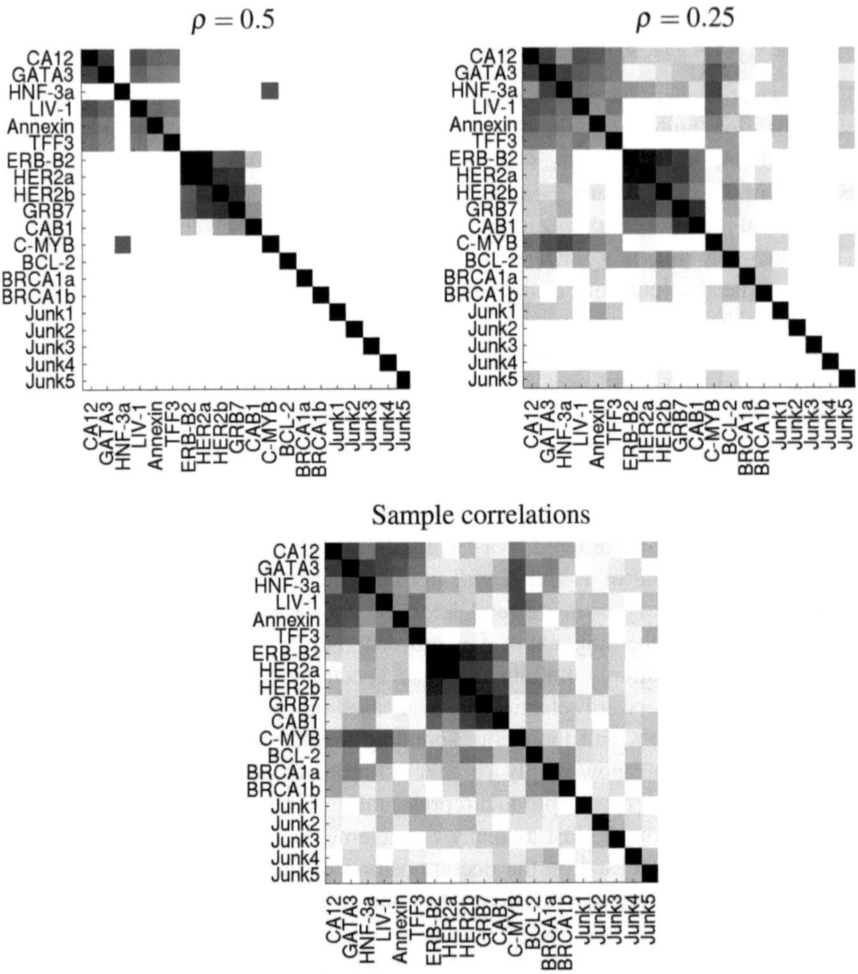

Fig. 2 Breast cancer gene expression data example in Sect. 4.2. Grey-scale heat maps show absolute values of elements in the estimated correlation matrix using the exploratory algorithm (*white*= 0 correlation, *black*= 1). The *first two frames* correspond to stopping the algorithm when the maximum absolute value of the residual correlation drops below $\rho = 0.5$ compared to $\rho = 0.25$, respectively. The *third frame* shows the full sample correlation matrix

clinically relevant cancer subtypes [3, 26, 33]. Several of the $q = 20$ genes, notably the leading 6 in Fig. 2 (CA12, GATA3, HNF-3α, LIV-1, Annexin, TFF3), are in part co-regulated in the ER network, some being directly transcribed by ER along with other factors. These genes vary across this subset of samples and are at relatively high levels of expression. These genes, as well as other breast cancer biomarker genes (C-MYB, BCL-2) that also interact with the ER network, play roles in multiple biological pathways; as a result, their inter-relationships in expression are more complicated than a simple one-dimensional ER factor would explain. Three of the variables (ERB-B2, HER2a, HER2b) are highly related read-outs of activity of the hormonal Her2 pathway (the first two are in fact different sequences from the same primary Her2 gene); other genes in the sample (GRB7, CAB1) are known to be regulated or co-regulated with Her2. Two additional gene sequences (BRCA1, BRCA2) relate to inherent susceptibility to breast cancer; their transcriptional relationships with ER and Her2 are poorly understood, although higher levels tend to be related to low ER and HER1 activity. To give a sense of robustness, five additional variables are included: the Junk genes represent random Gaussian noise.

After centering each of the $q = 20$ variables, the exploratory analysis was applied twice for a comparison of choice of stopping rule: we used thresholds of $|r_{i,j}| \geq 0.5$ and $|r_{i,j}| \geq 0.25$. A third analysis simply computes the sample correlation matrix and the corresponding eigenmatrix. Graphical summaries of the final estimates of the correlation matrix and the corresponding scaled eigenmatrix appear in Figs. 2 and 3, respectively. We can see the increase in sparsity in moving from no

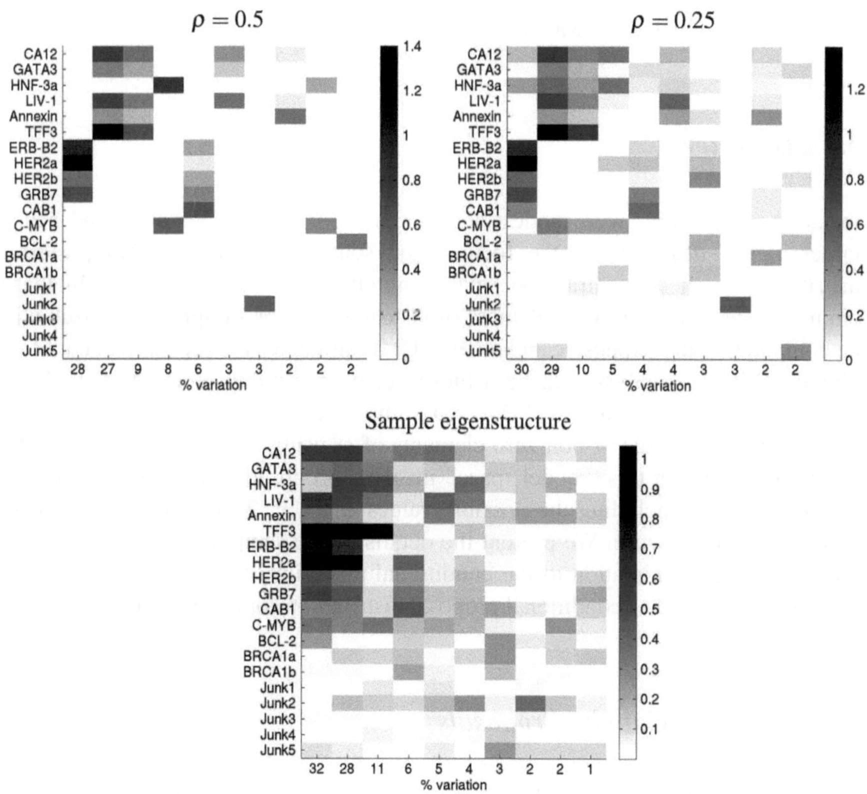

Fig. 3 Breast cancer gene expression data example in Sect. 4.2. Grey-scale heat maps show absolute values of elements in the first ten columns of the estimated scaled eigenmatrix $\boldsymbol{RD}^{1/2}$ corresponding to the correlation matrix in Fig. 2. The x-axes show the percent variation explained by each eigenvector (column) as implied by the empirical estimates of the d_j in each case

thresholding (the sample eigenmatrix) to a threshold of 0.25 and then 0.5, and how the sparse Givens construction—via this simple exploratory estimation method—naturally denoises the raw sample estimates. The major ER and Her2 "clusters" evident in the correlation matrices are sustained as we move up through the levels of thresholding, and the corresponding "factor loadings" structure represented in the eigenmatrices successively reduces the numbers and patterns of genes related to each factor (column). The most sparse structure in the first row shows that—assuming this level of sparsity—we uncover a dominant Her2 factor loaded on four of the Her2 cluster of genes, two main ER factors, and a few minor factors that each represent only modest levels of variation explained while contributing to the break-down of the complexity of expression relationships in the data.

5 Bayesian Analysis and Computation

We discuss and develop Bayesian computation for model fitting and exploration, presenting customized MCMC methods.

5.1 *Overview*

In target applications with modest and increasingly high values of q, and hence larger $m = q(q-1)/2$, the focus is on sparse structures so that posterior distributions will concentrate on smaller numbers of non-zero angles. In these circumstances, visiting every element of $\boldsymbol{\omega}$ using a Gibbs sampling approach will be computationally expensive and other MCMC strategies are recommended. Most effective MCMC analysis can be achieved using reversible jump Markov Chain Monte Carlo (RJ-MCMC) [12]. We have implemented such an approach based on exploring the space of non-zero elements of $\boldsymbol{\omega}$ using a birth/death RJ-MCMC. Each move through this "model space" involves proposed changes that introduce non-zero values, including the possible values $\omega = \pi/2$, and/or setting current non-zero values to zero. We present the details of the sampling algorithm by first outlining an approximation to the conditional posterior of a single, non-zero $\omega_{i,j}$ that we recommend as conditional proposal distribution for the MCMC.

5.2 *Wrapped Cauchy Proposals*

Consider any rotator pair (i,j) assuming $\omega_{i,j} \neq 0$. The conditional posterior is proportional to the conditional mixture prior, mixing a point mass at $\pi/2$ with $p_c(\cdot)$, multiplied by the conditional likelihood of the form discussed in the previous section—the conditional likelihood for $\omega_{i,j}$ given all other rotators and eigenvalues.

Our MCMC adopts a conditional proposal distribution for $\omega_{i,j}$ based on direct approximation. Specifically, we use a proposal with pdf

$$g(\omega) \equiv \beta_{\frac{\pi}{2}} I(\omega = \pi/2) + (1 - \beta_{\frac{\pi}{2}}) g_c(\omega)$$

where the continuous density $g_c(\cdot)$ is that of a wrapped Cauchy chosen to approximate the conditional posterior for $\omega_{i,j}$ conditional on $0 < |\omega_{i,j}| < \pi/2$; i.e., a Cauchy "wrapped" onto the interval $(-\pi/2, \pi/2)$ [10]. Specifically,

$$g_c(\omega) = \frac{1}{\pi} \frac{\sinh(2\sigma)}{\{\cosh(2\sigma) - \cos[2(x - \theta)]\}}$$

where (θ, σ) are chosen so that $g(\cdot)$ approximates the conditional posterior under prior $p_c(\cdot)$. The proposed values of (θ, σ) are based on direct numerical approximation. We set θ as the exact conditional posterior mode; this is easily evaluated numerically. Under any conjugate prior over non-zero values, which includes our recommended default prior $p_c(\cdot)$ in (5), note that $\log p(\omega_{i,j}|\boldsymbol{X}, -)$ is a quadratic form in $(\sin(\omega_{i,j}), \cos(\omega_{i,j}))$ on a bounded domain and can be evaluated along with any number of derivatives very quickly. Resulting numerical maximization is then routine and extremely efficient. At the solution θ, the curvature generates a value for the scale σ from

$$\frac{1}{\sigma^2} = -\frac{\partial^2}{\partial \omega_{i,j}} \log p(\omega_{i,j}|\boldsymbol{X}, -)\Big|_{\omega_{i,j}=\theta}.$$

The wrapped Cauchy form can be viewed as a diffuse posterior approximation—the result of an initial Laplace approximation subject to inflating the tails to ensure good coverage of the exact conditional posterior. To deal with cases in which the mode θ lies on the boundary, simply replacing $g_c(\cdot)$ with a $\text{Be}(\omega|0.25, 0.25)$ density has been empirically found to provides an effective, default proposal.

5.3 *Reversible Jump MCMC*

Denote all parameters of interest by $\boldsymbol{\Theta} = \{\mathscr{X}, \boldsymbol{\omega}, \boldsymbol{A}\}$ where, as introduced above, $\mathscr{X}$ is the set of pairs of indices (i,j) corresponding to included rotators with non-zero angles. In an overall MCMC, suppose we are at a current state at iterate t with parameters $\boldsymbol{\Theta}^{(t)} = \{\mathscr{X}^{(t)}, \boldsymbol{\omega}^{(t)}, \boldsymbol{A}^{(t)}\}$ with a current $z^{(t)} = |\mathscr{X}^{(t)}|$ rotators. Consider now either adding or removing a rotator index pair from $\mathscr{X}^{(t)}$. Set probabilities of adding a rotator (birth) and removing a rotator (death) at values denoted by p_B and p_D, respectively. For a proposed birth, randomly select an ordered pair,

$(i^*,j^*) \in \mathcal{M} \setminus \mathcal{Z}^{(t)}$ to index a proposed angle, and then generate a proposal $\omega^*_{i^*j^*}$ from $g(\omega_{i^*j^*})$ described in Sect. 5.2. This implies the following birth step accept/rejection ratio:

$$\alpha_B = \frac{p(\boldsymbol{X}|\omega^*_{i^*j^*}, -)p(\omega^*_{i^*j^*})(z^{(t)}+1)p_D}{p(\boldsymbol{X}|\omega^{(t)}_{i^*j^*}, -)p(0)g(\omega^*_{i^*j^*})(m-z^{(t)})p_B}. \tag{10}$$

For a proposed death step, choose an element from $\mathcal{Z}^{(t)}$ uniformly and set its corresponding angle to zero. The resulting rejection ratio is simply $\alpha_D = \alpha_B^{-1}$. We then set $\omega^{(t+1)}_{i^*j^*} = \omega^*_{i^*j^*}$ with probability $\min(1,\alpha_B)$. To facilitate better mixing, we do several reversible jump proposals in each MCMC iteration. This results in the updated (possibly, of course, also the same) set of rotator pairs $\mathcal{Z}^{(t+1)}$.

The MCMC next updates all non-zero angles indexed in $\mathcal{Z}^{(t+1)}$. For each pair $(i,j) \in \mathcal{Z}^{(t+1)}$, generate a proposal $\omega^*_{i,j}$ from $g(\omega_{i,j})$ and set $\omega^{(t+1)}_{i,j} = \omega^*_{i,j}$ with probability

$$\min\left\{1, \frac{p(\boldsymbol{X}|\omega^*_{i,j}, -)p(\omega^*_{i,j})g(\omega^{(t)}_{i,j})}{p(\boldsymbol{X}|\omega^{(t)}_{i,j}, -)p(\omega^{(t)}_{i,j})g(\omega^*_{i,j})}\right\}. \tag{11}$$

Since we update the elements of $\boldsymbol{\omega}^{(t)}$ in order, the recursive relationship between the conditional log likelihoods given in Eq. (8) makes computation extremely fast. This recursive update is initialized at

$$\boldsymbol{A}_{i_1j_1} = \boldsymbol{O}_{i_1j_1}(\omega^{(t)}_{i_1j_1})'R^{(t)}\boldsymbol{O}_{i_1j_1}(\omega^{(t)}_{i_1j_1}) \quad \text{and} \quad \boldsymbol{S}_{i_1j_1} = \boldsymbol{S}.$$

The log likelihood can then be optimized and evaluated quickly as described in the previous section. For $k > 1$ as we step through updates of rotator k, compute

$$\boldsymbol{A}_{i_kj_k} = \boldsymbol{O}_{i_kj_k}(\omega^{(t)}_{i_kj_k})'\boldsymbol{A}_{i_{k-1}j_{k-1}}\boldsymbol{O}_{i_kj_k}(\omega^{(t)}_{i_kj_k}) \quad \text{and}$$
$$\boldsymbol{S}_{i_kj_k} = \boldsymbol{O}_{i_{k-1}j_{k-1}}(\omega^{(t+1)}_{i_{k-1}j_{k-1}})'\boldsymbol{S}_{i_{k-1}j_{k-1}}\boldsymbol{O}_{i_{k-1}j_{k-1}}(\omega^{(t+1)}_{i_{k-1}j_{k-1}}).$$

Note that the recursions for $\boldsymbol{A}_{i_kj_k}$ and $\boldsymbol{S}_{i_kj_k}$ only involve taking linear combinations of two rows and columns, so we can avoid recomputing the entire eigenmatrix for every proposal. In words: (1) start with the sum of squares matrix and the eigenmatrix; (2) remove the first rotation by multiplying by its transpose; (3) perform a fast Metropolis move by exploiting the quadratic form of the likelihood; (4) decorrelate the sum of squares matrix with the new rotator and remove the next rotation from the eigenmatrix.

The final step is to update the entries of the diagonal precision matrix $\boldsymbol{A}$ from the current value $\boldsymbol{A}^{(t)}$. Let

$$\boldsymbol{B} = \boldsymbol{R}^{(t)\prime}\boldsymbol{S}\boldsymbol{R}^{(t)}.$$

Then for each $j = 1, \ldots, q$

$$p(a_j^{(t)}|\boldsymbol{X}, -) \propto \text{Ga}(a_j^{(t)}|(\eta_1 + n)/2, (\eta_2 + B_{j,j})/2)\, I(a_{j-1}^{(t)} < a_j^{(t)} < a_{j+1}^{(t)}) \quad (12)$$

where $Ga(x|a, b)$ denotes the pdf of the $Ga(a, b)$ distribution evaluated at x. Since the eigenvalues are constrained to be ordered, the conditional distributions are constrained as well. The resulting constrained gamma distribution is sampled using the inverse cdf method.

6 Simulation Study and Comparisons

We make a detailed, simulation-based comparison of the modelling approach with analysis using traditional Gaussian graphical modelling (GGM) [2, 7, 8, 19, 21, 30]. The GGM framework with decomposable graphs is directly comparable and stands as a current benchmark model context.

The simulation study was conducted using zero mean normal models in each of $p \in \{10, 20, 30, 40, 50, 75, 100\}$ dimensions, with a fixed sample size of $n = 150$ observations. Synthetic data sets generated from specific model classes were analyzed using the sparse Givens approach and the GGM approach, the latter using shotgun stochastic model search for the Bayesian analysis [19]. Each analysis was repeated for 100 simulation samples. The underlying models and synthetic data generation proceeded as follows:

1. Generate a target precision matrix $\boldsymbol{K} = \boldsymbol{U}'\boldsymbol{U}$ where $\boldsymbol{U}$ is upper triangular with:
   - $U_{i,i} = \sqrt{\nu_i}$ with $\nu_i \sim \chi^2_{p-i}$, $(i = 1, \ldots, p)$,
   - $U_{i,j} = u_{i,j} I(|u|_{i,j} > 1)$ where $u_{i,j} \sim N(0, 1)$, $(j > i,\ i = 2, \ldots, p-1)$, and
   - the $\nu_i, u_{i,j}$ are mutually independent.
2. Draw $n = 150$ observations $\boldsymbol{X}$ as a random sample from $N(0, \boldsymbol{K}^{-1})$.
3. Fit the sparse Givens model using 15,000 MCMC iterations. Discard the first 10,000 and save the final 5000 as a Monte Carlo sample for sparsity patterns and values of $\boldsymbol{K}$.
4. Fit the GGM model using 15,000 stochastic search iterations. Discard the first 10,000 and save the final 5000 graphs identified, their posterior probabilities and the parameters of the corresponding posteriors for $\boldsymbol{K}$ on each graph.

For prior distributions, the probability of including a "free" parameter was set to $2/(p-1)$. In the sparse Givens models, a free parameter is an angle; in GGMs, it is the probability of including a random edge. This specification aims to match the prior expectations of degrees of sparsity between the two approaches.

Comparisons are based on measuring agreement between the approximate posteriors and the "true" underlying data-generating distribution. For any precision matrix $\boldsymbol{K}_*$, we can directly compute the Kullback-Leibler (KL) divergence of the $N(0, \boldsymbol{K}_*^{-1})$ distribution from the true, underlying $N(0, \boldsymbol{K}^{-1})$ distribution. With both the MCMC posterior samples and the GGM search results, we can then approximately evaluate the posterior distribution for the KL divergence of the chosen model from the truth.

Figure 4 summarizes the posteriors for the KL divergences, aggregated across 100 repeat samples. We can see that in 20 dimensions, both methods perform similarly; this is not surprising since there is reasonable amount of data relative to the dimension. However, in 30 dimensions, the new sparse Givens approach is significantly better, and its dominance is progressively more pronounced as the dimension increases.

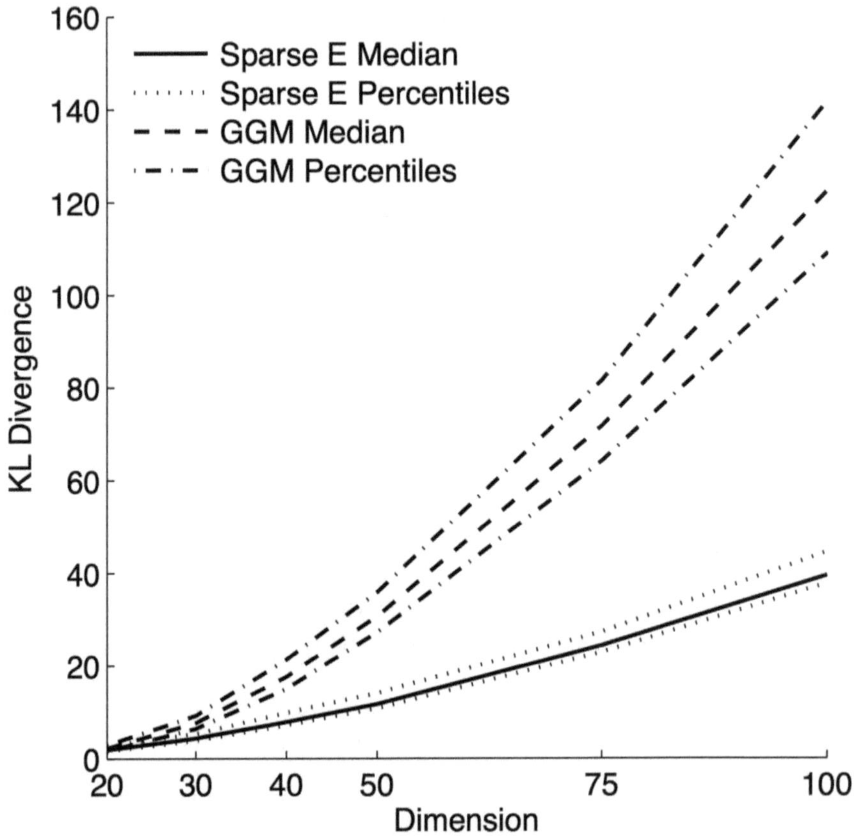

Fig. 4 Simulation study comparing GGM to the sparse Givens (labelled "Sparse E" in the figure) methodology. Shown are the medial, 10th and 90th percentiles of the posterior for (logged values of) the KL divergence from the fitted model to the true underlying data generating model

7 Mixtures of Sparse, Full-Rank Factor Models

Many applied contexts involve evident non-Gaussian structure as well as measurement error overlaid on the underlying dependency patterns we are interested in inferring via the sparse eigenmatrix models. The gene expression example of Sect. 4.2 is just one case-in-point. First, in the broader contexts of samples from the full breast cancer population, there is inherent non-Gaussianity representing heterogeneity in cancer states. This heterogeneity can be regarded as arising from a mixture of sub-populations, or "subtypes" that, in terms of expression data outcomes, are hugely overlapping [3, 26, 33]. More broadly, use of discrete mixtures of Gaussians is a well-established strategy for modelling what might be quite non-Gaussian distributional forms, whether or not there is an inherent in mixture components and discrimination/classification [4, 9, 35]. Second, measurement errors are ubiquitous. Again the gene expression example and broader context is a good example, as the experimental and data extraction contexts are well-known to overlay underlying biological variation with meaningful uncertainties that must be accommodated within a more general model in order to avoid obscuring relationships and leading to potential biases in resulting inferences [3, 24, 25, 27].

7.1 Mixture Models and Extension of MCMC Analysis

We address the above, general considerations with Gaussian mixture models overlaid with measurement errors. Each mixture component has a variance matrix modelled via the sparse Givens strategy; this can be directly interpreted as a sparse, full-rank latent factor model for underlying "structural" dependencies. As a result, the overall framework is a generalized, adaptively sparse model for "mixtures of (full-rank, sparse) factor analyzers" [28, 30].

Assume we observe n independent q-vector observations $\boldsymbol{Y} = \{\boldsymbol{y}_1, \ldots, \boldsymbol{y}_n\}$ where $\boldsymbol{y}_i = \boldsymbol{x}_i + \boldsymbol{\epsilon}_i$ with independent measurement errors $\boldsymbol{\epsilon}_i \sim N(\boldsymbol{0}, \boldsymbol{\Psi})$ having variance matrix $\boldsymbol{\Psi} = \text{diag}(\psi_1, \ldots, \psi_q)$. Suppose the latent signals $\boldsymbol{x}_i$ are independently drawn from a discrete mixture of multivariate normals having pdf

$$p(\boldsymbol{x}) = \sum_{c=1}^{C} w_c N(\boldsymbol{x}|\boldsymbol{\mu}_c, \boldsymbol{\Sigma}_c).$$

Equivalently,

$$\boldsymbol{y}_i|\gamma_i \sim N(\boldsymbol{\mu}_c, \boldsymbol{\Sigma}_c + \boldsymbol{\Psi}), \quad \text{where} \quad Pr(\gamma_i = c) = w_c,$$

involving the underlying latent mixture component indicators γ_i that are independently drawn from the multinomial distribution on cells $\{1 : C\}$ with the vector of cell probabilities $\boldsymbol{w} = (w_1, \ldots, w_C)'$.

We develop this mixture model under sparse Givens factor structures for each of the mixture components. That is, $\boldsymbol{\Sigma}_c = \boldsymbol{R}_c\boldsymbol{D}_c\boldsymbol{R}_c'$ where we model each of the $(\boldsymbol{R}_c, \boldsymbol{D}_C)$ with the prior structure of Sect. 3, independently across components c. This allows for differing degrees and patterns of sparsity as we move across components of the mixture, in the context of also accommodating realistic assessment of overlaid measurement errors. We couple this with conditionally conjugate normal priors for the $(\boldsymbol{\mu}_c|\boldsymbol{\Sigma}_c)$ independently across components, and a similarly conditionally conjugate Dirichlet prior for the mixture weights $\boldsymbol{w}$. The final component of prior specification is a set of q conditionally independent inverse gamma priors for the measurement error variances ψ_j, $j = 1 : q$.

The traditional MCMC analysis of multivariate normal mixtures [5, 22] is easily extended to apply here. Several points require note. At each iterate conditional on currently imputed values of the $\boldsymbol{x}_i$, we resample new values of the mixture component indicators γ_i for each of the $i = 1 : n$ observations. Conditional on these indicators, the imputed signal "data" vectors $\boldsymbol{x}_i$ are organized into C conditionally independent normal subgroups. The inherent component labelling issue is automatically addressed each iteration using the efficient component relabelling strategy of Cron and West [5]. The numbers of observations in each group define the conditional multinomial sample needed to draw new values of the mixture weights $\boldsymbol{w}$ from the implied conditional Dirichlet posterior. We then resample new group means $\boldsymbol{\mu}_c$ from the implied set of C conditional normal posteriors. Subtracting the group means from the values of the $\boldsymbol{x}_i$ within each group, we are then in a context of having C replicates of the normal, sparse Givens model. Hence we apply C parallel RJ-MCMC steps to draw new values of rotator index sets, angles and eigenvalues in each of the components. The final, additional component of the overall MCMC posterior simulation arises due to the additive measurement error structure of the model. Given the resampled parameters and component indicators, the implied conditional posterior for each $\boldsymbol{x}_i$ is normal, so easily sampled; given the new value of $\boldsymbol{x}_i$, we compute new synthetic residuals $\boldsymbol{\epsilon}_i = \boldsymbol{y}_i - \boldsymbol{x}_i$ that lead to a set of q, independent conditional posteriors for the ψ_i that are each of inverse gamma form.

Additional technical details of these steps appear in the Appendix, and in supporting material, we provide code implementing this MCMC algorithm.

7.2 A Broader Study in Breast Cancer Genomics

We analyse a set of $n = 295$ breast cancer gene expression sample that represent the full range of breast cancers; the data set uses the same 15 genes as in the example of Sect. 4.2, but now reflecting full population heterogeneity; variations in the expression levels of these 15 breast cancer related genes is much greater across this full set of 295 tumor samples. The $q = 20$-dimensional data set again includes five "Junk" genes generated as Gaussian noise, to add dimension for the evaluation of the model analysis.

As discussed in Sect. 4.2, breast cancer heterogeneity based on molecular markers related to ER and Her2 pathways is often regarded in terms of over-lapping cancer subtypes. The genes selected for this study relate to these pathways, and the variability across samples is certainly empirically consistent with at least three underlying components; see some scatter plots on a few genes in Fig. 5. We fit the sparse Givens, finite mixture model $C = 4$. Priors for residual measurement error variances are informed by a wealth of prior information from studies of gene expression data using Affymetrix microarrays in breast cancer and other contexts [3, 24–27, 31, 32]. Specifically, we adopt $\psi_j \sim InvGa(3.1, 0.17)$ with implied 95 % prior credible intervals for measurement error standard deviations of about $(0.15, 0.5)$. For the mixture weights $\boldsymbol{w}$, we take a uniform Dirichlet prior. For component locations, we take $\boldsymbol{\mu}_c | \boldsymbol{\Sigma}_c \sim N(\boldsymbol{0}, \tau \boldsymbol{\Sigma}_c)$ where τ is large to induce a rather diffuse marginal prior on mixture locations; the analysis summarized below has $\tau = 1000$. The prior over the sparse Givens parameters for each $\boldsymbol{\Sigma}_c$ takes $\beta_0 = 0.99$, $\beta_{\pi/2} = 0.25$, and $\kappa = 0$. This prior expresses an expectation of a fair degree of sparsity in each $\boldsymbol{R}_c$, coupled with a vague uniform prior on values of non-zero angles. Finally for $\boldsymbol{D}_c$, we have $\eta_1 = 1/1000$ and $\eta_2 = 1/1000$ representing an uninformative prior on the eigenvalues, up to the constraints imposed by their ordering.

For starting values, we first crudely partition the data using k-means clustering, then use the exploratory algorithm of Sect. 4.2 with a correlation threshold of 0.5. We run the MCMC for 200,000 iterations, discarding the first 100,000 for burn-in to ensure convergence, with a number of subjective assessments of this. The analysis identifies three main components with posterior means of components weights of $(0.564, 0.303, 0.125, 0.008)'$. Figure 5 shows some aspects of the posterior through scatter plots of data on a few selected genes. From the MCMC we compute estimates

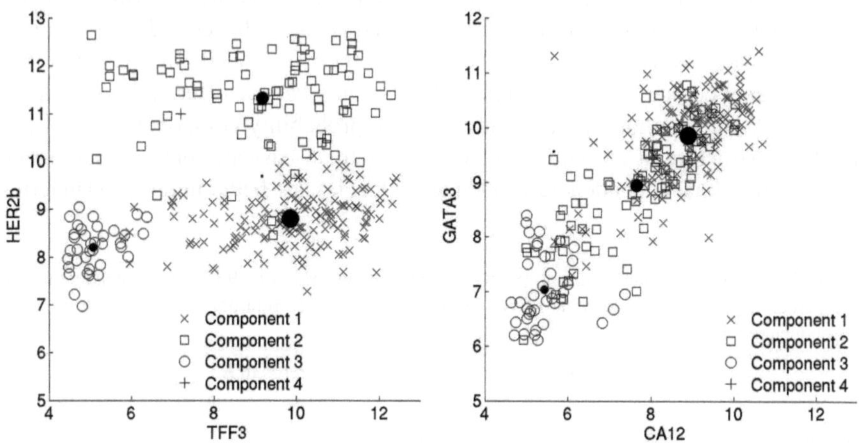

Fig. 5 Aspects of estimated component classification summaries in the analysis of the mixture model for the gene expression data. The *filled circles* correspond to the estimated means of the mixture components and their sizes are proportional to the estimated component weights

of the sample component classification probabilities $Pr(\gamma_i = c|\boldsymbol{Y})$ for each $i = 1 : n$, and allocate sample i to the most probable component for the purpose of this graphical display; the data points are plotted as symbols corresponding to their most probable component. The dominant identified component $c = 1$ represents cases with expression varying across high levels for genes linked to the ER pathway, including TFF3, CA-12 and GATA3 shown in Fig. 5, and with Her2 pathway genes varying at relatively low levels; these represent the broad luminal subtype of breast cancers [3, 26, 33]. The second main component $c = 2$ represents cases generally high in Her2 expression levels, with other genes varying across the spectrum; this corresponds to high-risk Her2 breast cancers that are generally targets for the Her2 receptor inhibiting drug herceptin. The third, smaller component $c = 3$ represent the so-called triple-negative/basal-like tumors, with generally low levels of activity of both ER and Her2 related genes. The patterns in the figure, and in those of other genes in the example, as well as the posterior estimates of relative sizes of these three main components, are quite consistent with the known cancer biology and relative probabilities of these three broad, and imprecisely defined clinical subtypes of tumors.

Table 1 summarizes the posterior for the number of non-zero angles in each mixture component and the sparsity of $\boldsymbol{R}_c$. The maximum number of rotators is 105 and the maximum sparsity of $\boldsymbol{R}$ is 210. The posterior favours a very sparse set of angles in each mixture component and the eigenstructure in each component is quite sparse as a result.

Figures 6 and 7 give graphical summaries generating insights into the inferred sparse structures underlying the $\boldsymbol{\Sigma}_c$ for each component $c = 1 : 4$. Figure 6 shows heat maps of approximate posterior probabilities of non-zero values in the precision matrices $\boldsymbol{K}_c = \boldsymbol{\Sigma}_c^{-1}$ indicating the nature of sparsity and the underlying graphical model structure. Component $c = 1$ has high probabilities on multiple edges linking pairs of ER related genes, Her2 related genes and tying in the two BRCA genes. Component $c = 2$ more sharply identifies a Her2-related cluster and a distinct ER-related cluster, with somewhat weaker links to the two related BRCA genes. The much sparser component $c = 3$ highlights links only between Her2 related genes.

Finally, we see that, appropriately, the low probability component $c = 4$ has really no structure at all, consistent with prior for a basically empty component. These conditional dependencies, and independencies, are better understood in terms

Table 1 Posterior medians and end-points of approximate posterior 95 % credible intervals for the percentage of sparse elements of $\boldsymbol{R}_c$ and of the number of rotators in each of the mixture components $c = 1, 2, 3$

	% non-zero rotators			% zeros in $\boldsymbol{R}$		
	2.5 %	50 %	97.5 %	2.5 %	50 %	97.5 %
Component 1	9.5	10.5	12.1	66.8	71.8	73.7
Component 2	8.4	10.0	11.0	74.5	82.6	87.4
Component 3	1.6	3.2	4.2	95.3	92.1	97.6

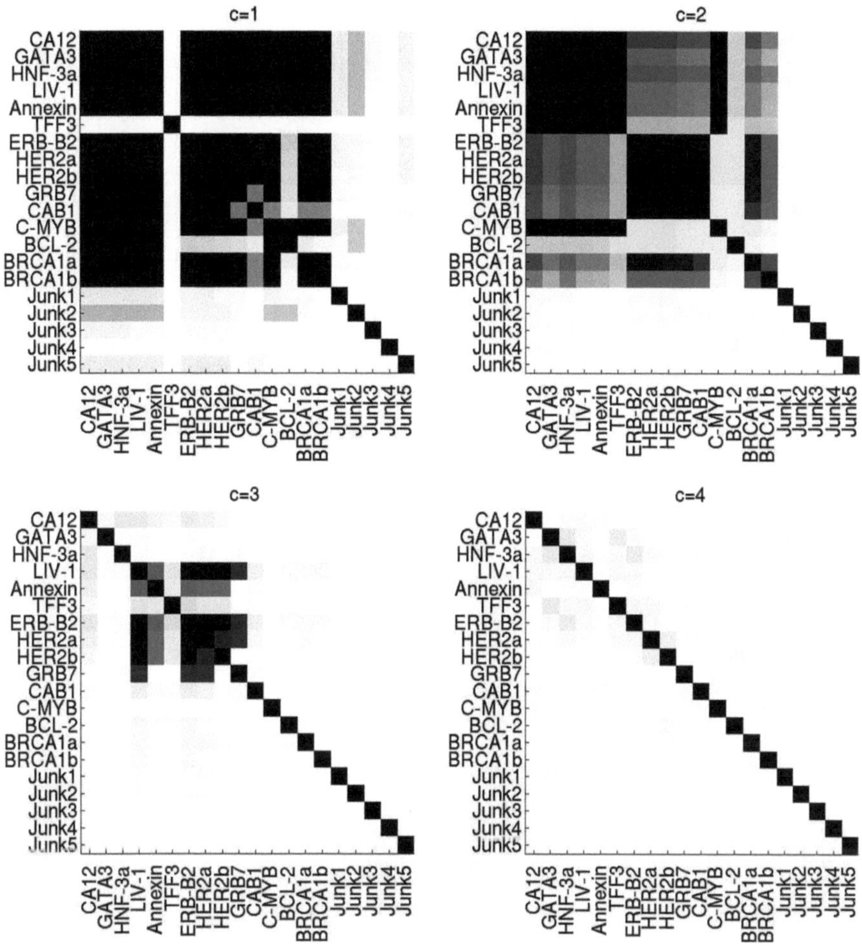

Fig. 6 Heat maps showing posterior probabilities of non-zero entries in $\boldsymbol{K}_c$ for each normal mixture component $c = 1 : 4$ in analysis of cancer gene expression data. Shading runs from *white*=0 to *black*=1 in each

of the estimated factor structure underlying eigenmatrices and eigenvalues of the sparse Givens models in each component; these are shown in the left column of Fig. 7 for the three main components. For the "high ER" tumors in component $c = 1$, we see one dominant and two subsidiary eigenvectors, indicating three "ER-related factors" based on non-zero loadings of the ER-related genes; these presumably reflect several dimensions of the underlying patterns of variability in these genes as a result of the complexity of the ER network. The second dominant eigenvector relates to the Her2 cluster. For the "high Her2" tumors in $c = 2$, we see the dominant factor is indeed linked to the Her2 gene cluster, while the fact that ER related genes vary across the scale in these tumors leads to a natural set of three

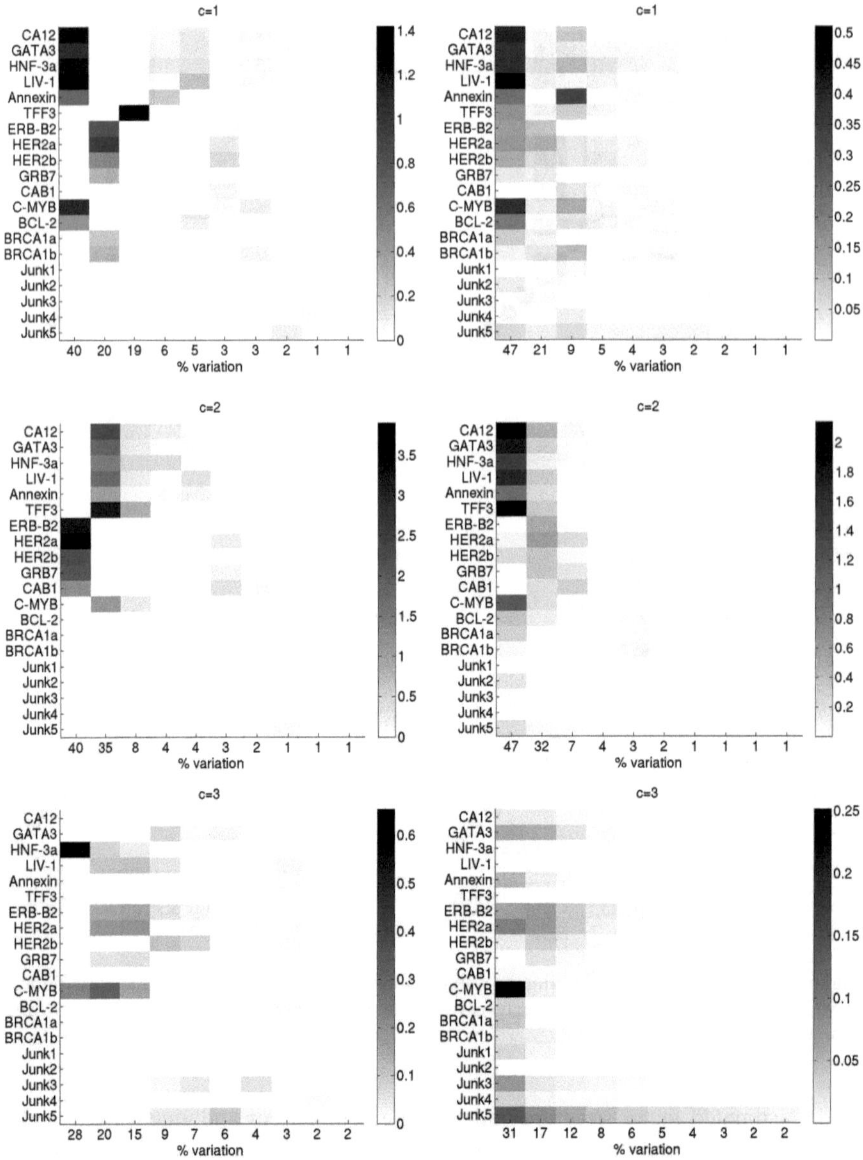

Fig. 7 Heat maps showing posterior means of the first ten columns of $\boldsymbol{R}_c\boldsymbol{D}_c^{1/2}$ for the three main mixture components in analysis of cancer gene expression data. *Left column*: sparsity model, and *Right column*: full non-sparse model. The percent variation explained by each eigenvector is indicated on the x-axes, based on posterior means of the d_j in each case

or four ER-related factors. For the triple negative/basal-like tumors in component $c = 3$, we see residual biological pathway activity highlighted involving HNF-3α and C-MYB genes, as well as important factors in both ER and Her2 pathways; although these two pathways are less active in tumors in this group, there is still meaningful variation among subsets of some of these genes.

For comparison, the right column in Fig. 7 shows the corresponding eigenstructure extracted from an analysis using traditional inverse Wishart priors on the $\boldsymbol{\Sigma}_c$, i.e., in the standard analysis with no sparsity. It is very clear how the sharp factor-based groupings in the sparse Givens mixture model "cleans-up" the much noisier standard results. In addition to cleaner and focused inference on dependency structures, we also found that the standard analysis—by comparison with the sparse model—generates over-diffuse estimates of the spread of mixture components and so less sharp classification of samples, as a result.

8 Additional Comments

In terms of modelling variations and extensions, one interesting question relates to the interpretation of the sparse Givens model as factor analysis. Our examples have stressed this interpretation from an applied viewpoint. Theoretically, the Givens model is a full-rank, orthogonal factor analysis model. We can imagine extensions to include reduced rank approximations that would be based on the use of priors giving positive probability to zero values among the d_i, relating more directly to alternative factor modelling frameworks [39].

We have experience in running the MCMC analysis for higher-dimensional variance matrices, including extensions of the gene expression examples with $q = 300$ genes. The overall performance of the MCMC is scalable, in terms of acceptance rates, while of course the running time and implementation overheads increase. In particular, as the number of rotators grows, a number of computational challenges arise. First, the numerical optimization to define Metropolis proposals $g_c(\omega_{i,j})$ becomes increasingly time consuming, so that one immediate area of research will be to explore more computationally efficient proposal strategies for the MCMC. Second, based on our positive experience with the exploratory analysis to define ad-hoc starting values for increasingly high-dimensional problems, one direction for improving the MCMC would be to consider alternatives to the birth/death strategy based on more aggressive local search in neighborhoods of "good" sparsity configurations. Some of the concepts and computational strategies underlying shotgun stochastic search in regression and graphical models [14–16, 20] may be of real benefit here. The potential for distributed computation, including using GPU hardware [13, 34, 35] is also of interest.

Supplementary Material

As noted in the text, code implementing the analyses reported here is (freely) available to interested readers at the authors' web site.

Acknowledgements This work was completed while the first author was a Ph.D. student in the Department of Statistical Science at Duke University. The research was partly supported by grants from the National Science Foundation [DMS-1106516] and the National Institutes of Health [1RC1-AI086032]. Any opinions, findings and conclusions or recommendations expressed in this work are those of the authors and do not necessarily reflect the views of the NSF or NIH.

Appendix: MCMC in Mixtures of Sparse Givens Models

Additional technical details of the MCMC algorithm in Sect. 7 are given here.

(a) *Starting values:* We use k-means clustering to define initial, crude classification of the data into C groups, giving starting values for component indicators $\boldsymbol{\gamma}$. Group means and proportions define starting values $\boldsymbol{\mu}_c$ and $\boldsymbol{w}_c$. Initial values for the Givens structures within each group are then created using the exploratory algorithm of Sect. 4. Beginning with the sample variance matrix of each group c, this algorithm produces a sparse Givens structure with starting values for the rotator pairs, angles and eigenvalues, and hence $\boldsymbol{R}_c$, $\boldsymbol{D}_c$ and $\boldsymbol{\Sigma}_c$. The measurement error variances ψ_j in $\boldsymbol{\Psi}$ are initialized at draws from the prior.

(b) *Rotator structure and angle updates:* For each cluster $c = 1 : C$ defined at the current iterate of the MCMC, we update the rotators selected and corresponding angles using the RJ-MCMC analysis of Sect. 5.3.

(c) *Latent data $\boldsymbol{X}$:* Each $\boldsymbol{x}_i$ is resampled from the complete conditional normal posterior whose mean vector $\boldsymbol{m}_i$ and variance matrix $\boldsymbol{M}_i$ are given by

$$\boldsymbol{m}_i = \boldsymbol{M}_i(\boldsymbol{\Psi}^{-1}\boldsymbol{y}_i + \boldsymbol{\Sigma}_{\gamma_i}^{-1}\boldsymbol{\mu}_{\gamma_i}) \quad \text{and} \quad \boldsymbol{M}_i^{-1} = \boldsymbol{\Psi}^{-1} + \boldsymbol{\Sigma}_{\gamma_i}^{-1}.$$

Note that the $\boldsymbol{\Sigma}_c^{-1}$ can be calculated trivially even in high dimensional cases simply by inverting the eigenvalues.

(d) *Measurement error variances ψ_j:* Each of the q elements of the diagonal matrix $\boldsymbol{\Psi}$ is resampled from a complete conditional given by

$$\psi_j^{-1} \sim Ga(\phi_a + n/2, \phi_b + \sum_{i=1}^{n} \epsilon_{ji}^2/2)$$

for $j = 1 : q$, where ϵ_{ji} is the j-the element of $\boldsymbol{y}_i - \boldsymbol{x}_i$.

(e) *Component indicators* $\boldsymbol{\gamma}$: The set of n component classification indicators $\boldsymbol{\gamma} = (\gamma_1, \ldots, \gamma_n)'$ are drawn from conditionally independent multinomials, each with sample size 1 and probabilities over the C cells defined by

$$Pr(\gamma_i = c|-) \propto w_c N(\boldsymbol{x}_i|\boldsymbol{\mu}_c, \boldsymbol{\Sigma}_c), \qquad c = 1 : C,$$

where $N(\boldsymbol{x}|\cdot, \cdot)$ denotes the multivariate normal pdf.

(f) *Component weights* $\mathbf{w}$: Resampled weights come from the complete conditional Dirichlet posterior with parameter $(\alpha_1, \ldots, \alpha_C)'$ and $\alpha_c = 1/C + n_c$ where

$$n_c = \sum_{i=1}^{n} I(\gamma_i = c), \quad c = 1 : C.$$

(g) *Component means* $\boldsymbol{\mu}_c$: Denote by $\bar{\boldsymbol{x}}_c$ the sample mean in group c given a current set of component indicators. Then the component means are sampled in parallel from the C conditional normal posteriors with means $(n_c + 1/\tau)^{-1} n_c \bar{\boldsymbol{x}}_c$ and variance matrices $(n_c + 1/\tau)^{-1} \boldsymbol{\Sigma}_c$, $c = 1 : C$.

(h) *Eigenvectors* $\boldsymbol{D}_c$: Finally, the complete conditional distributions of the diagonal elements of $\boldsymbol{D}_c = \boldsymbol{A}_c^{-1}$ are independent inverse gammas constrained by the ordering; see (12), applied to each of the C groups in parallel. These are sampled in sequence using the inverse cdf method.

References

1. Anderson, T.W., Olkin, I., Underhill, L.G.: Generation of random orthogonal matrices. SIAM J. Sci. Stat. Comput. **8**, 625–629 (1987)
2. Carvalho, C.M., West, M.: Dynamic matrix-variate graphical models. Bayesian Anal. **2**, 69–98 (2007)
3. Carvalho, C.M., Lucas, J.E., Wang, Q., Chang, J., Nevins, J.R., West, M.: High-dimensional sparse factor modelling - applications in gene expression genomics. J. Am. Stat. Assoc. **103**, 1438–1456 (2008)
4. Chan, C., Feng, F., Ottinger, J., Foster, D., West, M., Kepler, T.B.: Statistical mixture modelling for cell subtype identification in flow cytometry. Cytometry A **73**, 693–701 (2008)
5. Cron, A.J., West, M.: Efficient classification-based relabeling in mixture models. Am. Stat. **65**, 16–20 (2011)
6. Daniels, M., Pourahmadi, M.: Modeling covariance matrices via partial autocorrelations. J. Multivar. Anal. **100**, 2352–2363 (2009)
7. Dobra, A., Jones, B., Hans, C., Nevins, J.R., West, M.: Sparse graphical models for exploring gene expression data. J. Multivar. Anal. **90**, 196–212 (2004)
8. Dobra, A., Lenkoski, A., Rodriguez, A.: Bayesian inference for general Gaussian graphical models with application to multivariate lattice data. J. Am. Stat. Assoc. **106**, 1418–1433 (2012)
9. Escobar, M.D., West, M.: Bayesian density estimation and inference using mixtures. J. Am. Stat. Assoc. **90**, 577–588 (1995)
10. Fisher, N.I.: Statistical Analysis of Circular Data. Cambridge University Press, Cambridge (1993)

11. Fulkerson, D.R., Gross, O.A.: Incidence matrices and interval graphs. Pac. J. Math. **15**, 835–855 (1965)
12. Green, P.J.: Reversible jump Markov chain Monte Carlo computation and Bayesian model determination. Biometrika **82**, 711–732 (1995)
13. Gruber, L.F., West, M.: GPU-accelerated Bayesian learning in simultaneous graphical dynamic linear models. Bayesian Anal. - Advance Publication, 2 March 2015. http://projecteuclid.org/euclid.ba/1425304898 (2015). doi:10.1214/15-BA946
14. Hans, C., West, M.: High-dimensional regression in cancer genomics. Bull. Int. Soc. Bayesian Anal. **13**, 2–3 (2006)
15. Hans, C., Dobra, A., West, M.: Shotgun stochastic search in regression with many predictors. J. Am. Stat. Soc. **102**, 507–516 (2007)
16. Hans, C., Wang, Q., Dobra, A., West, M.: SSS: high-dimensional Bayesian regression model search. Bull. Int. Soc. Bayesian Anal. **24**, 8–9 (2007)
17. Hoff, P.D.: Simulation of the matrix Bingham-von Mises-Fisher distribution, with applications to multivariate and relational data. J. Comput. Graph. Stat. **18**, 438–456 (2009)
18. Huang, E.S., West, M., Nevins, J.R.: Gene expression profiles and predicting clinical characteristics of breast cancer. Horm. Res. **58**, 55–73 (2002)
19. Jones, B., West, M.: Covariance decomposition in undirected Gaussian graphical models. Biometrika **92**, 779–786 (2005)
20. Jones, B., Dobra, A., Carvalho, C.M., Hans, C., Carter, C., West, M.: Experiments in stochastic computation for high-dimensional graphical models. Stat. Sci. **20**, 388–400 (2005)
21. Lauritzen, S.L.: Graphical Models. Clarendon Press, Oxford (1996)
22. Lavine, M., West, M.: A Bayesian method for classification and discrimination. Can. J. Stat. **20**, 451–461 (1992)
23. Lopes, H.F., McCulloch, R.E., Tsay, R.: Cholesky stochastic volatility. Technical Report, University of Chicago, Booth Business School (2010)
24. Lucas, J.E., Carvalho, C.M., Wang, Q., Bild, A.H., Nevins, J.R., West, M.: Sparse statistical modelling in gene expression genomics. In: Do, K., Mueller, P., Vannucci, M. (eds.) Bayesian Inference for Gene Expression and Proteomics, pp. 155–176. Cambridge University Press, Cambridge (2006)
25. Lucas, J.E., Carvalho, C.M., Chi, J.T.A., West, M.: Cross-study projections of genomic biomarkers: an evaluation in cancer genomics. PLoS One **4**, e4523 (2009)
26. Lucas, J.E., Carvalho, C.M., West, M.: A Bayesian analysis strategy for cross-study translation of gene expression biomarkers. Stat. Appl. Genet. Mol. Biol. **8**(1) Article 11, 1–26 (2009)
27. Lucas, J.E., Carvalho, C.M., Merl, D., West, M.: In-vitro to in-vivo factor profiling in expression genomics. In: Dey, D., Ghosh, S., Mallick, B. (eds.) Bayesian Modelling in Bioinformatics, pp. 293–316. Taylor-Francis, New York (2010)
28. McLachlan, G., Peel, D., Bean, R.: Modelling high-dimensional data by mixtures of factor analyzers. Comput. Stat. Data Anal. **41**, 379–388 (2003)
29. Nakajima, J., West, M.: Bayesian analysis of latent threshold dynamic models. J. Bus. Econ. Stat. **31**, 151–164 (2013). doi:10.1080/07350015.2012.747847
30. Rodriguez, A., Lenkoski, A., Dobra, A.: Sparse covariance estimation in heterogeneous samples. Electron. J. Stat. **5**, 981–1014 (2011)
31. Seo, D.M., Wang, T., Dressman, H.K., Herderick, E.E., Iversen, E.S., Dong, C., Vata, K., Milano, C.A., Rigat, F., Pittman, J., Nevins, J.R., West, M., Goldschmidt-Clermont, P.J.: Gene expression phenotypes of atherosclerosis. Arterioscler. Thromb. Vasc. Biol. **24**, 1922–1927 (2004)
32. Seo, D.M., Goldschmidt-Clermont, P.J., West, M.: Of mice and men: sparse statistical modelling in cardiovascular genomics. Ann. Appl. Stat. **1**, 152–178 (2007)
33. Sørlie, T.: Molecular portraits of breast cancer: tumour subtypes as distinct disease entities. Eur. J. Cancer **40**, 2667–2675 (2004)
34. Suchard, M.A., Holmes, C., West, M.: Some of the *What?*, *Why?*, *How?*, *Who?* and *Where?* of graphics processing unit computing for Bayesian analysis. Bull. Int. Soc. Bayesian Anal. **17**, 12–16 (2010)

35. Suchard, M.A., Wang, Q., Chan, C., Frelinger, J., Cron, A., West, M.: Understanding GPU programming for statistical computation: studies in massively parallel massive mixtures. J. Comput. Graph. Stat. **19**, 419–438 (2010)
36. West, M.: Bayesian factor regression models in the "large p, small n" paradigm. In: Bernardo, J.M., Bayarri, M.J., Berger, J.O., David, A.P., Heckerman, D., Smith, A.F.M., West, M. (eds.) Bayesian Statistics 7, pp. 723–732. Oxford University Press, Oxford (2003)
37. West, M., Blanchette, C., Dressman, H.K., Huang, E.S., Ishida, S., Spang, R., Zuzan, H., Marks, J.R., Nevins, J.R.: Predicting the clinical status of human breast cancer utilizing gene expression profiles. Proc. Natl. Acad. Sci. **98**, 11462–11467 (2001)
38. Yang, R., Berger, J.O.: Estimation of a covariance matrix using the reference prior. Ann. Stat. **22**, 1195–1211 (1994)
39. Yoshida, R., West, M.: Bayesian learning in sparse graphical factor models via annealed entropy. J. Mach. Learn. Res. **11**, 1771–1798 (2010)

Combining Single and Paired End RNA-seq Data for Differential Expression Analyses

Zhi-Ping Feng, Francois Collin, and Terence P. Speed

Abstract Combining RNA-seq data from different platforms should increase the power to detect differentially expressed genes, but may not be straightforward. Here we show how RUVs, a recently published method for removing unwanted variation and normalizing RNA-seq data, can combine the counts of single and paired end read libraries from formalin fixed, paraffin embedded tumor samples to permit differential expression analysis. Seven other intra- or inter-platform normalization methods are also described and the results are compared with those from RUVs.

1 Introduction

RNA-seq is a useful tool for detecting changes in gene expression in biological samples. These include the identification of disease biomarkers that may be important in the detection of different types or subtypes of diseases, with implications for diagnosis, prognosis and therapy [1]. The sample preparation process for RNA-seq can change from platform to platform due to the rapid evolution of high throughput sequencing [2]. Combining sequence data from technical replicates (the same sample sequenced more than once using separate libraries) should increase the power to detect differentially expressed genes (DEGs) [3, 4] and reduce coverage bias if the biases in the component technologies are complementary and of similar magnitude [5–8]. However, combining the data from different platforms, in particular single end (SE) and paired end (PE) read libraries, is not straightforward as sample preparation methods and read alignment significantly influence sequencing results. As a consequence, the analyses are typically performed in such way that the

Z.-P. Feng • T.P. Speed (✉)
The Walter and Eliza Hall Institute of Medical Research, 1G Royal Parade, Parkville, VIC 3052, Australia
e-mail: feng@wehi.edu.au; terry@wehi.edu.au

F. Collin
Genomic Health, Inc, 101 Galveston Drive, Redwood City, CA 94063-4700, USA
e-mail: francois.collin@singularbio.com

A. Frigessi et al. (eds.), *Statistical Analysis for High-Dimensional Data*, Abel Symposia 11, DOI 10.1007/978-3-319-27099-9_8

counts from the SE and PE read libraries are analyzed separately, and then (1) the DEGs from the two platforms are combined by intersecting the two sets (taking into account the direction of change); or (2) a formal meta analysis combining the results is carried out.

In this chapter we describe and compare methods for combining the counts of technical replicate SE and PE read libraries from formalin fixed, paraffin embedded (FFPE) tumor samples for differential expression analysis. FFPE is the standard processing technique for tumor tissue used in modern pathology. Such tumor samples are available in large quantities, making them ideal material for retrospective studies. Unfortunately, the fixation process and the storage conditions of FFPE samples frequently leads to significant RNA degradation and variable sample quality, making it difficult to carry out reliable and reproducible gene expression profiling studies [9, 10].

2 Data

RNA was extracted from tumor tissue samples taken at the time of resection from a cohort of 136 breast cancer patients [11]. The samples had a mean storage time of 6.2 years prior to RNA extraction. They were associated with long-term phenotypic data that might yield insight in gene expression changes that occur during various disease states. Among the 136 patients, 26 experienced breast cancer recurrence or death due to breast cancer or unknown causes, and the 110 still alive without breast cancer recurrence or who died due to other known causes, were considered censored at the time of last follow-up or death [11].

Samples from the 136 study tumors were prepared using kit ScriptSeq V1 and were sequenced by SE sequencing. For 131 of these, there was enough material left over for the PE sequencing and in these cases the same sample was sequenced by PE sequencing. For the other five cases in which the samples were depleted following the SE sequencing run, another sample was prepared for the PE sequencing using kit ScriptSeq V2. All of the SE sequencing was done to 50 bp while the PE sequencing was done to 100 bp with an Illumina HiSeq 2000 sequencing machine [11]. These tumor RNA samples were originally screened by qRT-PCR in the biomarker discovery phase of the development of the 21 gene breast cancer recurrence risk assay [12–15]. Through these studies, 16 genes have been characterized as breast cancer-related genes and are used to compute the Onco*type* DX®Recurrence Score®result (Ki67, STK15, Survivin, CCNB1 or cyclin B1, MYBL2, GRB7, HER2, ER, PGR, BCL2, SCUBE2, MMP11 or stromelysin 3, CTSL2 or cathepsin L2, GSTM1, CD68, and BAG1) [12–15]. We refer to this set of genes as the Onco*type* DX genes. In an analysis of a large data set of microarray gene expression data, 83 cell proliferation genes have been identified as forming a highly co-expressed genes module (unpublished in-house study). This proliferation gene module does not include the five genes making up the proliferation gene group component of the 21-gene breast cancer recurrence risk assay (Ki67, STK15, Survivin, CCNB1 or cyclin B1, MYBL2).

RNA-seq analysis of these tumors provides us with the opportunity to determine whether the biomarker RNAs originally discovered by qRT-PCR can be rediscovered by RNA-seq, and to identify potential new RNA risk markers. Also, the previously identified Onco*type* DX genes and cell proliferation genes can be used to evaluate RNA-seq analysis methods, as they are potential positive controls, or examples of genes having expression patterns that are associated with recurrence.

3 Methods

We focused our analysis on the gene-level read counts for the genes assayed by both platforms. This common set comprises 19,732 Refseq genes, before the weakly expressed genes were removed. We removed 4353 genes that failed to have more than 0.5 count per million (cpm) in at least 50 % of the samples, leaving 15,379 genes (71.7 %) left for the differential expression analyses. The analyses were mainly based on the linear model (LM) of the voom-limma package [16] normalized with either the TMM [17] or RUVSeq [18] method.

Limma is an R/Bioconductor package that provides an integrated solution for analysing data from gene expression experiments, particularly for microarray and RNA-seq data. In limma, the data are fitted to a linear model and differential expression analysis is carried out using moderated t-statistics with empirical Bayes' shrinkage of the sample variances [19, 20]. Recently, limma has been expanded to include voom-limma for analysing RNA-seq data [16, 21]. Voom-limma estimates the mean-variance relationship robustly and generates a precision weight for each normalized observation. The counts and associated precision weights are then entered into the limma analysis pipeline. In voom-limma the read library sizes can be used as normalization factors. These sample-specific normalization factors are used to rescale the observed counts. In addition, empirical Bayes' shrinkage was used, as that protects against hypervariable genes and improves the power to detect DEGs [22].

RUVSeq is an R/Bioconductor package that uses factor analysis to remove unwanted variation from RNA-seq data [18]. In particular, we used RUVg or RUVs to estimate unwanted variation, and then included the estimate into the design matrix used by voom-limma. Genes not affected by the biological covariates of interest but affected by the unwanted variation in the same way as the rest of the genes were defined as negative control genes in RUVSeq [18].

The detailed methods are listed below:

3.1 SE-voom

Here only the counts from SE read libraries were considered, and the voom-limma package [16] was used to test for differential gene expression between the recurrent and non-recurrent samples, normalized using the TMM method [17].

3.2 SE-RUVg

The data from the SE read libraries were normalized with the RUVSeq package, in the context of differential expression analysis carried out with voom-limma. The control genes used in this method were the 290 of 537 human house keeping (HK) genes [23] having FDR > 0.5 in a preliminary SE-voom analysis.

3.3 PE-voom

Here the same analysis as in the SE-voom was carried out on the PE read libraries.

3.4 PE-RUVg

Here we proceeded as in SE-RUVg but with the PE data, and control with a set of 301 HK genes coming from the 537 HK genes having FDR > 0.5 in the preliminary PE-voom analysis.

3.5 RBE-voom

Using the data from the SE and PE libraries combined, the removeBatchEffect function in limma was used before the same analysis as in the SE-voom was carried out.

3.6 META-voom

In the META-voom analyses, we combined the results from SE-voom and PE-voom. The estimated log fold change (logFC) and the *p*-values derived from the SE-voom and the PE-voom analyses were combined as follows:

$$logFC^c = W^s logFC^s + W^p logFC^p \tag{1}$$

where $W^s > 0, W^p > 0$ and $W^s + W^p = 1$ are the weights inversely proportional to the estimated variances (SE^2) of the separate SE (s) and PE (p) estimates of logFC. The combined p-value is calculated based on Fisher's combined chi square: χ^2_4 for $-2ln(p^s) - 2ln(p^p)$, and FDR is the combined p-value adjusted by the Benjamini and Hochberg method [24].

3.7 RUVs-voom

Here the combined SE and PE data were used, together with the RUVs function from the RUVSeq package, and differential expression analysis was carried out using voom-limma. This RUV option makes use of the fact that every sample has a "duplicate" pair of sequencing libraries, one SE and one PE. RUVs makes use of the differences of the gene-level counts (log scale) to estimate unwanted variation, these being in effect 'negative control samples', as they contain no effects of interest [18]. A set of 249 negative control genes were also used, chosen as an intersection of the 290 control genes used in SE-RUVg and 301 control genes used in PE-RUVg. After estimating the unwanted variation using RUVs, this was included in the design matrix with voom-limma to find DEGs.

3.8 RUVs-edgeR

This option is analogous to the preceding one, but using the edgeR package [25, 26] instead of voom-limma at the step of differential expression analysis.

4 Results

The PE and SE reads were uniquely mapped to a set of 19,732 genes. Among these were 537 HK genes and 83 cell proliferation genes [11, 12]. The SE read library sizes ranged from 3.1M to 11.2M with a median of 5.8M counts, and for the PE from 8.5M to 31.5M, with a median of 26.5M counts. After removing weakly expressed genes, 15,379 genes (71.7 %) remained for DEG analysis.

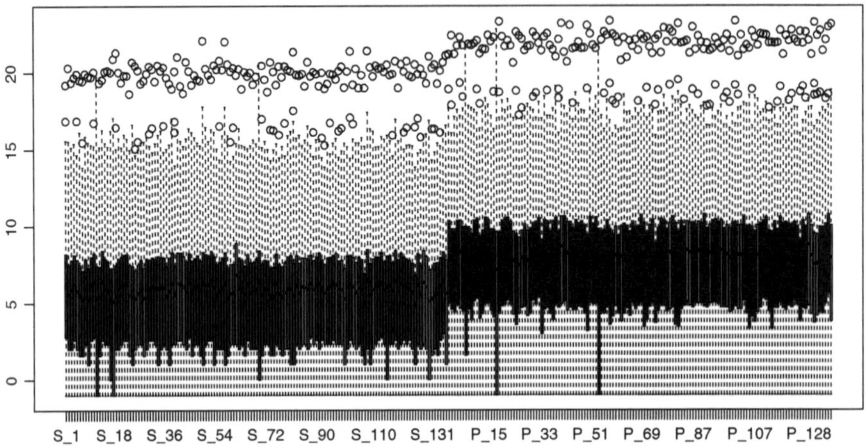

Fig. 1 Boxplot of the logged counts with offset 0.5 of the data from the SE and PE read libraries before normalization. The boxes in *blue* and *red* are the data from the SE libraries, representing the non-recurrent and recurrent samples, respectively. The boxes in *black* and *purple* are the data from the PE libraries, representing the non-recurrent and recurrent samples, respectively. This color scheme is kept the same in later plots. The batch effects can be seen clearly, as overall counts from the SE read libraries are lower than those from the PE libraries

4.1 Combined Data and Visualization

Before normalization the batch effects can be seen clearly from Fig. 1 (boxplot), and Fig. 6a (RLE plots) in Appendix 1. Overall the medians in both sets of plots are lower for SE than for PE read libraries. After normalization (Fig. 6b–g), the boxes in the RLE plots looked uniform, except for a few samples, especially from the PE read libraries prepared with Kit ScriptSeq V2.

After normalization with scaling methods such as the TMM [17] from limma or edgeR, or betweenLaneNormalization from EDAseq [27], the boxes in boxplots or RLE plots looked uniform (Fig. 6), but two batches can still be seen in the second principal component (Fig. 7). These need to be removed before or within the differential expression analysis. We used the removingBatchEffect (RBE) function in limma and RUVs in the RUVSeq package to normalize the data, and displayed plots of the first two principal components of the PCA after normalization in Figs. 2 and 7d–f. The RLE plots shown in Fig. 6d–g look uniform and very similar to Fig. 6b, c, but no obvious batch effects can be seen in Fig. 7d–f.

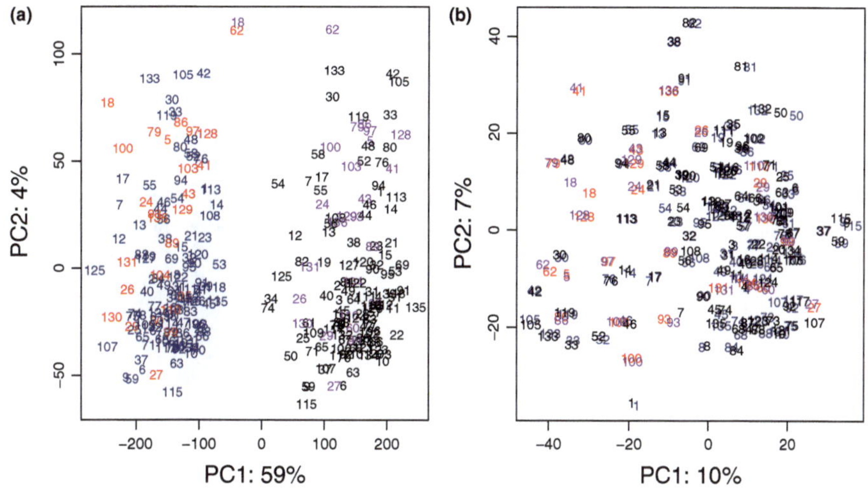

Fig. 2 The first two principal components (**a**) before normalization, (**b**) after normalization with RUVs with K=2. The color scheme is the same as Fig. 1, and the points are labeled with sample numbers. The points in Fig. 2b labeled with the same numbers but different colors are mostly overlapped, suggesting that the batch effects are largely removed by RUVs normalization

Table 1 Summary of the number of differentially expressed genes[a]

Method	p<0.05 (%)	FDR<0.05 (%)	FDR<0.05 Dx genes	FDR<0.05 proliferation
SE-voom	2602 (17)	231 (2)	3	17
SE-RUVg	3056 (20)	622 (4)	7	41
PE-voom	2563 (17)	120 (1)	2	6
PE-RUVg	3187 (21)	732 (5)	8	31
RBE-voom	4825 (31)	2661 (17)	11	71
META-voom	3601 (23)	1591 (10)	9	67
RUVs-voom	5254 (34)	3125 (20)	13	72
RUVs-edgeR	5200 (34)	3203 (21)	12	68

[a]The dashed line separates the results of intra-platform analyses from inter-platform analyses

4.2 *Differential Expression Analyses*

4.2.1 Results of Differential Expression Analyses with Different Methods

The main results concerning DEGs, Onco*type* Dx genes and cell proliferation genes detected by using eight different methods are summarized in Table 1. A histogram of p-values and a volcano plot from RUVs-voom (K=2) analysis are shown in Fig. 3. Further details are shown in Appendix 2.

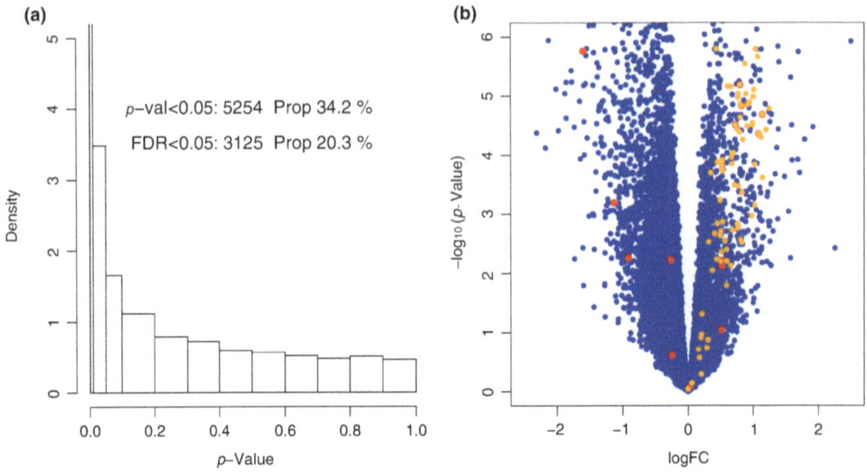

Fig. 3 Histogram of p-values (**a**) and volcano plot following tests of differential expression between recurrent and non-recurrent samples (**b**). The data were the combined SE and PE read libraries, and RUVs normalization with K=2 was used, together with voom-limma. The numbers of DEGs with either p-value < 0.05 or FDR < 0.05, are given, and the histogram breakpoints in (**a**) are at 0.001, 0.01, 0.05, 0.1, 0.2, 0.3, ..., 1.0. Onco*type* Dx genes are highlighted in *red* and cell proliferation genes in *orange* in (**b**)

In Appendix 2, Fig. 8a–i showed the plots of the mean-variance trends estimated by voom-limma, histograms of p-values and volcano plots for tests of differential expression between recurrent and non-recurrent samples for the data from the SE read libraries after three options of normalization ("none", "TMM" and "upperquartile") methods. Figure 9a–f showed histograms of p-values and volcano plots for the data from SE read libraries after normalization by RUVg and K=2, 3 and 4; Fig. 10a–i showed the plots analogous to Fig. 8, and Fig. 11a–f showed the plots analogous to Fig. 9, both sets for the data from the PE read libraries. Figure 12a–i show the plots similar to Fig. 8, but for combined SE and PE read libraries, using the removeBatchEffect function in limma. Figure 13a, b showed the results of the META-voom analysis. Figure 14a–i show the plots similar to Fig. 12, but for normalization with RUVs using K=1, 2, and 3. Figure 15a–i show the plots similar to Fig. 12 but differential expression analysis using edgeR. Finally, in Appendix 3 we display the toptable for the Onco*type* Dx genes after analyses by the different methods.

Other findings are the following. Many HK genes are identified as DEGs by using SE-voom or PE-voom. The negative control genes we used in SE-RUVg and PE-RUVg are therefore the subset of HK genes least likely to be DEGs detected by

SE-voom or PE-voom. Fewer DEGs can be identified by PE-voom than by SE-voom under FDR<0.05, but more can be detected by PE-RUVg than by SE-RUVg. More DEGs are identified by pooling data across the two platforms. The histograms of Figs. 8, 9, 10, 11, 12, 13, 14, and 15 shows that they are not uniformly distributed, which suggests that the assessments of significance may not be reliable. However, we will proceed as though they are, with caution.

From rows 1 and 2 of Table 1 we can see that after RUVg normalization, we find about 2 % more DEGs from the SE libraries, and from rows 3 and 4, that 4 % more from PE libraries than can be found using the TMM method. Similar results are obtained for Onco*type* Dx genes and cell proliferation genes.

We can also see from rows 5, 6, 7 and 8 of Table 1 that for the methods combining data or results, the numbers of DEGs are significantly increased at a p-value < 0.05 or FDR < 0.05, which indicates an increased power of detection of DEGs. RUVs-voom detected 3 % more DEGs than RBE-voom. All of these assertions rely on the p-values being valid. In row 6 of Table 1, the META-voom analysis appears to detect many fewer DEGs at a p-value of less than 0.05 or FDR less than 0.05 than the other methods.

4.2.2 Comparisons of the Differential Expression Analyses

Comparison of logFC and -log_{10}(p-$value$) derived by using the four different methods listed on rows 5–8 of Table 1 are shown in Fig. 4 and Figs. 16, 17, and 18.

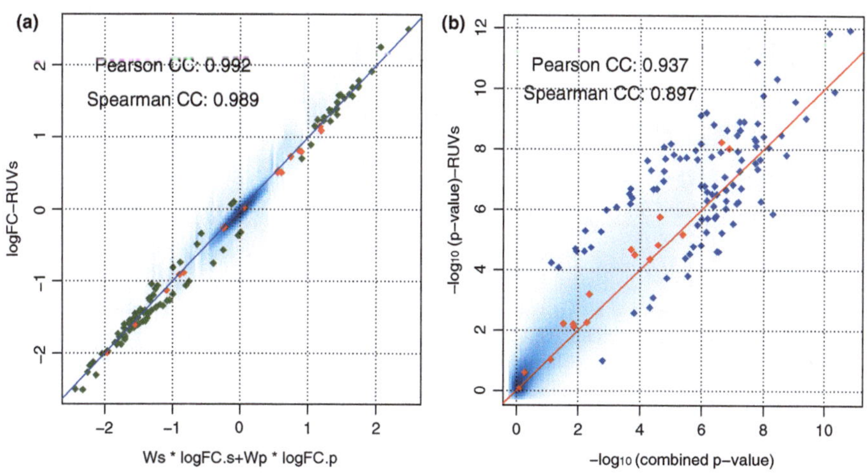

Fig. 4 Smoothed scatter plots comparing estimated logFC values (**a**) and $-log_{10}(p\text{-}value)$ (**b**) derived from RUVs-voom vs META-voom analysis. The correlation coefficients are given and the Onco*type* Dx genes are highlighted in *red*

The correlation coefficients are given in the figures, and they are very high when the same analysis pipeline was used.

Overlaps of the top 1000 DEGs (based on ranking by p-values) from RUVs-voom, RBE-voom and META-voom, RUVs-voom identifies more unique DEGs (Fig. 5a) in the top 1000 DEGs. With a p-value cutoff of 0.001 RUVs-voom identifies more down regulated unique DEGs, but fewer up regulated DEGs with same cutoff comparing the recurrent with non-recurrent samples (Fig. 5b, c). From Table 2 we can also see that the META-voom detects fewer DEGs than the other methods and RUVs-edgeR detects more DEGs than RUVs-voom. The DEGs detected with META-voom are mostly detected by RBE-voom analysis (99 %), but not vice versa (74 %).

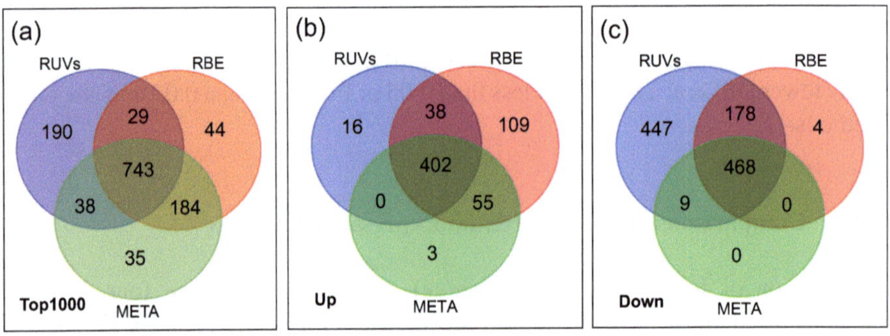

Fig. 5 Venn diagram comparing the results from each of the three indicated methods, *top* 1000 DEGs (ranked by p-values) (**a**), up (**b**) and down (**c**) regulated genes having p-value < 0.001, when comparing the recurrent and non-recurrent samples

Table 2 Agreement between DEGs found by different methods[a]

Method	RBE-voom (%)	RUVs-voom (%)	META-voom (%)	RUVs-edgeR (%)
RBE-voom	1254(100)	1086(87)	925(74)	956(76)
RUVs-voom	1086(70)	1557(100)	879(56)	1001(64)
META-voom	925(99)	879(94)	937(100)	789(84)
RUVs-edgeR	956(59)	1001(62)	789(49)	1614(100)

[a]In each cell is the number of DEGs with p-value < 0.001 by the methods with the row and column labels. The corresponding percentage of genes in each box is that found by the method of the row supported by the method of the column. For example, at a p-value <0.001, RUVs-voom identifies 1557 DEGs, 70 % of which are found by RBE-voom, 56 % by META-voom and 64 % by RUVs-edgeR

5 Discussion

5.1 *Efficiency of Normalization in the Context of Differential Expression Analyses*

About 2 % more DEGs were identified from the SE libraries after RUVg normalization (4 % more DEGs from the PE libraries) compared to those obtained using TMM normalization. SE-voom led to more DEGs than PE-voom, even though the SE libraries are smaller in size. This suggests that the data from PE libraries may be problematic. However, after RUVg normalization, PE-RUVg detects more DEGs than SE-RUVg, which suggests that RUVg normalization was effective at correcting for intra-platform batch effects. We know that the samples for PE sequencing were prepared using two different kits, and that those prepared using the ScriptSeq V2 kits were different from the rest.

The increase in effective sample size that resulted from an analysis of the combined data or a META analysis led to improved statistical power to detect DEGs when compared to an analysis of these SE or PE data alone. RUVs and RBE were both effective at removing the SE-PE differences, but RUVs seems slightly more efficient. With META analysis, fewer DEGs were identified at a given *p*-value than were using other methods. A good histogram of *p*-values for tests of differential expression should be flat with a spike at zero corresponding to the DEGs. The histograms of *p*-values for seven methods (Figs. 8, 9, 10, 11, 12, 13, 14, and 15, except for the META-voom analysis Fig. 13) all look very similar and not very far from uniformly distributed *p*-values, but all are systematically skewed towards zero. The distribution of *p*-values from the META analysis is different from the other seven, but also not ideal. As a result, we probably cannot rely on the *p*-values too much, in which case the small percentage differences (2 %, 4 %) between approaches should not be taken as definitive.

Values of logFC derived with LM version of RUVs, META analysis and RBE, are highly consistent (Figs. 4a and 16a) as are the $log_{10}(p\text{-values})$ (Figs. 4b and 16b), with more genes having a slightly smaller *p*-value in the RUVs-voom analysis than in META-voom and RBM-voom, which is consistent with the results listed in Table 1. The highly correlated logFC and *p*-values indicate a high concordance of DEGs detected by these methods (Table 2), with RUVs detecting slightly more unique genes in the top ranking DEGs.

The above results are also valid for the GLM versions of RUVs, RBE and META analysis (results not shown).

5.2 *Differential Expression Analysis Pipelines (LM Versus GLM) and the Influence of the Weakly Expressed Genes*

There are larger differences between the results of using different ways of finding DEGs than there are from different normalization methods using the same DE analysis pipeline. The correlation coefficient between the logFC derived with RUVs-voom and RUVs-edgeR is around 0.8 (Pearson 0.78, Spearman 0.86), and this drops when more weakly expressed genes are involved in the analysis (Figs. 17a and 18a). The correlation coefficient between the *p*-values derived from RUVs-voom and RUVs-edgeR is only about 0.7 (Pearson 0.66, Spearman 0.75). This concordance will improve after removing weakly expressed genes. Comparing results of the LM version of RUVs (or RUVg) with their GLM versions, we find that in both cases, the LM version is more robust against violations of the negative control gene assumption, and the influence of weakly expressed genes.

Although the LM-version of RUVs (or RUVg) usually detects fewer DEGs at a given *p*-value or FDR, this does not seem to be because it is less effective at removing the unwanted variation, but rather because the GLM based edgeR usually detects many more DEGs, especially when weakly expressed genes are involved in the analysis. However, many DEGs detected by edgeR with large logFC or small *p*-values (Figs. 17, 18 and 19) are not supported by a voom-limma analysis, especially among the weakly expressed genes (Fig. 19).

5.3 Negative Control Genes and Factors Contributing to Unwanted Variation for RUVg and RUVs

We can see from the volcano plots from the SE-voom, PE-voom and META analysis that many housekeeping (HK) genes are DEGs, which is not unexpected, given that the RNAs are extracted from cancer samples. Directly using all HK genes as negative control genes will violate the assumption of RUVg or RUVs that the negative control genes are not differentially expressed, and leads to different numbers of DEGs. But the changes are roughly of the same magnitude, and not dramatic, compared with the results obtained using empirically derived negative control genes [28, 29] (results not shown). Furthermore, RUVs seems more robust to the violation of the negative control gene assumption than RUVg.

The number of factors K of unwanted variation in RUVg and RUVs also influences the final results (see the number of DEGs labelled in the histograms from Figs. 9, 11, 14, and 15), although the differences are too subtle to be seen in the histograms. Less variation is removed with small K, while biologically interesting variation might be removed when K is too large. Here we used K=2 for RUVs, K=3 for SE-RUVg, and K=4 for PE-RUVg, which may be an indication that the overall data from the PE libraries has more unwanted variation than the data from the SE libraries. These results are consistent with the fact that two different kits were used for sample preparation for the PE sequencing. We understood that some samples had very low concentration in preparing PE sequencing libraries, such as sample 18 (almost used up) and sample 54. Large variations in the RLE plots from these libraries (Fig. 6) are likely due to the low sample input or over amplification. This within platform variation does not seem not to be corrected with the RBE-voom, which is a possible reason why RUVs-voom identifies a few more DEGs than RBE-voom.

With RUVs (or RUVg) normalization is done in the context of differential expression analysis rather on the expression levels. That is, RUVs and RUVg do not work from normalized data, but simply include a term for the unwanted variation in the linear or generalized linear model. Nevertheless, we have presented RLE and PCA plots of data described as normalized by these methods. These normalizations are obtained by subtracting the estimate of $W\alpha$ [18] in the LM or GLM. With RUVs, this is estimated without reference to the recurrence status of the sample, but this is not the case with RUVg. As a result, with RUVs this is a proper, "unsupervised" normalization, but with RUVg there is the possibility that the normalization enhances the difference between the recurrent and non-recurrent samples.

6 Conclusions

Combining the sequencing data from SE and PE libraries and removing their differences using RUVs or RBE, or combining the separate SE and PE results in a META analysis, increases the power to detect DEGs. RUVs is an effective method of removing the platform differences and identifying DEGs. RBE also removes the platform differences, but does not remove within platform batch effects. The differential expression analysis can make a big difference to the number of DEGs identified, but the results are more consistent after removal of weakly expressed genes.

Acknowledgements We thank Dr. Johann Gagnon-Bartsch and Dr. Davide Risso for providing the latest version of the RUV packages and Prof. Gorden Smyth for the explanation of variances estimation in edgeR and voom-limma.

Appendix 1: Visualizing the Data

Here we provide RLE and PCA plots before and after the normalizations. Relative Log Expression (RLE) plots (to mean) of the counts with offset 0.5 for the combined data from SE and PE libraries are shown in Fig. 6. Before normalization the batch effects can be seen clearly (the scale from −2.5 to 2.5, different from the rest of the plots). After normalization, the boxes looked uniform, except for few samples from the PE libraries, such as sample 18, 54 and 62. The batch effects cannot be fully removed with scaling normalization methods: TMM or betweenLaneNormalization, but can be removed with RBE and RUVs.

RLE Plot Before and After Normalization

See Fig. 6.

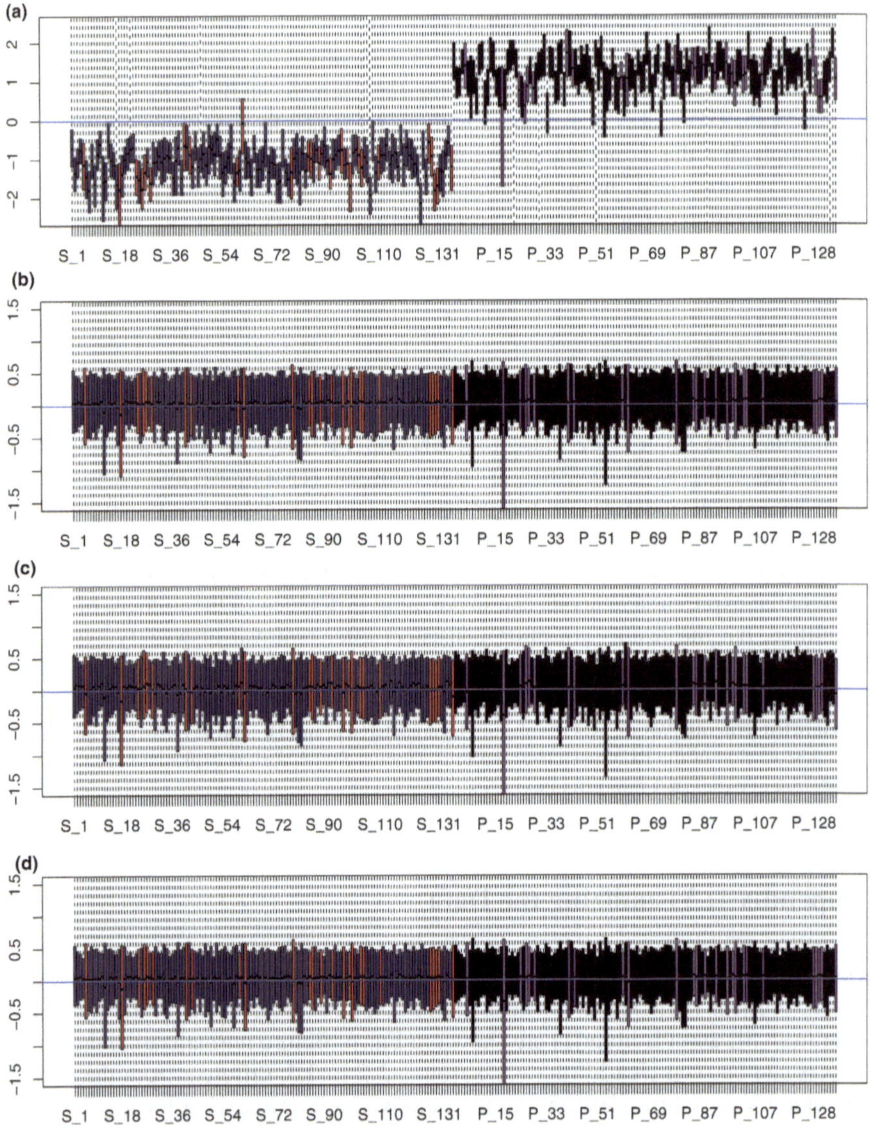

Fig. 6 (continued)

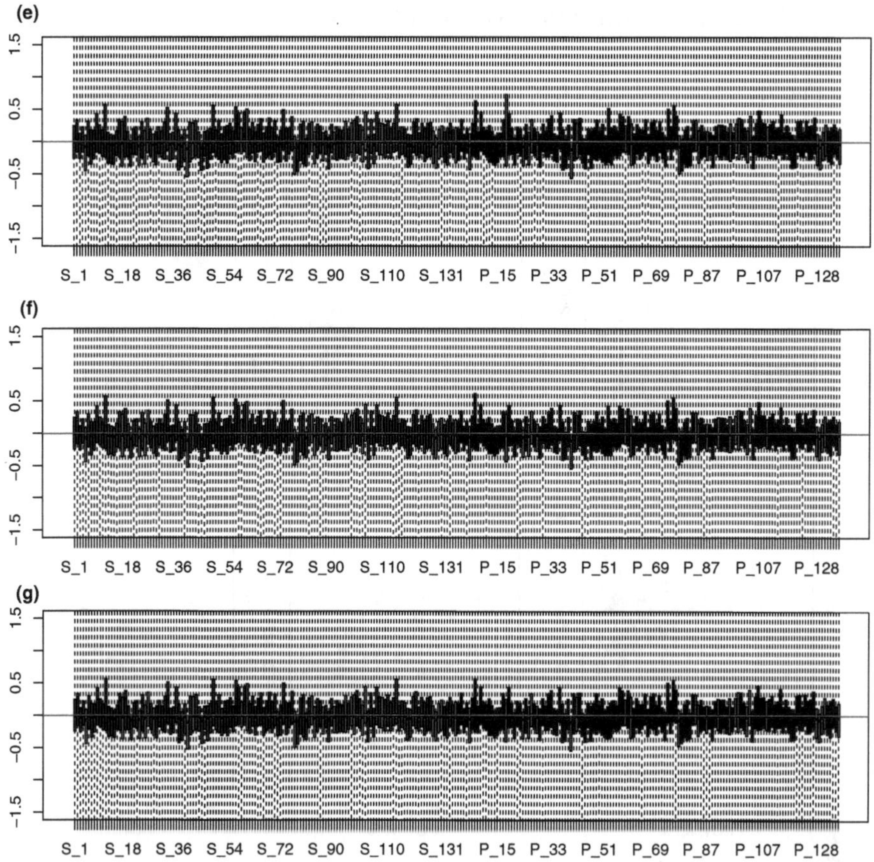

Fig. 6 RLE plots for the combined data from SE and PE read libraries (**a**) before normalization, (**b**) after TMM normalization (**c**) after betweenLane normalization (**d**) after RBE and TMM normalization and (**e**)–(**g**) after RUVs normalization (K=1, 2, and 3). The boxes in *blue* and *red* are the data from SE libraries for the non-recurrent and recurrent samples, respectively. The boxes in *black* and *purple* are the data from PE libraries for the non-recurrent and recurrent samples, respectively. The color scheme is kept the same in all the plots hereafter

PCA Plot Before and After Normalization

See Fig. 7.

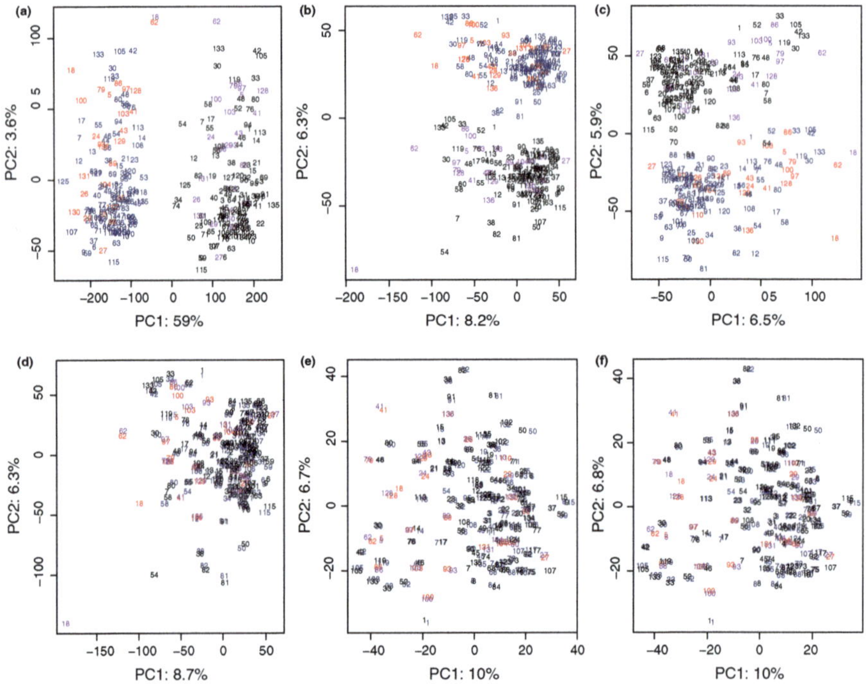

Fig. 7 The first two principal components (**a**) before normalization, (**b**) after TMM normalization, (**c**) after betweenLane normalization, (**d**) after RBE and TMM normalization, (**e**)–(**f**) after normalization with RUVs under K=1, and 2. The color scheme is the same as Fig.6, and the samples are numbered

Appendix 2: Differential Expression Analyses

Results of Differential Expression Analysis by Using Different Methods

Results of differential expression analysis are shown in Figs. 8, 9, 10, 11, 12, 13, 14, and 15.

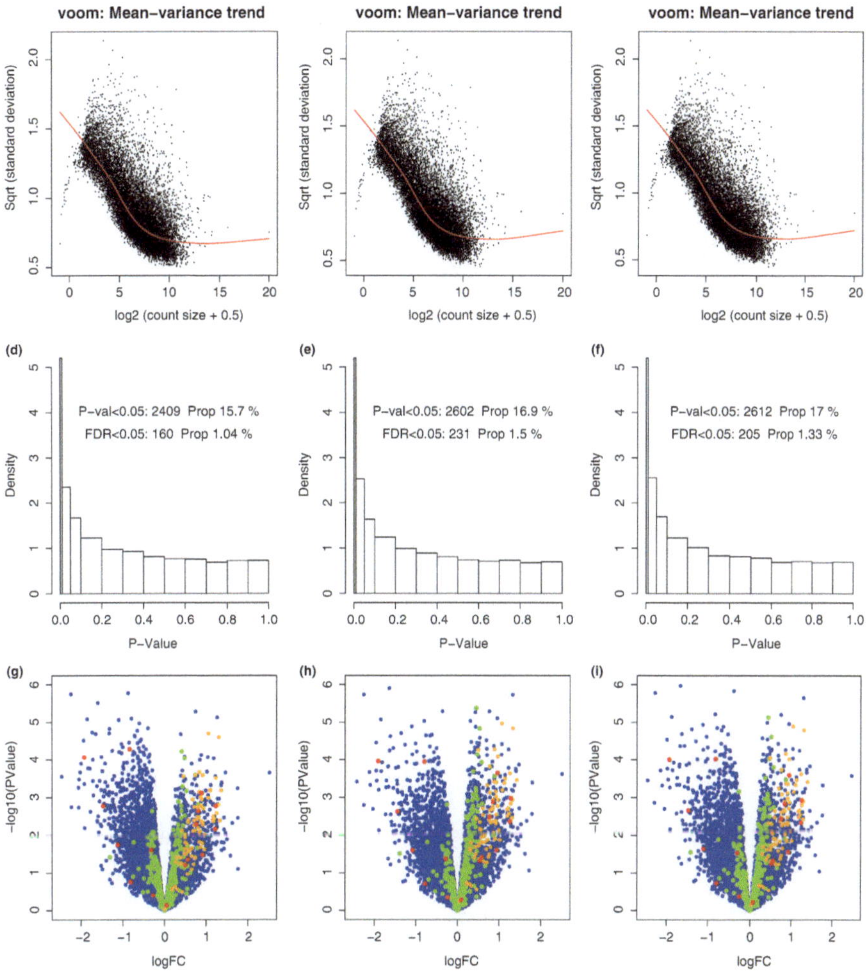

Fig. 8 Differential expression analysis with SE-voom. (**a**)–(**c**), the plots of the mean-variance trends estimated with limma-voom normalized with one of the options, "none", "TMM" and "upperquartile", (**d**)–(**f**) histograms of p-values (breakpoints are at 0.001, 0.01, 0.05, 0.1, 0.2, 0.3, ..., 1.0) and (**g**)–(**i**) volcano plots for tests of differential expression between samples of recurrence and non-recurrence for the data from the SE libraries after the three options of normalization. Sixteen Oncotype Dx genes are lighted in *red*, 537 house-keeping (HK) genes are in *green*, and the 83 cell proliferation genes are in *orange*. Many HK genes are DEGs based on this method. The numbers listed in (**e**) are used in Table 1

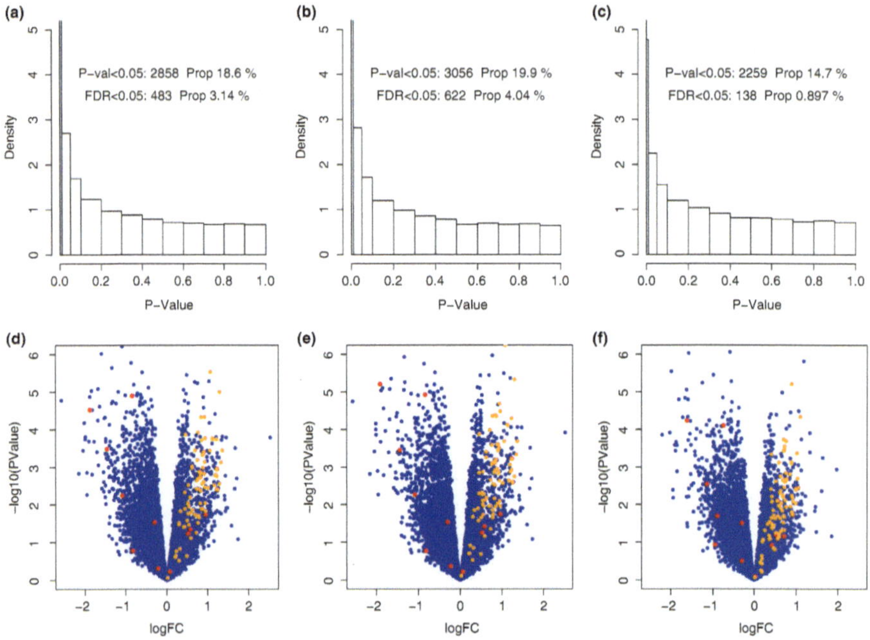

Fig. 9 Differential expression analysis with SE-RUVg and K=2, 3 and 4. Other details of (**a**)–(**f**) are the same as (d)–(i) of Fig. 8 , except for the normalization steps and negative control genes were removed during the test. More DEGs can be identified than using SE-voom under FDR<0.05. The numbers listed in (**b**) are used in Table 1

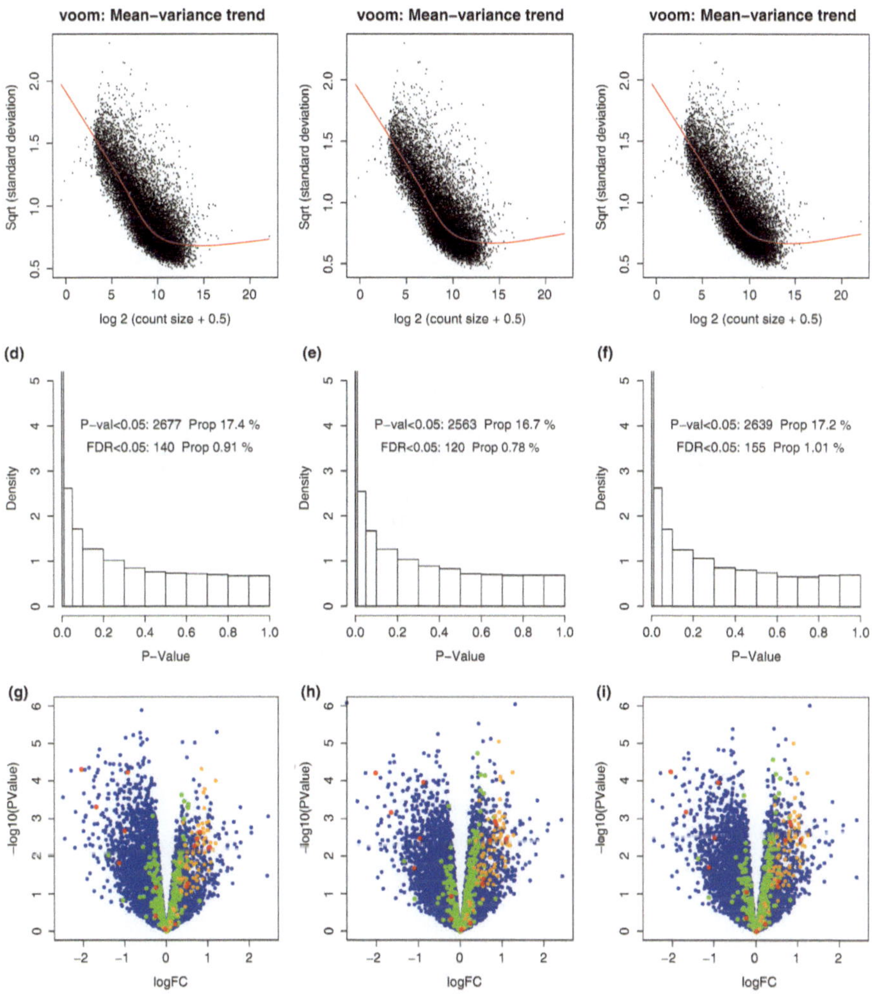

Fig. 10 Differential expression analysis with PE-voom. Other details are the same as in Fig. 8. Many HK genes are DEGs by using this method and fewer DEGs can be identified compared to SE-voom under FDR<0.05. The numbers listed in (**e**) are used in Table 1

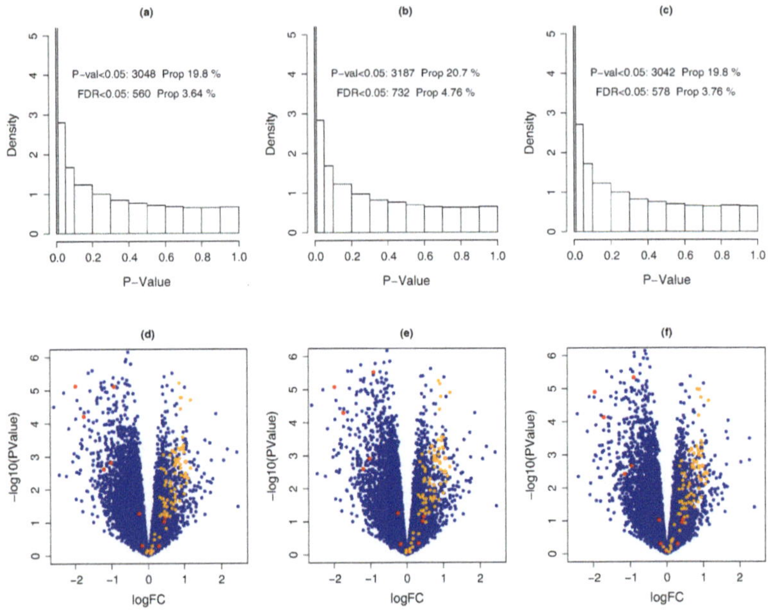

Fig. 11 Differential expression analysis with PE-RUVg and K=3, 4 and 5. Other details of (**a**)–(**f**) are the same as (d)–(i) of Fig. 9. The numbers listed in (**b**) are used in Table 1

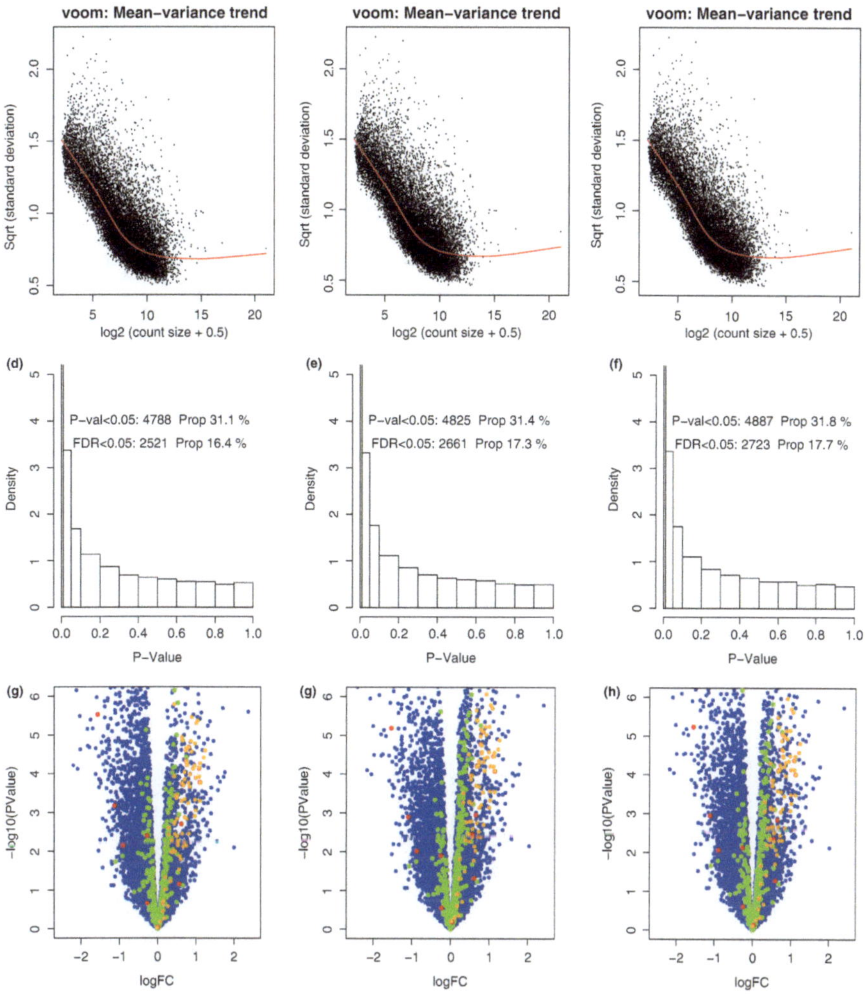

Fig. 12 Differential expression analysis with RBE-voom. Other details are the same as in Fig. 8. The numbers listed in (**e**) are used in Table 1

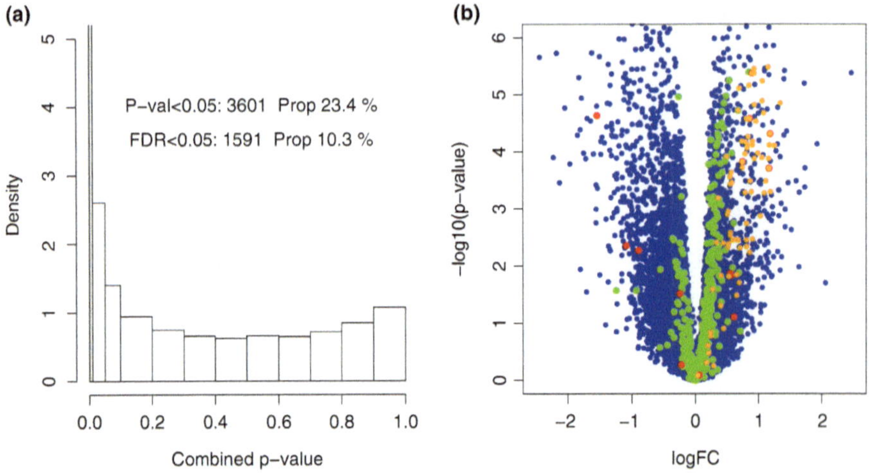

Fig. 13 Differential expression analysis with META-voom. Other details are the same as in Fig. 8e, h

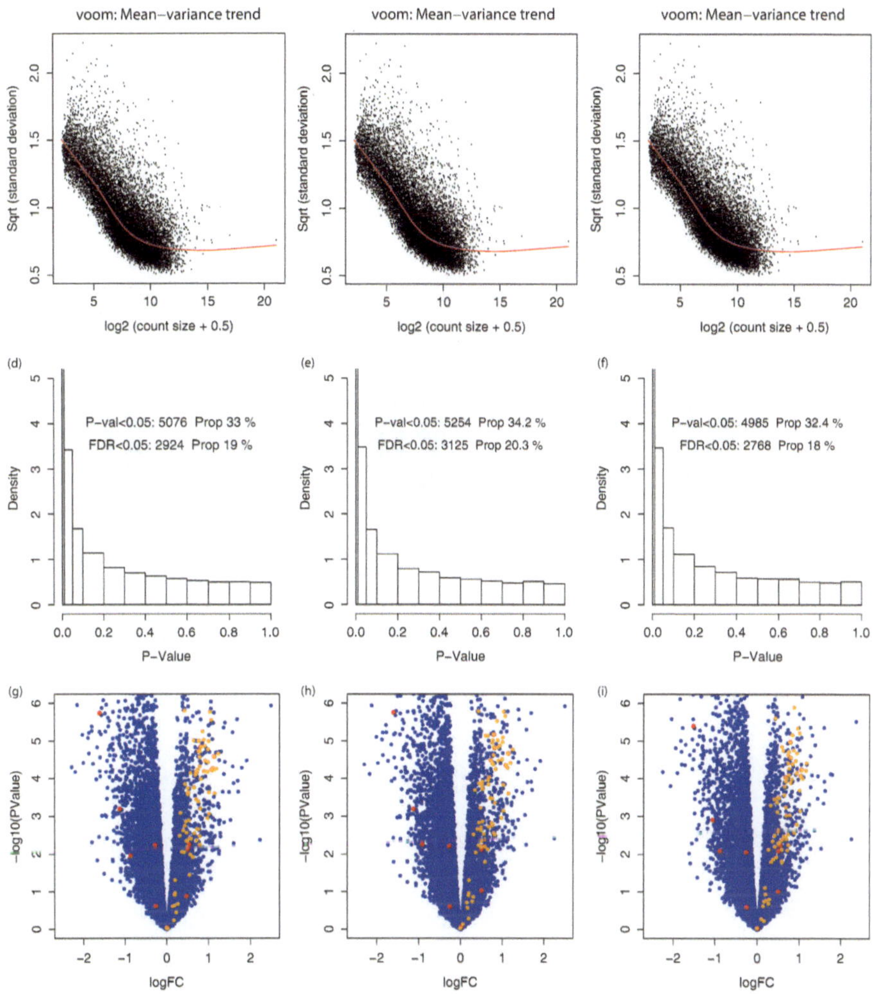

Fig. 14 Differential expression analysis with RUVs-voom and K=1, 2 and 3. Other details are the same as Fig. 8, except for the normalization steps. The numbers listed in (**e**) are used in Table 1

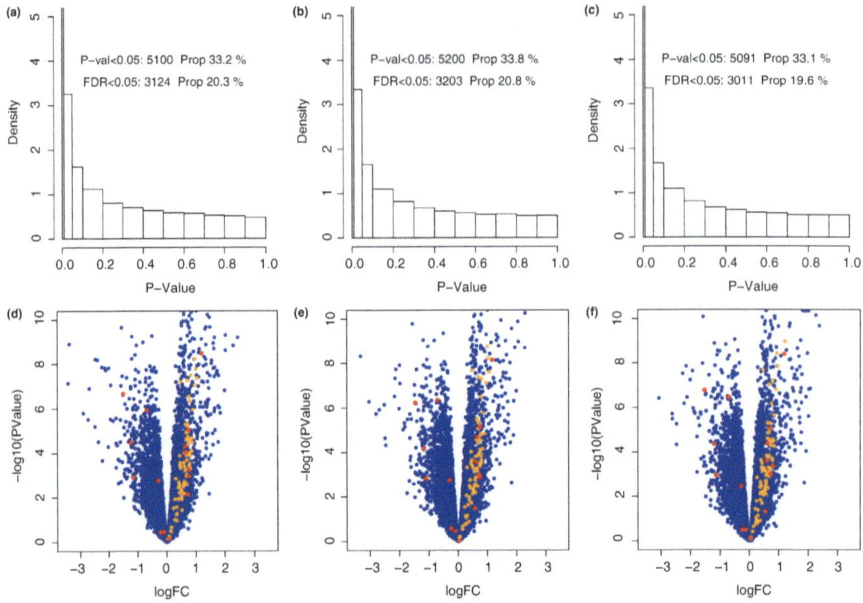

Fig. 15 Differential expression analysis with RUVs-edgeR and under K=1, 2 and 3. Other details are the same as Fig. 9. The numbers listed in (**b**) are used in Table 1

Comparison of the Results by Using Different Methods

Comparisons of the logFC or $-log_{10}$(p-value) derived by using RUVs-voom, RBE-voom and RUVs-edgeR are shown in Figs. 16, 17, 18, and 19.

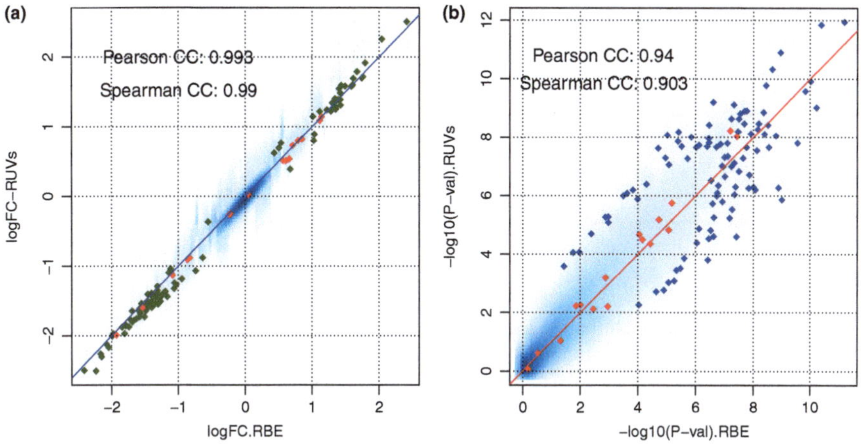

Fig. 16 Smoothed scatter plots show the correlation of logFC (**a**) or $-log_{10}$(p-value) (**b**) derived by using RUVs-voom and RBE-voom. The results of logFC or p-values determined by using these two methods are highly correlated, as indicated by the correlation coefficients listed

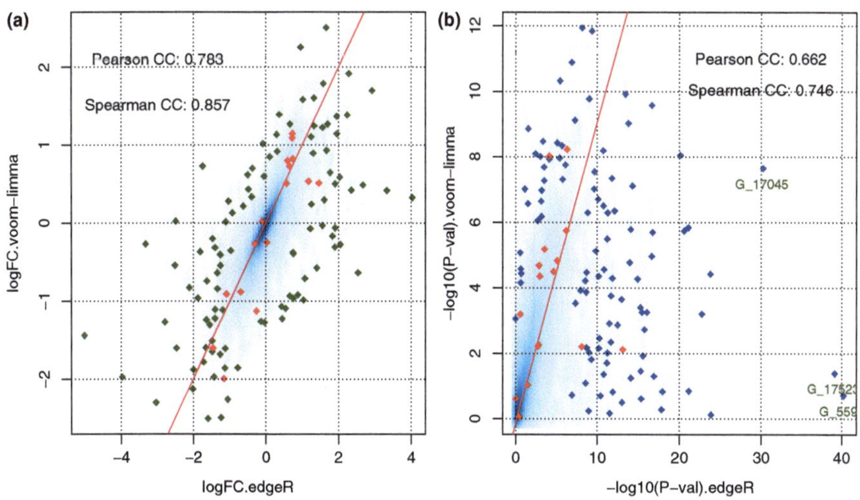

Fig. 17 Smoothed scatter plots show the correlation of logFC (**a**) or $-log_{10}$(p-value) (**b**) derived by using RUVs-voom and RUVs-edgeR after removing weakly expressed genes. The correlation of logFC or p-values determined by these two methods is lower than using the same differential expression analysis pipeline, but with different normalization methods. Some outlying genes are labelled

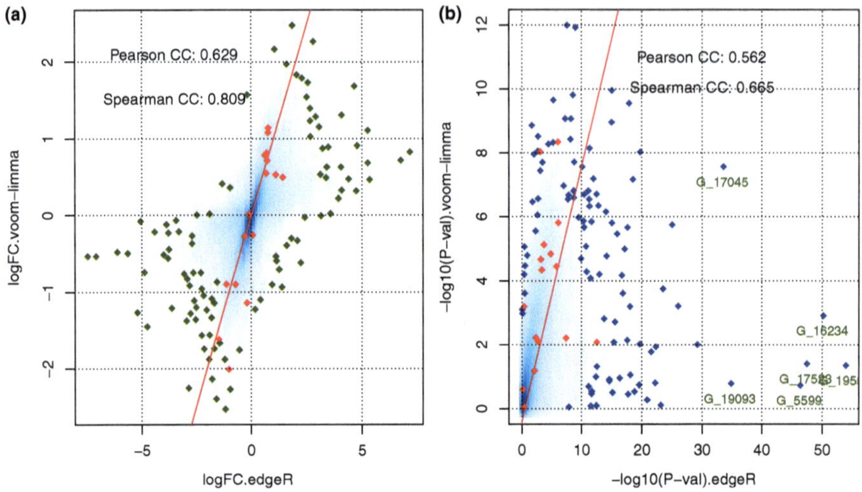

Fig. 18 Same as Fig. 17, but before the weakly expressed genes were removed. The correlations are lower than that showed in Fig. 17, which indicates that the correlation of logFC or *p*-values determined by using RUVs-voom and RUVs-edgeR can be increased by removing weakly expressed genes

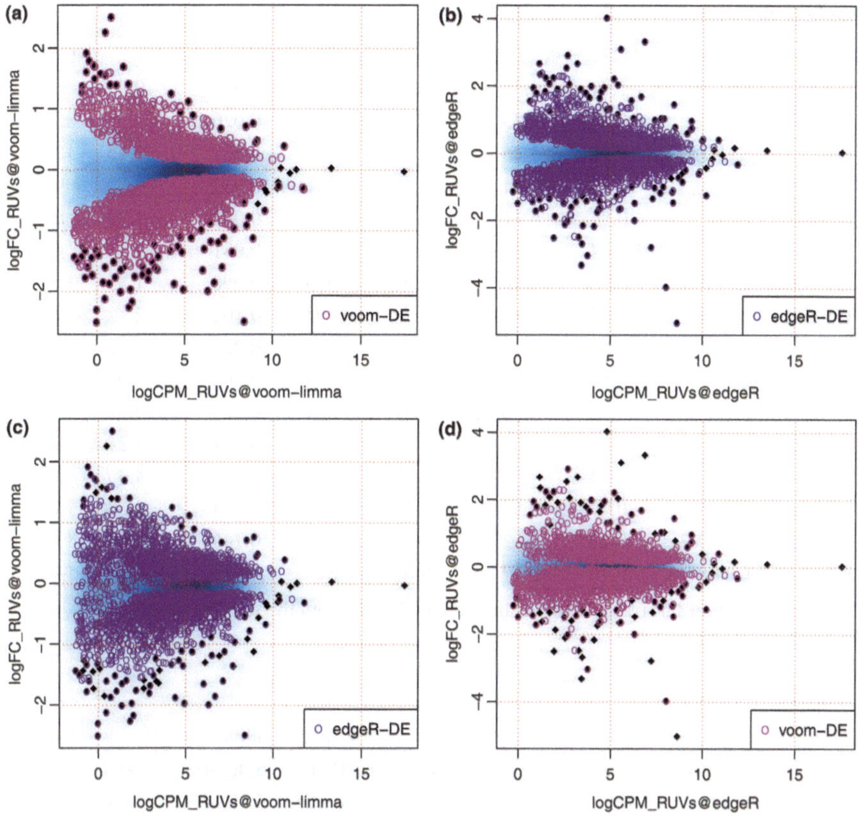

Fig. 19 Smoothed scatter plots of logFC for the differential expression between recurrent and nonrecurrent samples analyzed with RUVs (K=2) versus mean log expression of the data (MA plot), (**a**) and (**c**) with RUVs-voom, and (**b**) and (**d**) with RUVs-edgeR method. The genes having FDR<0.05 determined by using RUVs-voom are highlighted in *magenta* and RUVs-edgeR in *purple*. Some DEGs detected by edgeR with a large logFC are not confirmed by voom-limma and vice versa, especially for the weakly expressed DEGs

Appendix 3: Toptable of the Onco*type* DX Genes

Here we provide results of differential expression analyses for the Onco*type* DX genes. DEGs with FDR<0.05 are listed above the horizontal dashed line in each table (Tables 3, 4, 5, 6, 7, 8, 9, and 10).

Table 3 SE-voom

Gene	Name	logFC	AveExpr	t	*p*.value	adj.*p*.val	B	Order[a]
G18365	CEGP1	−1.91	6.31	−3.99	0.000	0.026	0.97	6
G1975	Bcl2	−0.79	7.35	−3.98	0.000	0.026	0.91	5
G14382	STK15	0.97	3.26	3.79	0.000	0.032	0.45	11
G19678	MYBL2	1.29	2.54	3.35	0.001	0.057	−0.89	9
G19220	Ki-67	0.86	6.21	3.28	0.001	0.062	−1.29	8
G2627	PR	−1.44	7.21	−3.10	0.002	0.081	−1.88	4
G1852	CCNB1	0.78	3.90	3.00	0.003	0.090	−1.89	10
G5065	SURV	1.27	1.11	2.90	0.004	0.102	−2.12	7
G1853	CTSL2	0.95	−0.60	2.27	0.025	0.225	−3.42	12
G18279	GRB7	0.59	3.87	2.09	0.038	0.266	−3.97	1
G10477	EstR1	−1.08	8.95	−2.27	0.025	0.225	−3.98	3
G6828	BAG1	−0.28	5.41	−2.05	0.042	0.274	−4.25	16
G896	HER2	0.54	7.53	2.01	0.047	0.290	−4.49	2
G23064	GSTM1	−0.77	−0.93	−1.32	0.190	0.524	−4.58	15
G12558	STMY3	−0.23	6.32	−0.75	0.454	0.746	−6.09	13
G12106	CD68	0.10	5.77	0.65	0.518	0.789	−6.11	14

[a] Order is based on survival analyses using qRT-PCR data from the same samples

Table 4 SE-RUVg

Gene	Name	logFC	AveExpr	t	*p*.value	adj.*p*.val	B	Order[a]
G18365	CEGP1	−1.91	6.31	−4.71	6.1E−06	5.0E−03	3.64	6
G1975	Bcl2	−0.84	7.35	−4.55	1.2E−05	5.1E−03	3.00	5
G14382	STK15	0.91	3.26	3.76	2.5E−04	1.8E−02	0.37	11
G2627	PR	−1.45	7.21	−3.67	3.5E−04	2.1E−02	−0.15	4
G19678	MYBL2	1.24	2.54	3.52	5.9E−04	2.7E−02	−0.39	9
G1852	CCNB1	0.81	3.90	3.45	7.5E−04	3.1E−02	−0.64	10
G19220	Ki-67	0.85	6.21	3.50	6.3E−04	2.8E−02	−0.65	8
G5065	SURV	1.25	1.11	3.08	2.5E−03	5.8E−02	−1.68	7
G10477	EstR1	−1.08	8.95	−2.83	5.4E−03	8.4E−02	−2.68	3
G1853	CTSL2	0.96	−0.60	2.40	1.8E−02	1.5E−01	−3.18	12
G6828	BAG1	−0.30	5.41	−2.21	2.9E−02	1.9E−01	−3.98	16
G18279	GRB7	0.58	3.87	2.10	3.8E−02	2.2E−01	−3.99	1
G23064	GSTM1	−0.82	−0.93	−1.38	1.7E−01	4.6E−01	−4.54	15
G896	HER2	0.52	7.53	1.93	5.6E−02	2.7E−01	−4.66	2
G12558	STMY3	−0.23	6.32	−0.79	4.3E−01	7.0E−01	−6.09	13
G12106	CD68	0.06	5.77	0.52	6.1E−01	8.2E−01	−6.22	14

Table 5 PE-voom

Gene	Name	logFC	AveExpr	t	p.value	adj.p.val	B	Order[a]
G18365	CEGP1	−2.02	6.27	−4.14	6.1E−05	3.1E−02	1.46	6
G1975	Bcl2	−0.88	7.24	−3.99	1.1E−04	3.1E−02	0.89	5
G2627	PR	−1.66	7.01	−3.48	6.8E−04	5.8E−02	−0.81	4
G14382	STK15	0.83	3.35	3.32	1.2E−03	6.9E−02	−0.98	11
G19220	Ki-67	0.85	6.21	3.26	1.4E−03	7.5E−02	−1.44	8
G19678	MYBL2	1.10	2.57	2.98	3.4E−03	9.8E−02	−1.86	9
G5065	SURV	1.09	2.94	2.95	3.7E−03	1.0E−01	−1.95	7
G23064	GSTM1	−0.97	4.01	−2.99	3.3E−03	9.6E−02	−1.98	15
G1852	CCNB1	0.71	3.81	2.95	3.8E−03	1.0E−01	−2.06	10
G10477	EstR1	−1.10	8.82	−2.34	2.1E−02	2.1E−01	−3.90	3
G18279	GRB7	0.53	4.09	1.95	5.3E−02	3.1E−01	−4.33	1
G896	HER2	0.56	7.57	2.08	4.0E−02	2.7E−01	−4.44	2
G6828	BAG1	−0.21	5.34	−1.59	1.1E−01	4.2E−01	−5.14	16
G1853	CTSL2	0.24	−0.02	0.52	6.0E−01	8.3E−01	−5.19	12
G12558	STMY3	−0.22	6.36	−0.73	4.6E−01	7.4E−01	−6.21	13
G12106	CD68	0.02	5.98	0.13	8.9E−01	9.6E−01	−6.43	14

Table 6 PE-RUVg

Gene	Name	logFC	AveExpr	t	p.value	adj.p.val	B	Order[a]
G1975	Bcl2	−0.91	7.24	−4.88	3.0E−06	2.6E−03	4.21	5
G18365	CEGP1	−1.98	6.27	−4.64	8.3E−06	3.2E−03	3.28	6
G2627	PR	−1.74	7.01	−4.19	5.0E−05	7.8E−03	1.56	4
G1852	CCNB1	0.68	3.81	3.55	5.3E−04	2.5E−02	−0.37	10
G14382	STK15	0.76	3.35	3.35	1.0E−03	3.4E−02	−0.93	11
G5065	SURV	1.06	2.94	3.31	1.2E−03	3.6E−02	−1.02	7
G23064	GSTM1	−1.02	4.01	−3.30	1.2E−03	3.7E−02	−1.16	15
G19220	Ki-67	0.80	6.21	3.27	1.4E−03	3.8E−02	−1.47	8
G19678	MYBL2	1.02	2.57	3.00	3.2E−03	5.7E−02	−1.82	9
G10477	EstR1	−1.20	8.82	−3.08	2.5E−03	5.2E−02	−2.11	3
G6828	BAG1	−0.25	5.34	−1.93	5.6E−02	2.6E−01	−4.65	16
G18279	GRB7	0.43	4.09	1.67	9.8E−02	3.4E−01	−4.90	1
G896	HER2	0.46	7.57	1.82	7.0E−02	2.9E−01	−4.99	2
G1853	CTSL2	0.31	−0.02	0.75	4.6E−01	7.1E−01	−5.16	12
G12558	STMY3	−0.18	6.36	−0.70	4.8E−01	7.3E−01	−6.31	13
G12106	CD68	0.03	5.98	0.26	7.9E−01	9.2E−01	−6.49	14

Table 7 RBE-voom

Gene	Name	logFC	AveExpr	t	*p*.value	adj.*p*.val	B	Order[a]
G18365	CEGP1	−1.93	6.29	−5.66	3.7E−08	1.6E−05	8.38	6
G1975	Bcl2	−0.83	7.30	−5.57	6.3E−08	2.3E−05	7.90	5
G2627	PR	−1.53	7.11	−4.60	6.5E−06	4.1E−04	3.59	4
G19220	Ki-67	0.84	6.21	4.56	7.9E−06	4.6E−04	3.41	8
G14382	STK15	0.79	3.31	4.38	1.7E−05	7.4E−04	2.72	11
G19678	MYBL2	1.11	2.55	4.21	3.4E−05	1.2E−03	2.05	9
G1852	CCNB1	0.71	3.86	4.07	6.1E−05	1.7E−03	1.53	10
G5065	SURV	1.14	2.02	4.00	8.3E−05	2.2E−03	1.25	7
G18279	GRB7	0.66	3.98	3.29	1.1E−03	1.3E−02	−1.11	1
G10477	EstR1	−1.09	8.89	−3.26	1.3E−03	1.4E−02	−1.22	3
G896	HER2	0.56	7.55	2.94	3.5E−03	2.8E−02	−2.12	2
G23064	GSTM1	−0.86	1.54	−2.61	9.7E−03	5.4E−02	−3.00	15
G6828	BAG1	−0.24	5.38	−2.51	1.3E−02	6.4E−02	−3.23	16
G1853	CTSL2	0.61	−0.31	1.99	4.8E−02	1.5E−01	−4.35	12
G12558	STMY3	−0.23	6.34	−1.07	2.8E−01	4.9E−01	−5.69	13
G12106	CD68	0.05	5.87	0.46	6.4E−01	7.9E−01	−6.14	14

Table 8 META-voom

Gene	Name	logFC	*p*.value	adj.*p*.val
G18365	CEGP1	−1.96	1.31E−07	5.77E−05
G1975	Bcl2	−0.83	2.33E−07	7.61E−05
G14382	STK15	0.90	4.19E−06	4.61E−04
G2627	PR	−1.55	2.30E−05	1.31E−03
G19220	Ki-67	0.86	2.62E−05	1.42E−03
G19678	MYBL2	1.19	4.81E−05	2.16E−03
G1852	CCNB1	0.74	1.49E−04	4.44E−03
G5065	SURV	1.17	1.94E−04	5.26E−03
G10477	EstR1	−1.09	4.36E−03	4.45E−02
G23064	GSTM1	−0.90	5.30E−03	5.08E−02
G896	HER2	0.55	1.35E−02	9.31E−02
G18279	GRB7	0.56	1.46E−02	9.76E−02
G6828	BAG1	−0.25	3.03E−02	1.54E−01
G1853	CTSL2	0.61	7.76E−02	2.82E−01
G12558	STMY3	−0.22	5.39E−01	8.57E−01
G12106	CD68	0.06	8.20E−01	9.95E−01

Table 9 RUVs-voom

Gene	Name	logFC	AveExpr	t	p.value	adj.p.val	B	Order[a]
G1975	Bcl2	−0.89	7.30	−6.01	5.9E−09	3.4E−06	10.01	5
G18365	CEGP1	−1.99	6.29	−5.93	9.4E−09	3.9E−06	9.59	6
G2627	PR	−1.60	7.11	−4.89	1.7E−06	1.3E−04	4.55	4
G14382	STK15	0.80	3.31	4.60	6.5E−06	3.2E−04	3.56	11
G19220	Ki-67	0.82	6.21	4.41	1.5E−05	5.6E−04	2.56	8
G5065	SURV	1.15	2.02	4.33	2.1E−05	6.9E−04	2.55	7
G1852	CCNB1	0.73	3.86	4.23	3.2E−05	9.2E−04	2.05	10
G19678	MYBL2	1.09	2.55	4.15	4.4E−05	1.2E−03	1.86	9
G10477	EstR1	−1.13	8.89	−3.46	6.3E−04	7.3E−03	−1.07	3
G23064	GSTM1	−0.91	1.54	−2.80	5.5E−03	3.2E−02	−2.32	15
G18279	GRB7	0.53	3.98	2.76	6.1E−03	3.5E−02	−2.77	1
G6828	BAG1	−0.27	5.38	−2.77	5.9E−03	3.4E−02	−2.91	16
G896	HER2	0.51	7.55	2.69	7.5E−03	4.0E−02	−3.27	2
G1853	CTSL2	0.51	−0.31	1.70	9.0E−02	2.2E−01	−4.35	12
G12558	STMY3	−0.25	6.34	−1.17	2.4E−01	4.2E−01	−6.07	13
G12106	CD68	0.02	5.87	0.19	8.5E−01	9.2E−01	−6.69	14

Table 10 RUVs-edgeR

Gene	Name	logFC	AveExpr	p.value	FDR	LR	Order[a]
G896	HER2	1.45	8.45	7.70E−14	3.20E−11	55.89	2
G18279	GRB7	1.17	4.87	7.10E−09	8.60E−07	33.51	1
G1975	Bcl2	−0.71	7.6	4.60E−07	2.60E−05	25.43	5
G2627	PR	−1.46	8.4	5.80E−07	3.10E−05	24.99	4
G19220	Ki-67	0.74	6.72	7.00E−06	2.30E−04	20.18	8
G1852	CCNB1	0.65	4.31	2.00E−05	5.00E−04	18.18	10
G18365	CEGP1	−1.17	7.69	6.70E−05	1.20E−03	15.9	6
G14382	STK15	0.6	3.82	2.70E−04	3.60E−03	13.27	11
G19678	MYBL2	0.72	3.51	1.00E−03	9.70E−03	10.79	9
G5065	SURV	0.73	3.39	1.30E−03	1.20E−02	10.32	7
G23064	GSTM1	−1.1	3.93	1.50E−03	1.30E−02	10.12	15
G6828	BAG1	−0.31	5.52	1.80E−03	1.40E−02	9.79	16
G1853	CTSL2	0.57	1.02	3.30E−02	1.10E−01	4.54	12
G10477	EstR1	−0.26	9.81	2.70E−01	4.60E−01	1.23	3
G12106	CD68	−0.11	6.1	3.40E−01	5.30E−01	0.89	14
G12558	STMY3	0.02	6.97	9.00E−01	9.50E−01	0.02	13

Glossary

RNA-seq A technology that uses the capabilities of next-generation sequencing to reveal a snapshot of RNA presence and quantity from a genome at a given moment in time.

RUVSeq Methods for removing unwanted variation and normalizing RNA-seq data.

RUVs Removing unwanted variation by using control samples (here differences of replicates).

RUVg Removing unwanted variation by using control genes.

Differentially expressed genes Genes expressed differently under given conditions.

FFPE sample formalin fixed and paraffin embedded sample.

qRT-PCR Real-time polymerase chain reaction.

Negative control genes Genes known to be not affected by the biological covariates of interest but affected by the unwanted variation in the same way as the rest of the genes.

Negative control samples Samples contain no biological effects of interest (here differences of replicates).

Positive control genes Genes known to be affected by the biological covariates of interest.

Onco*type* Dx Commercial diagnostic test that estimates the likelihood of disease recurrence in women with early-stage hormone estrogen receptor (ER) positive only breast cancer (prognostic significance).

edgeR Empirical analysis of digital gene expression data in R.

limma Linear models for microarray and RNA-seq mata.

EDAseq Exploratory data analysis and normalization for RNA-seq.

betweenLaneNormalization A between lane normalization method from EDAseq.

Principal component analysis A statistical procedure that uses an orthogonal transformation to convert a set of observations of possibly correlated variables into a set of values of linearly uncorrelated variables with certain optimal properties.

Volcano plot A scatter-plot of log fold-change versus significance ($-log_{10}$(*p*-value)) on the y- and x-axes, respectively.

Meta analysis Statistical methods for combining results from different studies.

References

1. van't Veer, L.J., Dai, H., van de Vijver, M.J., He, Y.D., Hart, A.A., Mao, M., Peterse, H.L., van der Kooy, K., Marton, M.J., Witteveen, A.T., Schreiber, G.J., Kerkhoven, R.M., Roberts, C., Linsley, P.S., Bernards, R., Friend, S.H.: Gene expression profiling predicts clinical outcome of breast cancer. Nature **415**, 530–6 (2002)
2. Grada, A., Weinbrecht, K.: Next-generation sequencing: methodology and application. J. Invest. Dermatol. **133**, e11 (2013)
3. Ching, T., Huang, S., Garmire, L.X.: Power analysis and sample size estimation for RNA-Seq differential expression. RNA **20**, 1684–1696 (2014)
4. Liu, Y., Zhou, J., White, K.P.: RNA-seq differential expression studies: more sequence or more replication? Bioinformatics **30**, 301–304 (2014)
5. Ross, M.G., Russ, C., Costello, M., Hollinger, A., Lennon, N.J., Hegarty, R., Nusbaum, C. Jaffe, D.B.: Characterizing and measuring bias in sequence data. Genome Biol. **14**, R51 (2013)
6. Battke, F., Nieselt, K.: Mayday SeaSight: combined analysis of deep sequencing and microarray data. PLoS One **6**, e16345 (2011)
7. Philippe, N., Bou Samra, E., Boureux, A., Mancheron, A., Ruffle, F., Bai, Q., De Vos, J., Rivals, E., Commes, T.: Combining DGE and RNA-sequencing data to identify new polyA+ non-coding transcripts in the human genome. Nucleic Acids Res. **42**, 2820–2832 (2014)
8. Wu, J.Q., Habegger, L., Noisa, P., Szekely, A., Qiu, C., Hutchison, S., Raha, D., Egholm, M., Lin, H., Weissman, S., Cui, W., Gerstein, M., Snyder, M.: Dynamic transcriptomes during neural differentiation of human embryonic stem cells revealed by short, long, and paired-end sequencing. Proc. Natl. Acad. Sci. U.S.A. **107**, 5254–5259 (2010)
9. Kashofer, K., Viertler, C., Pichler, M., Zatloukal, K.: Quality control of RNA preservation and extraction from paraffin-embedded tissue: implications for RT-PCR and microarray analysis. PLoS One **8**, e70714 (2013)
10. von Ahlfen, S., Missel, A., Bendrat, K., Schlumpberger, M.: Determinants of RNA quality from FFPE samples. PLoS One **2**, e1261 (2007)
11. Sinicropi, D., Qu, K., Collin, F., Crager, M., Liu, M.L., Pelham, R.J., Pho, M., Dei Rossi, A., Jeong, J., Scott, A., Ambannavar, R., Zheng, C., Mena, R., Esteban, J., Stephans, J., Morlan, J., Baker, J.: Whole transcriptome RNA-Seq analysis of breast cancer recurrence risk using formalin-fixed paraffin-embedded tumor tissue. PLoS One **7**, e40092 (2012)
12. Cobleigh, M.A., Tabesh, B., Bitterman, P., Baker, J., Cronin, M., Liu, M.L., Borchik, R., Mosquera, J.M., Walker, M.G., Shak, S.: Tumor gene expression and prognosis in breast cancer patients with 10 or more positive lymph nodes. Clin. Cancer Res. **11**, 8623–8631 (2005)
13. Paik, S., Tang, G., Shak, S., Kim, C., Baker, J., Kim, W., Cronin, M., Baehner, F.L., Watson, D., Bryant, J., Costantino, J.P., Geyer, C.E. Jr., Wickerham, D.L., Wolmark, N.: Gene expression and benefit of chemotherapy in women with node-negative, estrogen receptor-positive breast cancer. J. Clin. Oncol. **24**, 3726–3734 (2006)
14. Paik, S., Shak, S., Tang, G., Kim, C., Baker, J., Cronin, M., Baehner, F.L., Walker, M.G., Watson, D., Park, T., Hiller, W., Fisher, E.R., Wickerham, D.L., Bryant, J., Wolmark, N.: A multigene assay to predict recurrence of tamoxifen-treated, node-negative breast cancer. N. Engl. J. Med. **351**, 2817–2826 (2004)
15. Cronin, M., Sangli, C., Liu, M.L., Pho, M., Dutta, D., Nguyen, A., Jeong, J., Wu, J., Langone, K.C., Watson, D.: Analytical validation of the Oncotype DX genomic diagnostic test for recurrence prognosis and therapeutic response prediction in node-negative, estrogen receptor-positive breast cancer. Clin. Chem. **53**, 1084–1091 (2007)
16. Law, C.W., Chen, Y., Shi, W., Smyth, G.K.: Voom: precision weights unlock linear model analysis tools for RNA-seq read counts. Genome Biol. **15**, R29 (2014)
17. Robinson, M.D., Oshlack, A.: A scaling normalization method for differential expression analysis of RNA-seq data. Genome Biol. **11**, R25 (2010)
18. Risso, D., Ngai, J., Speed, T.P., Dudoit, S.: Normalization of RNA-seq data using factor analysis of control genes or samples. Nat. Biotechnol. **32**, 896–902 (2014)

19. Smyth, G.K.: Linear models and empirical Bayes methods for assessing differential expression in microarray experiments. Stat. Appl. Genet. Mol. Biol. **3**, Article 3, 1–25 (2004)
20. Smyth, G.K., Yang, Y.H., Speed, T.: Statistical issues in cDNA microarray data analysis. Methods Mol. Biol. **224**, 111–136 (2003)
21. Ritchie, M.E., Phipson, B., Wu, D., Hu, Y., Law, C.W., Shi, W., Smyth, G.K.: limma powers differential expression analyses for RNA-sequencing and microarray studies. Nucleic Acids Res. **43**(7), e47, 1–13 (2015)
22. Phipson, B., Lee, S., Majewski, I.J., Alexander, W.S., Smyth, G.K.: Technical report. Empirical Bayes in the presence of exceptional cases, with application to microarray data (2013)
23. Eisenberg, E., Levanon, E.Y.: Human housekeeping genes are compact. Trends Genet. **19**, 362–365 (2003)
24. Benjamini, Y., Hochberg, Y.: Controlling the false discovery rate: a practical and powerful approach to multiple testing. J. R. Stat. Soc. Ser. B **57**, 289–300 (1995)
25. Robinson, M.D., McCarthy, D.J., Smyth, G.K.: edgeR: a Bioconductor package for differential expression analysis of digital gene expression data. Bioinformatics **26**, 139–140 (2010)
26. McCarthy, D.J., Chen, Y., Smyth, G.K.: Differential expression analysis of multifactor RNA-Seq experiments with respect to biological variation. Nucleic Acids Res. **40**, 4288–4297 (2012)
27. Bullard, J.H., Purdom, E., Hansen, K.D., Dudoit, S.: Evaluation of statistical methods for normalization and differential expression in mRNA-Seq experiments. BMC Bioinf. **11**, 94 (2010)
28. Gagnon-Bartsch, J.A., Jacob, L., Speed, T.P.: Removing Unwanted Variation from High Dimensional Data with Negative Controls. Technical report. Available via DIALOG (2013), http://statistics.berkeley.edu/tech-reports/820
29. Gagnon-Bartsch, J.A., Speed, T.P.: Using control genes to correct for unwanted variation in microarray data. Biostatistics **13**, 539–552 (2012)

An Imputation Method for Estimating the Learning Curve in Classification Problems

Eric B. Laber, Kerby Shedden, and Yang Yang

Abstract The learning curve expresses the error rate of a predictive modeling procedure, when applied to a particular population, as a function of the sample size of the training dataset. It typically is a decreasing function with a positive limiting value (bounded below by the Bayes error rate). An estimate of the learning curve can be used to assess whether a modeling procedure is expected to become substantially more accurate if additional training data were obtained. Here, we consider an imputation-based procedure for estimating learning curves. We focus on classification, although the idea is applicable to other predictive modeling settings. Simulation studies indicate that useful estimates of learning curves can be obtained for roughly a four-fold increase in the size of the training set relative to the available data, and that the proposed imputation approach outperforms an alternative estimation approach based on parameterizing the learning curve. We illustrate the method with an application that predicts the risk of disease progression for people with chronic lymphocytic leukemia.

1 Introduction

Predictive models describe the relationship between a set of predictor variables and an outcome, and are used in areas ranging from personalized medicine to computational advertising. For example, in personalized medicine the aim may be to predict which patients with a particular disease are likely to respond favorably to a treatment based on information contained in a set of pre-treatment biomarkers [9]. Predictive models are developed using a training data set, and their "generalization

E.B. Laber (✉)
NC State University, Raleigh, NC, USA
e-mail: laber@stat.ncsu.edu

K. Shedden
University of Michigan, Ann Arbor, MI, USA
e-mail: kshedden@umich.edu

Y. Yang
LinkedIn, Mountain View, CA, USA
e-mail: tamahome728@gmail.com

A. Frigessi et al. (eds.), *Statistical Analysis for High-Dimensional Data*,
Abel Symposia 11, DOI 10.1007/978-3-319-27099-9_9

performance" is typically assessed with respect to a test set that is independent of the training data. Optimizing some measure of generalization performance is usually the first priority in predictive modeling, although issues such as model interpretability, and ease of implementation may also be important.

One common type of predictive modeling is binary classification, in which the outcome Y takes on one of two possible values. In classification problems, the expected misclassification rate is a natural measure of generalization performance. Suppose that we observe a training set of n feature-label pairs $\mathscr{D}_n = \{(X_i, Y_i)\}_{i=1}^n$. Using the training data $\mathscr{D}_n$, we can construct a classifier $\hat{c}_n$, say using logistic regression. The goal is to use the classifier $\hat{c}_n$ to predict the labels Y from the observed features X of unlabeled cases. The expected misclassification rate $\tau(n)$ of the classifier $\hat{c}_n$ is the expected proportion of incorrectly labeled features X averaged over both the feature-label distribution of test cases and the distribution of $\mathscr{D}_n$; that is,

$$\tau(n) \triangleq \mathbb{E}\{Y \neq \hat{c}_n(X)\} = E_{\mathscr{D}_n} E\{Y \neq \hat{c}_n(X) | \mathscr{D}_n\}, \tag{1}$$

where $\mathbb{E}$ denotes expectation taken with respect to both (X, Y) and the training data $\mathscr{D}_n$. Our primary focus here is to estimate the function $\tau(n)$, which has been termed the "learning curve" ([1, 7, 8], p. 243).

In practice, knowledge of the learning curve can contribute to both study design and interpretation of predictive modeling results. Study design questions arise naturally if the training data are acquired from a pilot study with a modest sample size. Such a study may produce encouraging evidence that a predictive relationship exists, raising hope that the performance can be improved merely through use of a larger training set. If we had a procedure indicating that this was indeed possible, we could use this as evidence to advocate for a larger study using the same features and predictive modeling approach. On the other hand, if the performance is unlikely to benefit from a larger training set, we should focus on identifying other predictive variables or modeling approaches. Note that in many applications, the "raw material" for constructing new variables is not in short supply. For example, screening studies for molecular biomarkers often employ assays that collect data for thousands of genes. If the initial modeling efforts focus on a set of candidate genes which appear unpromising based on an estimated learning curve, there are many additional variables to explore in the data in-hand.

Learning curves can also contribute to the interpretation of predictive modeling results. In many settings in which predictive modeling is applied, the variables naturally fall into domains. For example, many genomic approaches to cancer risk prediction base their predictions on the expression levels of genes associated with cell growth, division, proliferation, and other functional categories that have been linked to cancer. One way to assess the biological influence of genes in a particular functional category is through the predictive power based only on the given gene set. However, the apparent predictive performance as estimated by, say, cross validation, is partly determined by the power and sample size of the study that generated the data. It is thus not comparable across studies with different power. The true biological influence of a gene category should not depend on study design factors such as the sample size. A learning curve, if estimable from data, provides a way to assess the predictive power of a set of variables in a way that does not depend on the study design.

The rest of the paper is organized as follows. Section 2 reviews some previous work on learning curves. Section 3 describes three approaches to learning curve estimation, including one existing approach and two new approaches. Section 4 compares the performances of these approaches using simulated examples. Section 5 illustrates the imputation approach using a data set in which the goal is to predict the risk that a patient with chronic lymphocytic leukemia (CLL) will experience a poor outcome. Section 6 provides some concluding remarks.

2 Learning Curves

Learning curves have been an object of interest for several decades. Bounds on the learning curve follow from the work of Vapnik and Chervonenkis [16] and Vapnik [15]. These bounds have the power law form $a + b/m^{\alpha}$, where $\alpha = 1/2$ holds in the many parametric settings. The bounds are tight if nothing is known about the distribution of X and one takes a worst-case perspective. If information about the distribution of X is available or can be estimated from observed X values, tighter bounds can be obtained (e.g., [8]).

The problem we consider here is to estimate the learning curve rather than to bound it. Thus, we consider the setting in which data on (X, Y) are available, and we focus on estimating the learning curve with low bias and variance. To succeed at this, we must capture the general form of the function (e.g., the order at which the function τ changes with n), but also the relevant constants and lower order terms.

Our focus here is on binary classification, but for comparison we briefly consider the setting of linear regression using least-squares methods. In this case, an expression for the learning curve $\tau(n)$ can be derived explicitly. The generalization performance in this case is naturally assessed using the mean-square prediction error (MSPE) $\mathbb{E}[(Y - \hat{Y})^2]$ for a prediction $\hat{Y} = \hat{Y}(x)$ of the unobserved Y given its feature vector $X = x$. For training sets of sample size n, the expected MSPE is $\sigma^2(1 + \mathrm{tr}(CM)/n)$, where $M = E[(\mathbf{X}'\mathbf{X}/n)^{-1}]$ for the training design matrix $\mathbf{X}$ and $C = E[X^*X^{*\prime}]$ for the test set covariate vector X^*. The reduction in MSPE due to the use of a larger training set is reflected in the term $\sigma^2 c/n$, where $c = \mathrm{tr}(CM)$ captures both the complexity of the model and the similarity of the training and testing distributions of covariate vectors.

3 Approaches to Learning Curve Estimation

In this section, we describe three approaches to learning curve estimation. The first approach follows a proposal of Mukherjee et al. [10]. To our knowledge, the second and third approaches are new.

3.1 *Subsampling and Extrapolation*

In 2003, Mukherjee et al. described an approach to learning curve estimation based on parameterizing the learning curve. We are not aware that a name has been given to this method, and therefore we termed it "SUBEX" for "subsampling and extrapolation." The method parameterizes the learning curve as an inverse power law of the form $\tau(m) = a + bm^{-\alpha}$. As noted above, this expression is exact in the case of linear least squares regression. The unknown parameters in this expression are $a \in \mathbb{R}$ and b, $\alpha \geq 0$.

In the "subsampling" stage of the SUBEX algorithm, the parametric form $\tau(m) = a + bm^{-\alpha}$ is fit by first using cross-validation on subsamples of the data of various sizes $m' < m$ to obtain direct estimates of $\tau(m')$. For each m_j ($m_j < m$), independently subsample B subsets of the training data of size m_j, fit the classification model to each subset, and use the complementary $m - m_j$ samples to unbiasedly estimate the error rate. These B error rate estimates are then averaged to produce an estimate $\hat{\tau}(m_j)$ of $\tau(m_j)$. The parametric form for $\tau(m)$ is then fit to the set of points $\{(m_j, \hat{\tau}(m_j)), j = 1, \ldots, J\}$ to estimate a, b, and α using some form of nonlinear regression. For example, nonlinear least squares would estimate a, b and α by minimizing $\sum_{j=1}^{J} \left\{\hat{\tau}(m_j) - a - bm_j^{-\alpha}\right\}^2$, where the $m_j \leq m$ are a set of sample sizes on which the error rate is directly estimated. In the "extrapolation" stage of the SUBEX algorithm, the generalization performance for sample sizes $m' > m$ of interest are estimated as $\hat{\tau}(m')$.

As shown in Sect. 4, the SUBEX estimator can be positively biased, conveying an overly optimistic assessment of the generalization performance. One reason for this optimism is the asymmetry in the constraints placed on τ. The curve is constrained to be non-increasing, which is quite natural, but owing to the high variance in cross-validation estimators, the constraint is active on a non-negligible proportion of modest-sized training sets under simple generative models. By contrast, aside from being constrained to be non-negative, the curve is unrestricted in how rapidly it can decrease. Thus, when averaged over training sets, a negative bias in the learning curve results.

3.2 Imputation and Interpolation

The second approach we consider for estimating the learning curve uses data imputation and interpolation; we term this procedure "IMPINT." In this approach, one first estimates the joint distribution of the feature-label pair (X, Y). This estimation is generally performed by separately estimating the feature distribution p_X, and the conditional distribution $p_{Y|X}$ of the label Y given the feature X. After estimating the joint distribution $p_{XY}(x, y)$, one can synthesize data sets of any size. The ability to simulate such data sets allows direct estimation of any point on the learning curve. Specifically, one can generate an arbitrary number of training sets of a given sample size m from the estimated distribution $\hat{p}_{XY} = \hat{p}_X\hat{p}_{Y|X}$, build a classifier on each one, and then average their generalization performance over newly drawn feature-label pairs from $\hat{p}_{XY}$. The complete learning curve can be obtained via interpolation among the learning curve points that are directly estimated.

3.2.1 IMPINT for Logistic Regression

Suppose we observe a training set $\mathscr{D}_n$ of feature-label pairs $\{(X_i, Y_i)\}_{i=1}^n$ drawn *i.i.d.* from an unknown distribution with density $p_{X,Y}(x, y)$. The features, X, take values in $\mathbb{R}^p$, and the binary labels, Y, are coded to take values in $\{0, 1\}$. Define $\pi(x; \beta) \triangleq \text{expit}(x^\mathsf{T}\beta) = 1/(1 + e^{-x^\mathsf{T}\beta})$. The distribution $p_{X,Y}(x, y)$ factors into the product $p_{Y|X}(y|x)p_X(x)$. Under the logistic regression model, the conditional distribution of $Y|X$ has the form $p_{Y|X}(y|x) = \pi(x; \beta^*)^y\{1 - \pi(x; \beta^*)\}^{1-y}$, with $\beta^* \in \mathbb{R}^p$ denoting the unknown true parameter value. The marginal distribution of the label X, denoted by $p_X(x)$, is left unspecified for now.

The conditional error rate for a particular training set $\mathscr{D}_m$ is

$$R(\mathscr{D}_m; \beta^*) \triangleq \int \Big[\pi(x; \beta^*)1\{x^\mathsf{T}\hat{\beta}_m \le \kappa\} + (1 - \pi(x; \beta^*))1\{x^\mathsf{T}\hat{\beta}_m > \kappa\}\Big] p_X(x)dx, \tag{2}$$

where $\hat{\beta}_m = \hat{\beta}_m(\mathscr{D}_m)$ is the maximum likelihood estimator of β^* and the classification rule is given by $\hat{c}_m(x) = 1\{x^\mathsf{T}\hat{\beta}_m \ge \kappa\}$ for some threshold $\kappa \in \mathbb{R}$. Using (1), we can express the learning curve as

$$\tau(m) = \mathbb{E}R(\mathscr{D}_m, \beta^*) = \int R(\mathscr{D}_m, \beta^*) \prod_{i=1}^{m} p_X(x_i)p_{Y|X}(y_i)dx_idy_i. \tag{3}$$

If β^* and $p_X(x)$ were both known, one could compute $\tau(m)$ for each m using (3) using Monte Carlo methods as follows: (1) use β^* and $p_X(x)$ to generate B training sets of size m, say $\mathscr{D}_m^{(1)}, \mathscr{D}_m^{(2)}, \ldots, \mathscr{D}_m^{(B)}$; (2) fit a logistic regression model to each training set to obtain estimator $\hat{\beta}_m^{(b)}$ of β^*; (3) generate a large test set, say $\mathscr{D}_*$; and (4) compute

$$\tau(m) \approx \frac{1}{BN}\sum_{b=1}^{B}\sum_{(X,Y)\in\mathscr{D}_*}\left[\pi(X;\beta^*)\cdot 1\{X^{\intercal}\hat{\beta}_m^{(b)} \le \kappa\} + (1-\pi(X;\beta^*))\cdot 1\{X^{\intercal}\hat{\beta}_m^{(b)} > \kappa\}\right]$$

$$\approx \frac{1}{BN}\sum_{b=1}^{B}\sum_{(X,Y)\in\mathscr{D}_*}\left[Y\cdot 1\{X^{\intercal}\hat{\beta}_m^{(b)} \le \kappa\} + (1-Y)\cdot 1\{X^{\intercal}\hat{\beta}_m^{(b)} > \kappa\}\right]. \qquad (4)$$

The IMPINT estimate of $\tau(m)$, which we denote by $\hat{\tau}_{II}(m)$, is formed by applying the approximation given in (4) over imputed training and testing sets generated using an imputation model fit to the complete observed training data $\mathscr{D}_n$. Let $\hat{p}_X(x)$ denote an estimator of $p_X(x)$ and $\hat{\beta}_n$ denote the maximum likelihood estimator of β^*. Use $\hat{p}_X(x)$ and $\hat{\beta}_n$ to generate B training sets of size m, $\hat{\mathscr{D}}_m^{(1)}, \hat{\mathscr{D}}_m^{(2)}, \ldots, \hat{\mathscr{D}}_m^{(B)}$, and large test set $\hat{\mathscr{D}}_*$ be a large test set. The IMPINT estimator is

$$\hat{\tau}_{II}(m) \triangleq \frac{1}{BN}\sum_{b=1}^{B}\sum_{(X,Y)\in\hat{\mathscr{D}}_*}\left[Y\cdot 1\{X^{\intercal}\hat{\beta}_m^{(b)} \le \kappa\} + (1-Y)\cdot 1\{X^{\intercal}\hat{\beta}_m^{(b)} > \kappa\}\right], \qquad (5)$$

where $\hat{\beta}_m^{(b)} = \hat{\beta}_m^{(b)}(\hat{\mathscr{D}}_m^{(b)})$ denotes the maximum likelihood estimator based on the bth imputed training set $\hat{\mathscr{D}}_m^{(b)}$.

We found that the number of imputed data sets required to ensure that the IMPINT estimate is smoothly non-increasing can be relatively large. As a practical matter, it is more computationally efficient to use a smaller value of B (e.g. $B \approx$500–1000), and then feed the resulting estimate through a monotone smoother (e.g., Friedman and Tibshirani [6]; alternatively a parametric model could be fit as in Mukherjee et al. [10]). We found that the use of a monotone smoother reduces variance without introducing detectable additional bias.

3.2.2 Modeling the Feature Distribution

The model $\hat{p}_X$ for p_X can be obtained using any appropriate modeling approach for multivariate data. Labeled data is not needed to estimate $p_X(x)$, hence, if additional unlabeled features are available they can be used to improve the estimation of $p_X(x)$. If X is high dimensional, estimating this joint distribution fully nonparametrically is challenging. Fundamentally, the generalization error rate at a given point x in the feature space is a function of how well the limiting classification rule $c(x)$ matches the distribution $p_{Y|X=x}$, and how accurately $c(x)$ is estimated by $\hat{c}_n(x)$. Some possible approaches are demonstrated in the simulation studies and real data analysis below.

To avoid model mis-specification, it is tempting to simply use the empirical distribution function of X in place of p_X. However, in our experience, this approach does not work well with continuous covariates. In particular, the estimated learning curve tends be substantially biased downward. This may occur because points in the training set have positive mass in the testing population. Thus, the model is not relied upon to interpolate probabilities between observed X points; see [4] for a discussion of the role played by the distance between training and testing sets in classification.

3.3 Bias Reduction for Learning Curve Estimates

We found that a simple bias reduction substantially improves the performance of the learning estimates obtained from imputed data. This leads to a modified IMPINT approach, which we call BRIE for "Bias Reduced Imputation Estimator." To motivate this approach, consider what happens when we estimate $p_{Y|X}$ using the best-fitting regression model (e.g., a fitted logistic regression model). This will overstate the strength of the relationship between X and Y, particularly when the true relationship is weak (e.g., if Y and X are independent, then $\hat{p}_{Y|X}$ will still exhibit a relationship). Thus, the IMPINT estimator tends to be an optimistic estimator of $\tau(m)$, in the sense that it systematically overstates predictive accuracy. A simple bias correction addresses this problem.

We observed empirically (see Sect. 4) that for any positive integer k, the estimator $\hat{\tau}_{II}(m) - \hat{\tau}_{II}(m+k)$ exhibits little bias as an estimator of $\tau(m) - \tau(m+k)$. That is, the IMPINT estimator is nearly unbiased for the increments of the learning curve but not necessarily for its overall level. An explanation for this observation parallels the intuition behind the bootstrap as follows. The asymptote of the learning curve $\lim_{m\to\infty} \tau(m)$ is the Bayes error rate and thus depends exclusively on $p_X(x)$ and β^*. However, the increments of τ, in addition to depending on β^* and $p_X(x)$, depend on the sampling properties of the estimator $\hat{\beta}_m$ as well as the convergence behavior of $\hat{\beta}_m$ to its limiting value β^*. The increments of the IMPINT learning curve estimator $\hat{\tau}_{II}(n)$ are determined by the sampling properties of $\hat{\beta}_m^{(b)}$ as an estimator of $\hat{\beta}_n$ as well as the manner by which $\hat{\beta}_m^{(b)}$ approaches its limiting value. Thus, if the sampling properties of $\hat{\beta}_m^{(b)}$ about $\hat{\beta}_n$ accurately reflect the sampling properties of $\hat{\beta}_n$ about β^* and if $\hat{p}_X(x)$ is a reasonable estimator of $p_X(x)$, then the increments of $\hat{\tau}_{II}$ will approximate the increments of τ.

If one can accurately estimate the increments of the learning curve, all that remains is to find an unbiased estimator of the learning curve at a single training set size. This is provided by the leave-one-out cross-validation (LOOCV) estimator of the expected test error based on the complete observed training set $\mathscr{D}_n$, which provides an unbiased estimator of $\tau(n-1)$. Let $\hat{\tau}_{CV}(n-1)$ denote the LOOCV estimator of $\tau(n-1)$. The BRIE is then given by $\hat{\tau}_B(m) \triangleq \hat{\tau}_{II}(m) + \{\hat{\tau}_{CV}(n-1) - \hat{\tau}_{II}(n-1)\}$. Thus, BRIE is simply a shifted version of the IMPINT estimator.

The choice to use the LOOCV estimator of the misclassification rate is not essential. Noting that $\tau(n) \approx \tau(n-1)$, one could employ any unbiased (or nearly unbiased) estimator of the expected test error $\tau(n)$ to recenter the uncorrected estimator of the learning curve. There are also other ways to achieve this bias correction. For instance, the MLE $\hat{\beta}_n$ of β derived from the training set may be rescaled by a factor $c < 1$, producing a shrunken coefficient vector β which can be calibrated to make the IMPINT estimator nearly unbiased at $\tau(n)$. We found that this approach gives similar results to those obtained using the simple additive bias correction.

3.3.1 Relationship of IMPINT/BRIE to Other Statistical Procedures Using Imputation

Here we discuss the relationship between the IMPINT and BRIE procedures and two well-known statistical procedures that use model-based imputation: the parametric bootstrap [5] and multiple imputation [12].

The parametric bootstrap is most commonly used when performing inference on the parameters of a model. The learning curve is implicitly a function of the generating model and therefore of its parameters. Common applications of the parametric bootstrap include estimating standard errors, and bias reduction [3]. The parametric bootstrap as most commonly applied draws samples of the same size as the training data set, whereas the IMPINT procedure relies on imputing data sets of various sample sizes, all greater than the training set sample size. In the IMPINT procedure, we are using a parametric bootstrap-like procedure to define a sampling population for a sample that is larger than our observed sample size, and to approximate the integral in (3). The bias reduction step of BRIE has no obvious analogue in the parametric bootstrap.

Multiple imputation is often used to address estimation and inference challenges that arise due to missing data, or in settings where the data are partially-observed by design. The emphasis on the term "multiple" in "multiple imputation" reflects both the desire to empirically estimate an expected value (over the imputation distribution), and to obtain standard errors for estimates obtained from imputed data sets that reflect the additional uncertainty resulting from the imputation. In the setting of estimating the learning curve τ at a single point $\tau(m+n)$ $(m > 0)$, we can view the "complete data" as having size $n+m$ and we are imputing the "missing" m samples. Again, the bias reduction step of BRIE does not have an obvious analogue in multiple imputation.

4 Empirical Studies

In this section we examine the performance of the SUBEX, IMPINT, and BRIE procedures in terms of bias and variance, using a series of simulation studies. For each example we used 1000 Monte Carlo iterations, $B = 1000$ imputed data sets, and an imputed test set $\mathcal{D}_*$ of size 5000. All initial training sets are of size $n = 50$

and we estimate $\tau(m)$ for $m = 75, 100, 150$, and 200 using this initial training set. Thus, we are attempting to extrapolate substantially beyond the initial training set size.

For our simulation studies, we consider the following class of models. The distribution of the features X is a p-variate normal distribution with $AR(1)$ variance-covariance matrix Σ given by $\Sigma_{i,j} = r^{|i-j|}$. The true parameter vector β^* is a p-vector of ones. Thus, this class of models is determined by the dimension of the model p and the level of dependence between the features which is governed by the parameter $r \in (-1, 1)$.

Figure 1 shows a few examples of learning curves generated using this class of models. The left hand side of Fig. 1 shows the learning curve $\tau(m)$ based on training sets of size $n = 50$, for p fixed at 15 and $r = 0.0, 0.25, 0.50$, and 0.75. The figure shows that as r increases, both the learning rate and the asymptotic error rate (i.e., the Bayes error rate) decrease (differences in the learning rate are most evident for sample sizes less than 100). These changes are mostly driven by the fact that as the positive correlation r increases, the distribution of $|X^{\mathsf{T}}\beta^*|$ becomes stochastically larger, and thus fewer points lie near the optimal decision boundary $\{x \in \mathbb{R}^p : x^{\mathsf{T}}\beta^* = 0\}$. The right hand side of Fig. 1 shows the learning curve $\tau(m)$ based on training sets of size $n = 50$ for r fixed at 0.10 and $p = 10, 15, 20$, and 25. The figure shows, as would be expected, that the learning curve becomes steeper as the dimension of the problem increases (the raw values of τ_m are difficult to compare across values of p since the Bayes error rate changes with p). We use these examples to examine bias and variance properties of the BRIE and SUBEX estimator.

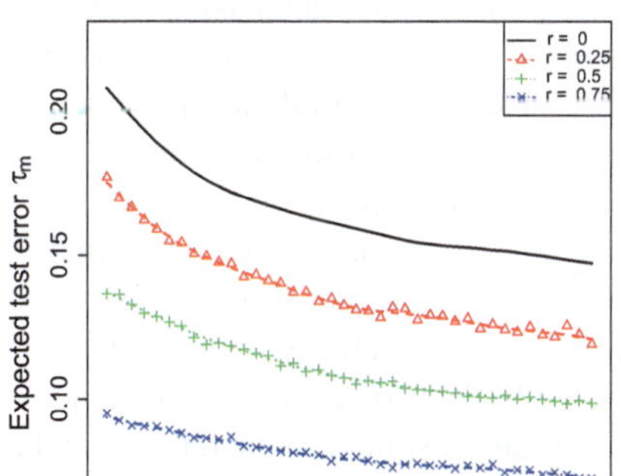

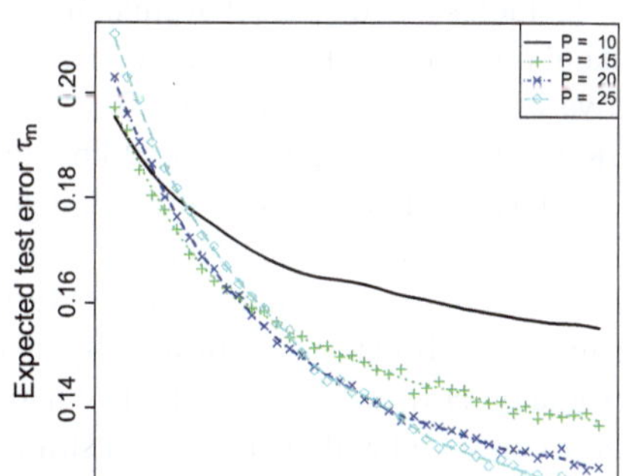

Fig. 1 *Left*: Learning curves $\tau(m)$ for training sets of size $n = 50$, for the $AR(1)$ normal model with $p = 15$ and $r = 0, 0.25, 0.5, 0.75$. *Right*: Learning curves $\tau(m)$ for training sets of size $n = 50$ for the $AR(1)$ normal model with $r = 0.10$ and $p = 10, 15, 20, 25$

4.1 Task One: Estimating the Improvement in Expected Error Rate

We first consider the task of estimating the improvement in expected error rate if additional training data are obtained. That is, our goal is to estimate $\delta(n, m) \triangleq \tau(n) - \tau(m)$ for $m \geq n$. Note that the plug-in BRIE estimate of $\delta(n, m)$, $\hat{\delta}_B(n, m) \triangleq \hat{\tau}_B(n) - \hat{\tau}_B(n)$, is equal to the plug-in IMPINT estimate of $\delta(n, m)$. Estimation of $\delta(n, m)$ is an easier problem than estimating the entire learning curve $\tau(m)$, as it only requires estimating the shape but not the absolute level of the learning curve. This quantity may be of interest to a researcher who cares more about relative improvement, e.g. 5 % point reduction in expected error rate, than in the absolute error rates, e.g., a reduction from 12 to 7 %.

Tables 1 and 2 show the estimated expected values and standard deviations for the BRIE (IMPINT) and SUBEX estimators, on a class of eight models as described at the beginning of this section. The BRIE exhibits substantially smaller bias and standard deviation than the SUBEX estimator in all instances, and provides useful estimates even when extrapolating from $n = 50$ to $m = 200$, a four-fold increase in sample size. The reduction in variability in BRIE relative to SUBEX presumably results from the variance in SUBEX resulting from the use of the LOOCV estimator $\hat{\tau}_{CV}(n-1)$, which is well-known to be highly variable [2, 4, 13, 14]. The bias in the SUBEX estimator could be due to the true value of τ not following an inverse power law exactly, or could be due to the asymmetric constraints imposed on the fitted curve, as discussed previously.

In Tables 1 and 2, the marginal distribution $p_X(x)$ was estimated using maximum likelihood for a normal model with unknown mean vector μ and unknown variance-covariance matrix Σ given by $\Sigma_{i,j} = \sigma^2 \rho^{|i-j|}$. Thus, this simulation provides the BRIE estimator the advantage of knowing the form of the covariance matrix.

Tables 3 and 4 show the analogous results when $\hat{p}_X(x)$ is modeled as a multivariate normal distribution with unconstrained variance-covariance matrix. The usual plug-in estimator of the covariance is used. The tables show that the BRIE estimator still exhibits substantially smaller bias and variability than the SUBEX estimator. However, the standard deviation of the BRIE is on average about twice as large compared with using the constrained covariance estimate as in Tables 1 and 2.

4.2 Task Two: Estimating the Learning Curve

Next we consider the more difficult task of estimating the full learning curve, not just its increments. Our goal is to estimate $\tau(75)$, $\tau(100)$, $\tau(150)$, and $\tau(200)$ using a training set size of $n = 50$. As in the previous section, we use the SUBEX estimator as a baseline for comparison.

Tables 5 and 6 show the estimated expected values and standard deviations for the BRIE and the SUBEX estimator of the learning curve on the same eight models

Table 1 Mean and standard deviation of the BRIE and SUBEX estimator for estimating the improvement in the expected error rate when the training set size is increased to $n = 50$ to $m = 75$ and $m = 100$

p	r	$\delta(50, 75)$	$\hat{\delta}_B(50, 75)$, SD	$\hat{\delta}_S(50, 75)$, SD	$\delta(50, 100)$	$\hat{\delta}_B(50, 100)$, SD	$\hat{\delta}_S(50, 100)$, SD
10	0.10	0.0173	0.0145, 0.00477	0.0254, 0.0296	0.0249	0.0209, 0.00613	0.0415, 0.0486
15	0.10	0.0232	0.0253, 0.00362	0.0297, 0.0323	0.0362	0.0376, 0.00461	0.0484, 0.0531
20	0.10	0.0266	0.0327, 0.00382	0.0383, 0.0397	0.0415	0.0497, 0.00499	0.0625, 0.0650
25	0.10	0.0294	0.0328, 0.00347	0.0400, 0.0384	0.0475	0.0498, 0.00450	0.0653, 0.0630
15	0.00	0.0210	0.0263, 0.00344	0.0296, 0.0321	0.0372	0.0390, 0.00440	0.0483, 0.0527
15	0.25	0.0222	0.0226, 0.00375	0.0272, 0.0317	0.0300	0.0340, 0.00478	0.0444, 0.0520
15	0.50	0.0100	0.0169, 0.00462	0.0235, 0.0287	0.0180	0.0259, 0.00615	0.0383, 0.0471
15	0.75	0.00590	0.00986, 0.00478	0.0147, 0.0166	0.00824	0.0151, 0.00651	0.0238, 0.0271

The BRIE estimator used a multivariate normal model with the restriction that $\Sigma_{ij} = \sigma^2 \rho^{|i-j|}$ to estimate $p_X(x)$. The BRIE estimator is seen to be significantly less biased than the SUBEX estimator, as well as, possessing smaller standard deviation across training sets

Table 2 Mean and standard deviation of the BRIE and SUBEX estimator for estimating the improvement in the expected error rate when the training set size is increased to $n = 50$ to $m = 150$ and $m = 200$

p	r	$\delta(50, 150)$	$\hat{\delta}_B(50, 150)$, SD	$\hat{\delta}_S(50, 150)$, SD	$\delta(50, 200)$	$\hat{\delta}_B(50, 200)$, SD	$\hat{\delta}_S(50, 200)$, SD
10	0.10	0.0322	0.0268, 0.00679	0.0616, 0.0727	0.0388	0.0285, 0.00686	0.0742, 0.0880
15	0.10	0.0484	0.0497, 0.00496	0.0720, 0.0794	0.0563	0.0556, 0.00490	0.0870, 0.0963
20	0.10	0.0614	0.0673, 0.00523	0.0930, 0.0971	0.0699	0.0765, 0.00541	0.112, 0.117
25	0.10	0.0684	0.0674, 0.00484	0.0973, 0.0943	0.0823	0.0767, 0.00469	0.117, 0.124
15	0.00	0.0487	0.0512, 0.00478	0.0719, 0.0789	0.0576	0.0571, 0.00476	0.0868, 0.0956
15	0.25	0.0459	0.0456, 0.00506	0.0660, 0.0778	0.0525	0.0515, 0.00487	0.0797, 0.0943
15	0.50	0.0313	0.0356, 0.00684	0.0570, 0.0705	0.0357	0.0410, 0.00673	0.0687, 0.0855
15	0.75	0.0150	0.0210, 0.00763	0.0351, 0.0405	0.0189	0.0244, 0.00791	0.0421, 0.0490

The BRIE estimator used a multivariate normal model with the restriction that $\Sigma_{ij} = \sigma^2\rho^{|i-j|}$ to estimate $p_X(x)$. The BRIE estimator is seen to be significantly less biased than the SUBEX estimator, as well as, possessing smaller standard deviation across training sets

Table 3 Mean and standard deviation of the BRIE and SUBEX estimator for estimating the improvement in the expected error rate when the training set size is increased to $n = 50$ to $m = 75$ and $m = 100$

p	r	$\delta(50, 75)$	$\hat{\delta}_B(50, 75)$, SD	$\hat{\delta}_S(50, 75)$, SD	$\delta(50, 100)$	$\hat{\delta}_B(50, 100)$, SD	$\hat{\delta}_S(50, 100)$, SD
10	0.10	0.0173	0.0100, 0.00206	0.0254, 0.0296	0.0249	0.0140, 0.00330	0.0415, 0.0486
15	0.10	0.0232	0.0209, 0.00670	0.0297, 0.0323	0.0362	0.0314, 0.00865	0.0484, 0.0531
20	0.10	0.0266	0.0240, 0.00372	0.0383, 0.0397	0.0415	0.0372, 0.00519	0.0625, 0.0650
25	0.10	0.0294	0.0256, 0.00748	0.0400, 0.0384	0.0475	0.0404, 0.0102	0.0653, 0.0630
15	0.00	0.0210	0.0217, 0.00704	0.0296, 0.0321	0.0372	0.0325, 0.00910	0.0483, 0.0527
15	0.25	0.0222	0.0184, 0.00620	0.0272, 0.0317	0.0300	0.0280, 0.00806	0.0444, 0.0520
15	0.50	0.0100	0.0140, 0.00568	0.0235, 0.0287	0.0180	0.0215, 0.00750	0.0383, 0.0471
15	0.75	0.00590	0.00879, 0.00413	0.0147, 0.0166	0.00824	0.0135, 0.00554	0.0238, 0.0271

The BRIE estimator used an unrestricted multivariate normal model to estimate $p_X(x)$. The BRIE estimator is seen to be significantly less biased than the SUBEX estimator, as well as, possessing smaller standard deviation across training sets

Table 4 Mean and standard deviation of the BRIE and SUBEX estimator for estimating the improvement in the expected error rate when the training set size is increased to $n = 50$ to $m = 150$ and $m = 200$

p	r	$\delta(50, 150)$	$\hat{\delta}_B(50, 150)$, SD	$\hat{\delta}_S(50, 150)$, SD	$\delta(50, 200)$	$\hat{\delta}_B(50, 200)$, SD	$\hat{\delta}_S(50, 200)$, SD
10	0.10	0.0322	0.0202, 0.00476	0.0616, 0.0727	0.0388	0.0240, 0.00563	0.0742, 0.0880
15	0.10	0.0484	0.0421, 0.00939	0.0720, 0.0794	0.0563	0.0477, 0.00918	0.0870, 0.0963
20	0.10	0.0614	0.0519, 0.0101	0.0930, 0.0971	0.0699	0.0603, 0.00998	0.112, 0.117
25	0.10	0.0684	0.0578, 0.0118	0.0973, 0.0943	0.0823	0.0682, 0.0118	0.117, 0.124
15	0.00	0.0487	0.0435, 0.00991	0.0719, 0.0789	0.0576	0.0492, 0.00974	0.0868, 0.0956
15	0.25	0.0459	0.0381, 0.00878	0.0660, 0.0778	0.0525	0.0436, 0.00857	0.0797, 0.0943
15	0.50	0.313	0.0298, 0.00839	0.0570, 0.0705	0.0357	0.0345, 0.00836	0.0687, 0.0855
15	0.75	0.0150	0.0188, 0.00636	0.0351, 0.0405	0.0189	0.0218, 0.00650	0.0421, 0.0490

The BRIE estimator used an unrestricted multivariate normal model to estimate $p_X(x)$. The BRIE estimator is seen to be significantly less biased than the SUBEX estimator, as well as, possessing smaller standard deviation across training sets

Table 5 Mean and standard deviation of the BRIE and SUBEX estimator for estimating the learning curve when the training set size is increased from $n = 50$ to $m = 75$ and $m = 100$

p	r	$\tau(75)$	$\hat{\tau}_B(75)$, SD	$\hat{\tau}_S(75)$, SD	$\tau(100)$	$\hat{\tau}_B(100)$, SD	$\hat{\tau}_S(100)$, SD
10	0.10	0.179	0.184, 0.0634	0.166, 0.0735	0.172	0.179, 0.0619	0.152, 0.0828
15	0.10	0.174	0.175, 0.0636	0.141, 0.0755	0.161	0.164, 0.0639	0.127, 0.0832
20	0.10	0.176	0.177, 0.0679	0.154, 0.0831	0.161	0.163, 0.0678	0.136, 0.0926
25	0.10	0.181	0.187, 0.0715	0.174, 0.0851	0.163	0.172, 0.0713	0.151, 0.0994
15	0.00	0.187	0.190, 0.0655	0.169, 0.0831	0.171	0.179, 0.0664	0.151, 0.0940
15	0.25	0.155	0.158, 0.0610	0.147, 0.0739	0.147	0.148, 0.0610	0.134, 0.0814
15	0.50	0.126	0.126, 0.0581	0.110, 0.0686	0.118	0.118, 0.0582	0.100, 0.0748
15	0.75	0.0891	0.0861, 0.0507	0.0744, 0.0505	0.0868	0.0814, 0.0508	0.0683, 0.0527

The BRIE estimator used a multivariate normal model with the restriction that $\Sigma_{ij} = \sigma^2 \rho^{|i-j|}$ to estimate $p_X(x)$. The BRIE estimator is seen to be significantly less biased than the SUBEX estimator, as well as, possessing smaller standard deviation across training sets

Table 6 Mean and standard deviation of the BRIE and SUBEX estimator for estimating the learning curve when the training set size is increased from $n = 50$ to $m = 150$ and $m = 200$

p	r	$\tau(150)$	$\hat{\tau}_B(150)$, SD	$\hat{\tau}_S(150)$, SD	$\tau(200)$	$\hat{\tau}_B(200)$, SD	$\hat{\tau}_S(200)$, SD
10	0.10	0.164	0.173, 0.0647	0.139, 0.0911	0.158	0.169, 0.0651	0.133, 0.0945
15	0.10	0.149	0.153, 0.0643	0.113, 0.0905	0.141	0.146, 0.0644	0.107, 0.0930
20	0.10	0.141	0.148, 0.0676	0.120, 0.100	0.133	0.139, 0.0674	0.112, 0.103
25	0.10	0.143	0.155, 0.0710	0.130, 0.111	0.129	0.144, 0.0707	0.122, 0.114
15	0.00	0.160	0.167, 0.0670	0.134, 0.101	0.151	0.161, 0.0674	0.127, 0.103
15	0.25	0.131	0.137, 0.0611	0.121, 0.116	0.124	0.131, 0.0613	0.116, 0.0917
15	0.50	0.106	0.101, 0.0583	0.919, 0.0795	0.101	0.105, 0.0583	0.0886, 0.0811
15	0.75	0.0800	0.0761, 0.0508	0.0625, 0.0550	0.0761	0.0730, 0.0508	0.0597, 0.0561

The BRIE estimator used a multivariate normal model with the restriction that $\Sigma_{ij} = \sigma^2\rho^{|i-j|}$ to estimate $p_X(x)$. The BRIE estimator is seen to be significantly less biased than the SUBEX estimator, as well as, possessing smaller standard deviation across training sets considered in the preceding section. Like the results for estimating the improvement in error rate, the BRIE shows only negligible bias for estimating the learning curve, while the bias for SUBEX is substantial. BRIE also has a smaller variance than SUBEX, but the advantage is substantially smaller than in the case of estimating learning curve increments. This is likely due to the fact that the bias correction used in the BRIE method is based on the highly variable leave-one-out cross validation estimator of $\tau(n-1)$.

In practice, learning curve estimates are useful to the extent that they can distinguish between substantially different possible true learning curve patterns. For estimating learning curve increments, with an increase in sample size from 50 to 150 (Table 4, left columns), the range of possible true increments is roughly 0.05 (0.015 to 0.0684). The standard error for the BRIE estimate of these quantities is around 0.01, so the range of possible outcomes in our simulations is at least five times greater than the standard error. For estimating the learning curves themselves, the analogous results in Table 6 (left columns) show a range of 0.08 in the true values, and a standard error of 0.05–0.07. Thus the maximum observed difference is only slightly greater than the standard error, suggesting that the practical value of estimators of the learning curve may be limited, while useful information can be obtained from estimates of the learning curve increments. This point is underscored in the example considered in the next section.

5 Example: Four Year Survival Probability for CLL

We next demonstrate the BRIE approach to estimating learning curves using data from a study of prognostic factors for outcomes of patients with chronic lymphocytic leukemia (CLL). The duration between the time that a subject entered a study and the time the subject required treatment (TTFT), a surrogate for disease progression, was obtained for 209 CLL subjects in a prospective study [11]. For this analysis, the TTFT outcomes were dichotomized according to whether treatment was needed within 4 years of diagnosis. Eleven potential prognostic markers were used to predict this outcome using logistic regression. The markers are: ZAP70%, p53 status, CD38%, IgVH mutation status, age at diagnosis, Rai stage at diagnosis, number of positive lymph node groups, subchromosomal losses, chromosomal losses, subchromosomal gains, and chromosomal gains. This set of predictor variables includes binary (p53, IgVH), ordered categorical (Rai stage), count (chromosomal/subchromosomal losses and gains, positive lymph node groups), and continuous (ZAP70%, CD38%, age) measures.

We calculated the BRIE estimator of the learning curves using two different models for the marginal distribution $p_X(x)$ of predictor variables. The first approach, which we denote "GM", used a Gaussian mixture. Here we stratified the training data into four groups, according to the joint pattern of values for the two binary variables (p53 and IgVH). Within each such group, the mean of the other nine non-binary variables was calculated, and a pooled covariance matrix for these nine variables over the four groups (centered at their respective means) was calculated. The GM model for the predictor variables was a four component Gaussian mixture, where the four components correspond to the four strata determined by the joint values of p53 and IgVH. The mixture components had means equal to the four stratum means in the training data, a common covariance structure equal to the pooled covariance matrix from the data, and marginal frequencies equal to the empirical frequencies of the four subgroups of training data defined by p53 and IgVH.

The second approach to modeling the covariate distribution, which we denote "GC", used a Gaussian copula. Here all data were converted to normal scores, then the correlation matrix of the normal scores was calculated. To produce simulated data from this model, we simulated Gaussian vectors according to this covariance matrix, then transformed each component of these vectors with the corresponding inverse normal scores function. The resulting model for simulated data has marginal distributions exactly equal to the univariate empirical distributions of the training set, and dependence which approximates the training set dependence.

The results are given in Table 7. Four different training set sizes are used (50, 75, 100, 150). For each training set size n, we sampled n observations without replacement from the overall CLL data set of 209 observations. These n observations were used for three purposes: to estimate the misclassification error rate using cross-validated logistic regression, to fit a logistic regression model for $p_{Y|X}(y|x)$, and to fit models for the predictor variable distribution $p_X(x)$ using the GM and GC approaches. Together, $p_X(x)$ and $p_{Y|X}(y|x)$ were used to define the data-generating population $p^*_{Y,X}(y,x) = p_{Y|X}(y|x)p_X(x)$. We then generated data sets of size n, $2n$, and $3n$ from $p^*_{Y,X}(y,x)$, fit another logistic regression model to each of these data sets, and evaluated the accuracy of these fitted rules relative to the data-generating population $p^*_{Y,X}(y,x)$. This process was repeated 1000 times and averaged to produce the results in Table 7.

Table 7 Learning curve analysis for the CLL data

			$\hat{\tau}_{II}$				
	n	CV	n	$2n$	$3n$		
GM	50	0.2775	0.2210	0.1968	0.1881	0.0242	0.0329
GM	75	0.2636	0.2342	0.2157	0.2096	0.0185	0.0246
GM	100	0.2580	0.2340	0.2201	0.2150	0.0139	0.0190
GM	150	0.2363	0.2364	0.2264	0.2227	0.0100	0.0137
GC	50	0.2775	0.2181	0.1922	0.1828	0.0259	0.0353
GC	75	0.2636	0.2387	0.2196	0.2130	0.0191	0.0257
GC	100	0.2580	0.2467	0.2316	0.2263	0.0151	0.0204
GC	150	0.2363	0.2470	0.2358	0.2321	0.0112	0.0149

Columns 7 and 8 show the gain in accuracy when the training set sample size increases from n to $2n$ (i.e. $\hat{\tau}_{II}(2n) - \hat{\tau}_{II}(n)$), and from n to $3n$ (i.e. $\hat{\tau}_{II}(3n) - \hat{\tau}_{II}(n)$), respectively

Table 7 shows that improvement in prediction accuracy of only 2–3 % may occur when increasing the training set sample size by factors of 2–3 in this setting. This result is stable over the two approaches to modeling the predictor variables. As expected, the magnitudes of the gain are greatest for smaller training set sizes, and when the increment in training set size is larger (i.e. when comparing $\hat{\tau}_{II}(3n) - \hat{\tau}_{II}(n)$ to $\hat{\tau}_{II}(2n) - \hat{\tau}_{II}(n)$). Overall, this analysis suggests that only a small improvement in accuracy is likely to result from increasing the training set size in this setting. To achieve more substantial gains in accuracy, more informative markers, or a better modeling approach for capturing the information in these 11 markers should be sought.

As expected, $\hat{\tau}_{II}$ underestimates the error rate, especially when the true error rate is high. This is a consequence of overfitting, since the strength of association in the fitted logistic regression model $\text{expit}P(Y = 1|X = x) = \hat{\beta}'x$ will tend to be stronger that the strength of association in the true model. In particular, if Y and X are independent in the true model, the fitted model will still have some association. As expected, this tendency diminishes as the sample size grows. As a result, $\hat{\tau}_{II}(m)$ tends to increase with m, whereas the CV error, and presumably the true error, decrease with n. We note that for larger sample sizes, the copula model for $p_X(x)$ produces BRIE curve estimates that more closely resemble the cross-validation results.

As noted above, $\hat{\tau}_{II}$ is generally too variable to be useful, so we focus on the accuracy gain, as shown in the final two columns of Table 7. Since we have 209 data points to work with, we directly apply cross-validation on subsamples up to size 209 to provide a direct cross-validation based estimate that is known to be nearly unbiased. For example, under the GC model, the error rate is predicted to drop from 0.2181 to 0.1828 when the training set sample size grows from 50 to 150, a gain of 0.0353. According to the cross-validation estimates, the gain is 0.2775 − 0.2363 = 0.0412. Similarly, when the training set sample size grows from 75 to 150, the predicted gain in classification accuracy using the GC model for $p_X(x)$ is 0.0191, and the corresponding estimate from cross-validation is 0.0273.

6 Discussion

We have discussed three relatively simple approaches for estimating the learning curve of a classifier. SUBEX methods rely on a parametric model of the learning curve, and use unbiased estimates of the classification error rate for sample sizes smaller than the observed training set size to estimate the model parameters. The IMPINT and BRIE methods model the data generating distribution, from which the learning curve can be estimated at arbitrary sample sizes without the need to model the learning curve. The BRIE approach incudes an additional bias reduction step to reduce the tendency of the plug-in estimate of the data-generating model to overstate the strength of the predictive relationship.

Learning curve estimation is a challenging problem, and no method considered here gives highly accurate results. However, we see through example that gains in predictive performance ranging from a low of 0.02 to a high of 0.07 can be observed for three-fold increases in the training set size (Table 4, column 2). In practice it will not be immediately obvious whether we are at the low end or the high end of this range, so having a means to predict the possible gain in performance would be valuable. Knowing that a gain of 0.07 can be achieved may lead to a very different strategy for follow-up research compared to knowing that a gain of only 0.02 should be expected. In the example, the BRIE approach estimates the gain in predictive performance nearly unbiasedly, with a standard error of at most 0.01. This provides us with power to confidently assess whether we are at the low end or the high end of the range of possible gains in performance.

The SUBEX and IMPINT/BRIE approaches differ in several major ways, any of which could impact their performances. One potential drawback of the SUBEX approach is that the inverse power law model for τ may not be able to represent the true learning curve. An exact analytic expression for τ is unlikely to exist, necessitating the use of convenience parameterizations such as the inverse power law. Another concern for SUBEX is its use of cross-validation, which is known to have high variance [4]. This variance may propagate to the learning curve estimate. The IMPINT method is not subject to these limitations, but concerns may arise about the need to estimate the data generating model, which is not necessary for the SUBEX approach.

As noted above, the SUBEX approach models the learning curve, while the IMPINT approach models the full data distribution. The learning curve is a simpler object than the data distribution, hence SUBEX seems to require fewer assumptions. However, the learning curve is not directly observed. Any appropriate statistical modeling framework can be used to obtain an estimate of the data generating model, and diagnostic and other tools are available to assess the fit of the model. Analogous tools for assessing the appropriateness of the learning curve model used by the SUBEX procedure are not readily available. Furthermore, the errors in the SUBEX procedure will be amplified by the need to extrapolate beyond the range of sample sizes that are directly estimated using subsampling. No analogous source of extrapolation variance seems to be present in the IMPINT/BRIE approach.

Learning curves have the potential to become a useful tool in applied statistics. One relevant analogy is to the widely-practiced fields of power analysis and sample size planning. In that setting, preliminary estimates of effect sizes are used to assess the power for various study designs. Learning curves can be viewed as a power analysis tool to be used when the research aims involve prediction rather than estimation and hypothesis testing. In classical power analysis, a range of possible population structures are usually considered rather then basing the determination of power entirely on a noisy point estimate from a small pilot study. In learning curve estimation, it is similarly advisable to consider a range of possibilities for key population parameters when attempting to delineate those situations where substantial gains in predictive performance are expected to occur.

Acknowledgements Eric Laber acknowledges support from NIH grant P01 CA142538 and DNR grant PR-W-F14AF00171. Kerby Shedden acknowledges support from NSF grant NSF-CDSE-MSS-1316731.

References

1. Amari, S., Fujita, N., Shinomoto, S.: Four types of learning curves. Neural Comput. **4**, 605–618 (1992)
2. Breiman, L., Spector, P.: Submodel selection and evaluation in regression. The x-random case. Int. Stat. Rev. **60**(3), 291–319 (1992)
3. Davison, A.C., Hinkley, D.V.: Bootstrap Methods and Their Applications. Cambridge Series in Statistical and Probabilistic Mathematics. Cambridge University Press, Cambridge (1997)
4. Efron, B.: Estimating the error rate of a prediction rule: improvement on cross-validation. J. Am. Stat. Assoc. **78**(382), 316–331 (1983)
5. Efron, B., Tibshirani, R.J.: An Introduction to the Bootstrap. CRC Press, Boca Raton (1994)
6. Friedman, J., Tibshirani, R.: The monotone smoothing of scatterplots. Technometrics **26**(3), 243–250 (1984)
7. Hastie, T., Tibshirani, R., Friedman, J.H.: The Elements of Statistical Learning. Springer, New York (2009)
8. Haussler, D., Kearns, M., Sebastian Seung, H., Tishby, N.: Rigorous learning curve bounds from statistical mechanics. Mach. Learn. **25**, 195–236 (1996)
9. Insel, T.R.: Translating scientific opportunity into public health impact: a strategic plan for research on mental illness. Arch. Gen. Psychiatry **66**(2), 128 (2009)
10. Mukherjee, S., Tamayo, P., Rogers, S., Rifkin, R., Engle, A., Campbell, C., Golub, T.R., Mesirov, J.P.: Estimating dataset size requirements for classifying dna microarray data. J. Comput. Biol. **10**(2), 119–142 (2003)
11. Ouillette, P., Collins, R., Shakhan, S., Li, J., Peres, E., Kujawski, L., Talpaz, M., Kaminski, M., Li, C., Shedden, K., Malek, S.N.: Acquired genomic copy number aberrations and survival in chronic lymphocytic leukemia. Blood **118**(11), 3051–3061 (2011)
12. Rubin, D.B.: Multiple Imputation for Nonresponse in Surveys, vol. 81. Wiley, New York (2004)
13. Snapinn, S.M., Knoke, J.D.: An evaluation of smoothed classification error-rate estimators. Technometrics **27**(2), 199–206 (1985)
14. Toussaint, G.: Bibliography on estimation of misclassification. IEEE Trans. Inf. Theory **20**, 472–479 (1974)
15. Vapnik, V.N.: Estimation of Dependences Based on Empirical Data. Springer, New York (1982)
16. Vapnik, V.N., Chervonenkis, A.Y.: On the uniform convergence of relative frequencies of events to their probabilities. Theory Probab. Appl. **16**, 264–280 (1971)

Bayesian Feature Allocation Models for Tumor Heterogeneity

Juhee Lee, Peter Müller, Subhajit Sengupta, Kamalakar Gulukota, and Yuan Ji

Abstract Tumor samples are composed of subclones that evolve stochastically by acquiring mutations and by selection of those that are beneficial to the survival of the organism or local environment. This process results in the often observed heterogeneity of tumor samples. We review some recent work on a new class of feature allocation models for statistical inference on this tumor heterogeneity. We use next-generation sequencing data. The developed methods identify cell subpopulations (subclones) in tumor samples and allow us to cluster samples based on these identified subclones. We characterize subclones by latent haplotypes that are defined as a scaffold of single nucleotide variations (SNVs) on the same homologous genome. That is, each subclone is defined by a unique set of SNVs. We formally represent these sets of SNVs in a binary matrix with columns corresponding to subclones and entries indicating the presence or absence of a set of SNVs that characterize each subclone. We use a simplified version of the Indian buffet process (IBP) as a prior model on this latent binary matrix. In a model extension we develop a categorical IBP that allows us to incorporate copy number variants (CNVs) in addition to SNVs to jointly define subclones. We illustrate the proposed methods with several data analyses.

J. Lee
UCSC, Santa Cruz, CA, USA
e-mail: juheelee@soe.ucsc.edu

P. Müller (✉)
UT Austin, Austin, TX, USA
e-mail: pmueller@math.utexas.edu

S. Sengupta • Y. Ji • K. Gulukota
NorthShore University HealthSystem, Evanston, IL, USA
e-mail: subhajit06@gmail.com; jiyuan@uchicago.edu; KGulukota@northshore.org

A. Frigessi et al. (eds.), *Statistical Analysis for High-Dimensional Data*,
Abel Symposia 11, DOI 10.1007/978-3-319-27099-9_10

1 Introduction

1.1 Background

We review a model-based Bayesian approach to inference on tumor heterogeneity (TH) based on next generation sequencing (NGS) data. We use data on single nucleotide variants (SNV) as well as copy number variations (CNV). The review is based on original work reported in [15, 16] and [30].

Genomics research is now addressing questions down to the cellular level, including questions such as whether cells in a biological sample possess the same genome or whether there exist distinct subclones with unique and distinct DNAs. Traditional theory assumes that cells in a somatic tissue all have the same genetic contents. This view is now being challenged, especially under disease conditions, such as cancer. In particular, it has been shown that not all cells in a tumor share the same genome [5, 13, 18, 25]. Figure 1 illustrates how such TH can arise as a result of multiple somatic mutations over the lifetime of a tumor, with each mutation occurring in only a fraction of cells. The process leads to a somatically mosaic sample with multiple subclones. This is known as tumor heterogeneity (TH). Each subclone is characterized by a set of specific somatic mutations. This could be a set of SNVs, or it could be structural mutations, such as CNVs. For example, Fig. 1 shows how a normal clone evolves into three different tumor subclones after 360 days and how each subclone is characterized by its unique set of SNVs (in red) and CNVs (in brown) at three loci. Green indicates no mutation. The figure also

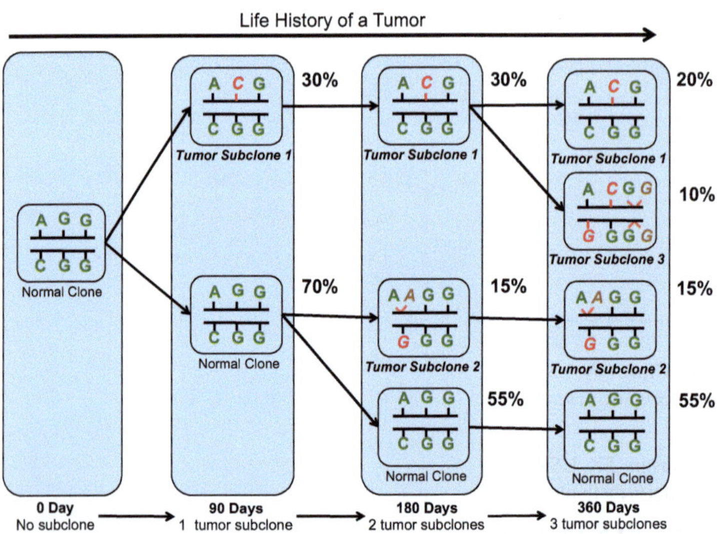

Fig. 1 The figure illustrates the accumulation of variants (SNVs and CNVs) over the life time of a tumor. Each new variant gives rise to two new subclones (cell subpopulations) of tumor cells

illustrates how the make up of the cell population as a composition of the subclones changes, as indicated by the percentages on the figure. Knowing the changes in subclonal structure over time, including the cellular fraction of each subclone (the percentages in the figure), can eventually, in future research, provide the basis for precise and targeted cancer treatment [11, 13, 14, 21]. Therefore, it is important to understand the basic biology of genetic heterogeneity for improved medical decisions on cancer treatment.

Next-generation sequencing (NGS) experiments have been successfully utilized in various genomic studies. NGS enables scientists to examine genetic contents at the single nucleotide level, thus providing opportunities for statistical inference for subclonal genetics. Such inference turns out to be challenging and requires sophisticated tools. A key challenge is the identification of subclones in tissue samples and the differentiation of samples based on these identified subclones.

Recent literature proposes methods of subclone reconstruction using either CNVs, SNVs or both [9, 20, 22, 28, 31]. For example, some methods [20] restrict analysis to copy-neutral regions and regions without loss of heterozygosity and only consider SNVs, and leaving it therefore impossible to reveal subclonal CNV structure. Some approaches use statistical models for (non-overlapping) clustering of SNVs, using, for example inference based on the Dirichlet process (DP) model. While such inference is useful to discover clusters of mutations with similar frequencies, it cannot directly infer subclones which are characterized by overlapping sets of mutations. Compare Fig. 1. Subclones are characterized by (overlapping) subsets of SNVs. Post-hoc computation or awkward constraints are needed to produce the desired clonal inference. Recent attempts in bioinformatics community, while promising, have fallen short of providing consolidated inference mainly due to lack of appropriate statistical models. We aim to fill the gap in the current literature by constructing a Bayesian feature allocation model to perform subclone reconstruction from NGS data.

1.2 Data

In [15] and [16] we develop feature allocation models (FEAMs) to reveal subclonal genetic structure of a biological sample, using NGS data. In NGS, including whole-genome sequencing (WGS) or whole-exome sequencing (WES), DNA sequences of short reads from tumor samples are recorded along with their alignment to the reference genome. At certain positions of the genome, some or all of the mapped reads will show a sequence different from what is in the reference genome (SNVs). In addition, at some positions of the genome more or fewer reads are mapped than at other positions in a sample (CNVs). The raw experimental data comprise the total number of reads ($\boldsymbol{N} = [N_{st}]$, $s = 1, \dots, S$ and $t = 1, \dots, T$) that are mapped to locus s in sample t and the number of those reads ($\boldsymbol{n} = [n_{st}]$) indicating a

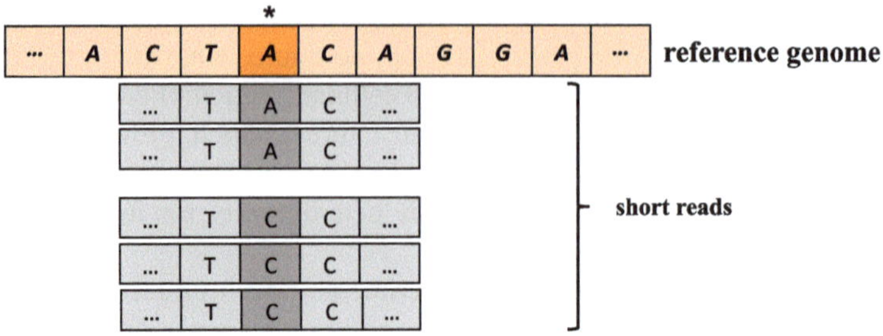

Fig. 2 An illustration of NGS data. The illustration shows that five short reads are mapped to a position marked with * and among them three reads indicate variation at the position, that is, $N_{st} = 5$ and $n_{st} = 3$

variation from the reference sequence. Figure 2 illustrates an example of DNA-Seq data where $N_{st} = 5$ and $n_{st} = 3$ are observed at the locus marked with (*). In [16], we utilized the proportion of short reads bearing a variant sequence at each genomic locus, called the VAF (n_{st}/N_{st}) to construct the haplotypes in the samples. If a tumor sample is homogeneous (i.e., having a single clone) with no CNV, the VAF values of all the loci should be close to 0, 0.5 or 1, reflecting the three possible homozygous and heterozygous alleles (i.e., AA, AB, BB) at any locus. VAF values different from those three values imply heterogeneity of the cellular genome in the tumor sample.

1.2.1 Inferring TH Based on SNVs

We briefly introduce the main elements of the modeling approach. Details are coming up later. We use a binary random matrix (**Z**) to define haplotypes in tumor samples based on SNVs and to quantify heterogeneity across the sample. Figure 3 illustrates an example of **Z** which defines five haplotypes ($C = 5, c = 0, \ldots, 4$) with 10 loci ($S = 10, s = 1, \ldots, S$). We represent the arrangement of SNVs like the could occur, for example, in the last column of Fig. 1 as a binary matrix. Each column, $z_c = (z_{1c}, \ldots, z_{Sc})$ is a binary vector whose elements indicate which haplotype c possesses an SNV at locus s. In the figure, black (white) indicates $z_{sc} = 1$ ($z_{sc} = 0$). For example, locus 1 in Fig. 3 possesses a variant sequence in the two haplotypes $c = 0$ and $c = 1$ (that is, $z_{10} = 1$ and $z_{11} = 1$). On the other hand, locus 9 possesses variant sequences in four haplotypes: $c = 0, 1, 2$ and 4. To proceed with Bayesian inference we need to construct a prior probability model $p(\mathbf{Z})$ for the unknown quantity **Z**. We use a feature allocation model, specifically, a variation of the Indian buffet process (IBP). See, for example, [8] for a recent review of the IBP. In the language of feature allocation models the haplotypes are the features and the loci are the experimental units that select the features. Each tumor sample is composed of these haplotypes. The haplotypes are not directly observed. The number of haplotypes and mixing proportions of the haplotypes for the samples are

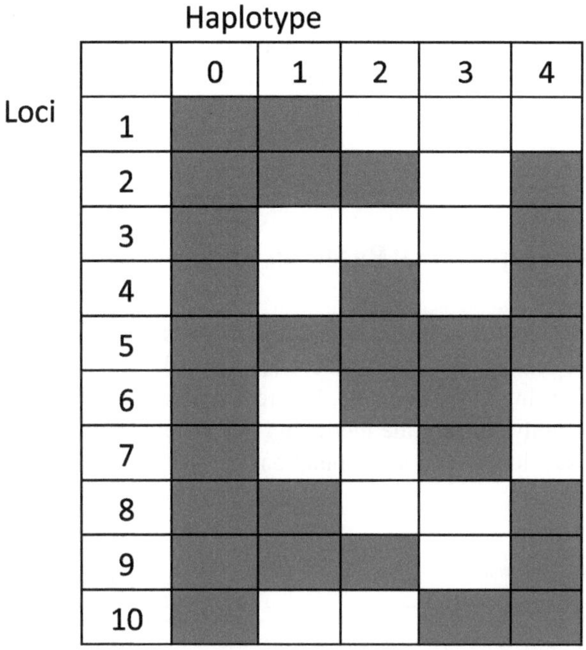

Fig. 3 An illustration of cell types (binary latent features) in columns. A *black/white* block indicates a variant/reference DNA sequence at the corresponding SNV (*row*) for the haplotype (*column*)

also unknown. We deconvolute the observed SNV frequencies for each sample as a composition of latent haplotypes. The details of this development are described in Sect. 2 with some real data example.

1.2.2 TH Based on CNVs and SNVs

Next we define an extension of the model to jointly model SNVs and CNVs. [15] develop such a model, using a categorical IBP (cIBP) for the joint modeling. This model characterizes subclones with SNVs and CNVs as integer vectors corresponding to subclone-specific copy numbers and numbers of variant alleles. A subclone is genetically characterized by both, subclonal sequence variants (i.e., SNVs) and structural variants (i.e., CNVs). For an accurate estimation of subclonal variant allele fractions, subclonal copy numbers need to be accounted for. The proposed model combines both variants and facilitates improved inference on TH. We define a subclone as a set of mutation calls and copy numbers at each of the loci of the recorded SNV's. Having more than one subclone within a sample implies heterogeneity in the sample. Posterior inference under the proposed model provides the desired full description of subclonal genetic structure, including the number of subclones, subclonal copy numbers and the numbers of alleles that possess variant sequences, as well as the cellular fractions of subclones that constitute each sample.

The remainder of the paper is organized as follows: Sect. 2 describes our initial attempt of a Bayesian feature allocation model for TH based on SNV developed in [16]. Section 3 describes another Bayesian feature allocation model extended for joint modeling of SNV and CNV in [15]. The last section concludes with a final discussion.

2 Modeling Haplotypes Based on SNV

We review the model developed in [16] and show some data examples. In [16] we proposed a feature allocation model [1, 2] to describe tumor heterogeneity based on SNVs using DNA-Seq data. Figure 4 illustrates an hypothetical example explaining the motivation for the model in [16]. Panel (a) of the figure shows that there are two subclones (cell subpopulations) in the tumor sample with different

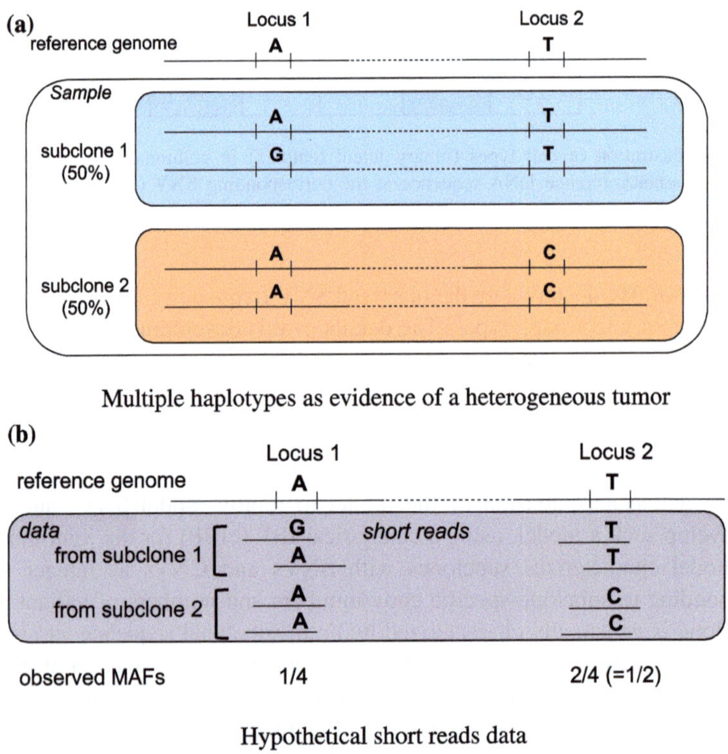

Fig. 4 An hypothetical example explaining how NGS data can be used to infer heterogeneous tumor samples. (**a**) shows that there are two subclones (cell subpopulations) in the tumor sample with different haplotypes consisting of two SNVs. (**b**) shows hypothetical short reads for this sample and observed VAFs assuming the equal proportions of the two subclones

haplotypes consisting of two loci: for subclone 1, there are two haplotypes, AT and GT. For subclone 2 there is only one haplotype, AC due to SNV. Thus, there are a total of three haplotypes in the tumor sample, implying heterogeneous cell populations (a population of homogeneous cells in a diploid organism would only support up to two haplotypes). Here sequence G for locus 1 and sequence C for locus 2 are mutations. Panel (b) shows hypothetical sequencing data of the sample in (a) assuming equal proportions of the two subclones. The short reads counts provide observed VAFs at the two loci. Those observed VAFs are used for statistical inference. In particular, we reconstruct the latent haplotypes in the sample and estimate the proportions of the sample over the identified haplotypes. The details of the model are described and some data analyses are reported below.

2.1 Models

2.1.1 Sampling Model

Suppose that T samples have been sequenced in an NGS experiment. Suppose that we have collected reads mapping data on S loci for the T samples using bioinformatics pipelines such as GATK and Samtools. Let $\boldsymbol{N}$ and $\boldsymbol{n}$ denote $S \times T$ matrices of the counts that are recorded in an NGS experiment, with N_{st} and n_{st} denoting the total number of reads and the number of reads that bear a mutated sequence, respectively, at locus s for tissue sample t, $s = 1, \ldots, S$ and $t = 1, \ldots, T$. We assume a binomial sampling model for n_{st} conditional on N_{st},

$$n_{st} \overset{indep}{\sim} \text{Bin}(N_{st}, p_{st}). \tag{1}$$

Figure 2 illustrates the model in (1) with $n_{st} = 3$ and $N_{st} = 5$. Conditional on N_{st}, the observed counts n_{st} are independent across s and t.

2.1.2 Prior Model

Recall that C denotes the (latent) number of distinct haplotypes. For a given C, a sample is considered as a mixture of C different haplotypes. Later we discuss a probability model for unknown C. Then p_{st} can be described as a sum of latent binary indicators, z_{sc} with weights, w_{tc};

$$p_{st} = w_{t0}p_0 + \sum_{c=1}^{C} w_{tc}z_{sc} \equiv \epsilon_{t0} + \sum_{c=1}^{C} w_{tc}z_{sc}. \tag{2}$$

Here, w_{tc} denotes the proportion of haplotype c in sample t. $z_{sc} \in \{0, 1\}$ indicates occurrence of SNV at locus s in haplotype c. In particular, $z_{sc} = 1$ indicates that haplotype c bears a variant sequence at locus s. Collecting the latent indicators z_{sc} in a $(S \times C)$ binary matrix, Z, we characterize C haplotypes using SNV occurrences at S loci in the observed T samples. In addition to C haplotypes in $\mathbf{Z}$, we introduce a background haplotype, labeled as haplotype $c = 0$ to account for experimental noise and haplotypes that appear with negligible abundance. Assuming equal relative frequency of SNV occurrence at all loci, we let $z_{sc} = 1$, $c = 0$ and all s and p_0 represent the relative frequency of SNV at a locus in the background haplotype. w_{tc}, $c = 0$ denotes the proportions of the background haplotype in sample t. Putting z_{s0}, p_0 and w_{t0} together, we obtain $\epsilon_{t0} = w_{t0}p_0z_{s0} = w_{t0}p_0$ in (2). The prior on $\boldsymbol{w}_t = (w_{t0}, \ldots, w_{tC})$ is defined later. For p_0, we assume $p_0 \sim \text{Be}(a_{00}, b_{00})$ with $a_{00} \ll b_{00}$ to inform a small p_0 value a priori. Joint inference on C, Z and $\boldsymbol{w}_t$ explains tumor heterogeneity.

We formally build a prior probability model for C, z_{sc} and w_{tc}. We start the prior construction with a prior for the number of haplotypes, C and propose prior distributions for z_{sc} and w_{tc} conditional on C. We consider a geometric distribution, $C \sim \text{Geometric}(r)$ where $\text{E}(C) = 1/r$. Conditional on C, we use a feature allocation model for a binary matrix $\mathbf{Z}$. We introduce feature-specific selection probabilities, μ_c, $c = 1, \ldots, C$ conditional on C and define the model of $\mathbf{Z}$ conditional on μ_c, that is, for $c = 1, \ldots, C$ and $s = 1, \ldots, S$,

$$\mu_c \mid C \overset{iid}{\sim} \text{Be}(\alpha/C, 1), \tag{3}$$

$$z_{sc} \mid \mu_c \overset{iid}{\sim} \text{Ber}(\mu_c). \tag{4}$$

A limiting distribution of $\mathbf{Z}$ defined in (3) and (4) by sending $C \to \infty$ is the Indian buffet process (IBP) [7, 29].

Next, we consider a prior distribution for w_{tc}. $\boldsymbol{w}_t = (w_{t0}, \ldots, w_{tC})$, $0 \leq w_{tc} \leq 1$ and $\sum_{c=0}^{C} w_{tc} = 1$, describes abundances of $(C + 1)$ haplotypes defined by $\mathbf{Z}$ in sample t. This implies that tumor samples are composed with common haplotypes but the relative weights in the composition are different across tissue samples, leading to sample-specific p_{st} as shown in (8). We assume Dirichlet priors for the relative weights w_{tc}, $\boldsymbol{w}_t \mid C \overset{iid}{\sim} \text{Dir}(a_0, a, \ldots, a)$ for $t = 1, \ldots, T$.

Recall the binomial sampling likelihood (1) with success probability, p_{st}. Given C, $\mathbf{Z}$ and $\boldsymbol{w}$, we define p_{st} in (2). In words, p_{st} is determined by C, $\mathbf{Z}$ and $\boldsymbol{w}_t$ with the earlier describing the latent haplotypes, and the latter specifying the relative abundance of each haplotype in sample t.

2.1.3 Posterior Inference

Let $\boldsymbol{x} = (\mathbf{Z}, \boldsymbol{w}, p_0)$, where $\boldsymbol{w} = \{w_{tc}\}$. Markov chain Monte Carlo (MCMC) posterior simulation proceeds by repeatedly carrying out transition probabilities that update the parameters in $\boldsymbol{x}$. MCMC posterior simulation for $\boldsymbol{x}$ conditional on C is straightforward. Gibbs sampling transition probabilities are used to update

z_{sc}, and Metropolis-Hastings transition probabilities are used to update $\boldsymbol{w}$ and p_0. In particular, the reparameterization of a Dirichlet random variable with $(C+1)$ independent Gamma random variables can be used in updating $\boldsymbol{w}$.

The number of haplotypes, C determines the dimensions of $\boldsymbol{Z}$ and $\boldsymbol{w}$ and the construction of transition probabilities that involve a change of C is more challenging, since the dimension of $\boldsymbol{Z}$ and $\boldsymbol{w}$ changes as C varies. We use a reversible jump (RJ) MCMC algorithm for posterior simulation [6]. We first define a proposal distribution $q(C, \tilde{C})$ for C, and then introduce a proposal distribution $q(\tilde{\boldsymbol{x}} \mid \tilde{C})$ for $\boldsymbol{x}$ conditional on the proposed $\tilde{C}$. The latter potentially involves a change in dimension of the parameter vector. We found that high posterior correlation of $\boldsymbol{Z}$ and $\boldsymbol{w}$ conditional on C greatly complicated the construction of a practicable RJ scheme. To overcome this, we use an approach similar to [3]. We split the data into a small training set $(\boldsymbol{n}', \boldsymbol{N}')$ with $n'_{st} = b_{st} n_{st}$, $N'_{st} = b_{st} N_{st}$, and a test data set, $(\boldsymbol{n}'', \boldsymbol{N}'')$ with $n''_{st} = (1 - b_{st}) n_{st}$ etc. In the implementation we use $b_{st} \sim \text{Be}(25, 975)$. Let $p_1(\boldsymbol{x} \mid C) = p(\boldsymbol{x} \mid \boldsymbol{n}', C)$ denote the posterior distribution under C using the training sample. We use p_1 in two instances. First, we replace the original prior $p(\boldsymbol{x} \mid C)$ by $p_1(\boldsymbol{x} \mid C)$ and, second, we also use it as proposal distribution $q(\tilde{\boldsymbol{x}} \mid \tilde{C}) = p_1(\tilde{\boldsymbol{x}} \mid \tilde{C})$. The test data is then used to evaluate the acceptance probability. The strategy can be characterized as model comparison by fractional Bayes factors [23] and is related to a similar approach proposed in [3] for model comparison with intrinsic Bayes factors. Both are originally proposed for model comparison with noninformative priors, but can be modified to facilitate MCMC across models as we need it here.

We summarize the joint posterior distribution, $p(C, \boldsymbol{Z}, \boldsymbol{w}, p_0 \mid \boldsymbol{n})$ by factorizing it as $p(C \mid \boldsymbol{n}) p(\boldsymbol{Z} \mid \boldsymbol{n}, C)\, p(\boldsymbol{w}, p_0 \mid \boldsymbol{n}, C, \boldsymbol{Z})$. Based on the available posterior Monte Carlo sample we (approximately) evaluate the marginal posterior distribution for C and determine the maximum a posteriori (MAP) estimate $C^\star$. We then estimate $\boldsymbol{Z}$ conditional on $C^\star$ as follows; For any two matrices, $\boldsymbol{Z}$ and $\boldsymbol{Z}'$, $1 \le c, c' \le C^\star$, let $\mathscr{D}_{cc'}(\boldsymbol{Z}, \boldsymbol{Z}') = \sum_{s=1}^{S} |z_{sc} - z'_{sc'}|$, that is, the difference between two columns, c and c', one from each of the two matrices. We then define a distance $d(\boldsymbol{Z}, \boldsymbol{Z}') = \min \sum_{c=1}^{C^\star} \mathscr{D}_{c,\pi_c}(\boldsymbol{Z}, \boldsymbol{Z}')$, where π_c is a permutation of $\{1, \ldots, C^\star\}$ and the minimum is over all possible permutations. A posterior point estimate for $\boldsymbol{Z}$ is defined as

$$\boldsymbol{Z}^\star = arg \min_{\boldsymbol{Z}'} \int d(\boldsymbol{Z}, \boldsymbol{Z}') dp(\boldsymbol{Z} \mid \boldsymbol{n}, C^\star) \approx arg \min_{\boldsymbol{Z}'} \frac{1}{L} \sum_{\ell=1}^{L} d(\boldsymbol{Z}^{(\ell)}, \boldsymbol{Z}'),$$

for a posterior Monte Carlo sample, $\{\boldsymbol{Z}^{(\ell)}, \ell = 1, \ldots, L\}$. Finally, we report posterior point estimates $\boldsymbol{w}^\star$ and $p_0^\star$ for $\boldsymbol{w}$ and p_0 conditional on $C^\star$ and $\boldsymbol{Z}^\star$.

2.2 *Pancreatic Cancer Data*

NGS data were obtained from exome sequencing of $T = 5$ samples of pancreatic ductal adenocarcinoma (PDAC) patients at Northshore hospital and analyzed in [16]. PDAC is a particularly aggressive tumor with median survival of less than a

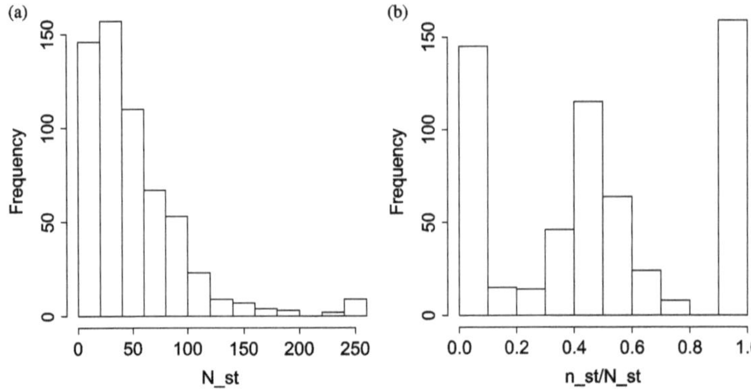

Fig. 5 Pancreatic cancer data: the *left panel* shows a histogram of the total number of mapped reads, N_{st} (**a**), and the *right panel* shows a histogram of the empirical fractions, n_{st}/N_{st} (**b**)

year. We extracted genomic DNA from each tissue and constructed an exome library from these DNA using Agilent SureSelect capture probes. The exome library was then sequenced in paired-end fashion on an Illumina HiSeq 2000 platform. About 60 million reads—each 100 bases long—were obtained. Since the SureSelect exome was about 50 Mega bases, raw (pre-mapping) coverage was about 120 fold. We then mapped the reads to the human genome (version HG19) [4] using BWA [17] and called variants using GATK [19]. Post-mapping, the mean coverage of the samples was between 60 and 70 fold.

A total of nearly 115,000 SNVs and small indels were called within the exome coordinates. A bioinformatics filtering was performed to restrict our attention to SNVs (1) that occur within genes that are annotated to be related to PDAC in the KEGG pathways database [10], (2) that make a difference to the protein translated from the gene, and (3) that exhibit significant coverage in all samples. This filtering left us with $S = 118$ loci for $T = 5$ tumor samples. A summary of the data is presented in Fig. 5. As shown in panel (a) of the figure, the binomial likelihood is very informative due to the large N_{st} values.

To fit the proposed model, we specified the priors by letting $r = 0.2$, $\alpha = 1$, $a = 1$, $a_0 = 1$, $a_{00} = 5$ and $b_{00} = 95$. We generated $b_{st} \sim \text{Be}(25, 975)$ to split the data into a small training and test sets. We ran MCMC posterior simulation over 35,000 iterations, discarding an initial transient of 10,000 iterations.

The resulting posterior inference is summarized in Fig. 6. Panel (a) shows the marginal posterior distribution for C. The posterior mode is $C^{\star} = 4$. The posterior point estimate of $\boldsymbol{Z}$ conditional on $C^{\star}$ is shown in Fig. 6b and the corresponding posterior point estimate of $\boldsymbol{w}$ in Fig. 6c. Here, green (light grey) represents a variant sequence and red (dark green) represents a reference sequence. We find that each sample has two or three two dominant haplotypes, that is, two green (light grey) columns for each row in the heatmap. Haplotypes 2, 3, 4 are shared by different sets of the five samples. For example, sample 2 has a large scaled abundance level for haplotypes 1, 2 and 3. Sample 4 is mainly dominated by haplotypes 1 and 3.

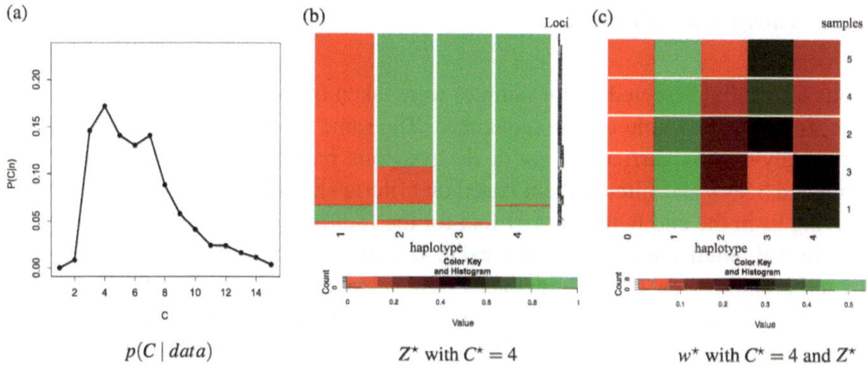

Fig. 6 Pancreatic cancer data: the posterior distribution of C in (**a**), the heatmaps of $\boldsymbol{Z}^\star$ and $\boldsymbol{w}^\star$ with $C^\star = 4$ in (**b**) and (**c**), respectively. Note that for $c = 0$, $p_0^\star z_{t0}^\star$ is illustrated in the first column of panel (**c**)

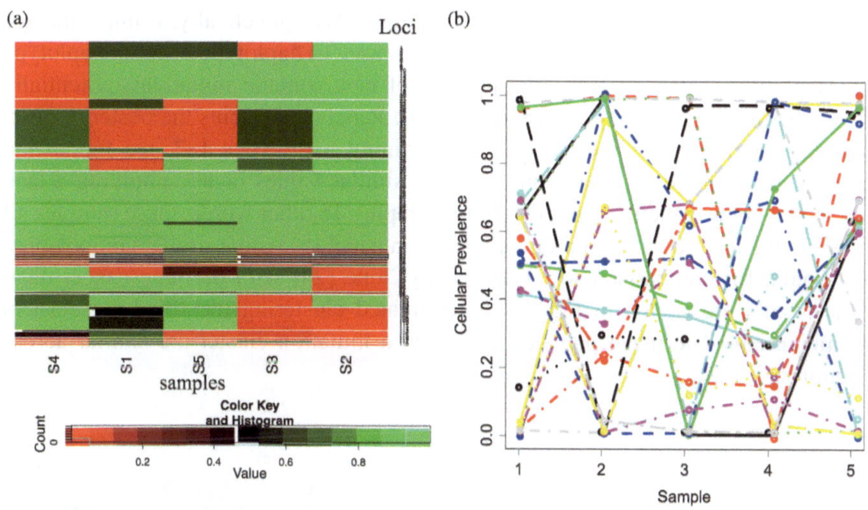

Fig. 7 Pancreatic cancer data: estimated cellular prevalence of loci clusters over samples by PyClone. (**a**) Heatmap of cellular prevalence. (**b**) Mean prevalence for each cluster

These results indicate that while tumors are unique, there are haplotypes shared by different patients. The results also clearly show that each tumor (in this data) is made of more than one haplotype: usually two or three dominant haplotypes and other minor types. To our knowledge, this is the first attempt to analyze the internal clonal composition of multiple PDAC tumor samples based on NGS data.

For comparison, we also evaluated tumor heterogeneity for the same pancreatic cancer data using PyClone [24]. The results are shown in Fig. 7. The posterior estimated clustering includes 24 loci clusters, shown in panel (a). The estimated mean cellular prevalences of each cluster across the five samples are shown in (b). The estimated mean cellular prevalences vary substantially across samples.

2.3 Lung Cancer Data

Four surgically dissected tumor samples were taken from the same patient with lung cancer and were whole-exome sequenced. The same bioinformatics pre-processing and analysis was carried out as in the previous pancreatic cancer example. We obtained SNVs and filtered them based on criteria similar to the previous example, leaving us in the end with $S = 101$ loci for the four intra-tumor samples.

We estimated the proposed Bayesian feature allocation model with the same hyperparameters as in the previous PDAC data analysis. Figure 8 summarizes the inference results. Panel (a) shows the marginal posterior distribution for C, identifying a posterior mode at $C^\star = 3$, that is three distinct haplotypes. Panel (b) shows the posterior point estimate, $\boldsymbol{Z}^\star$, conditional on $C^\star = 3$. The figure shows which loci possess SNV for each of the three haplotypes. Haplotype 3 contains the smallest number of mutations (green or light grey bars), implying that haplotype 3 might be the parental tumor cells. Haplotypes 1 and 2 are descendants of haplotype 3 with additional somatic mutations. Phylogenetically, a simple lineage can be hypothesized, with haplotype 3 as the parent of haplotype 1 and\or haplotype 2. Haplotype 2 possesses a large number of new somatic mutations, potentially representing a type of aggressive tumor cells. Panel (c) presents the posterior point estimate of $\boldsymbol{w}$, $\boldsymbol{w}^\star$ with $C^\star$ and $\boldsymbol{Z}^\star$. Examining haplotypes 1–3, we found that interestingly, all four tumor samples share similar values of $\boldsymbol{w}_t^\star$, implying a lack of spatial heterogeneity across the tumor samples. In other words, these samples all possess the inferred three tumor haplotypes in panel (b) with a similar composition.

Again, for comparison we also used PyClone [24] with the lung cancer data. The results are shown in Fig. 9. The estimated clustering identified six clusters of mutations. The mean prevalences within a mutation cluster are similar across samples.

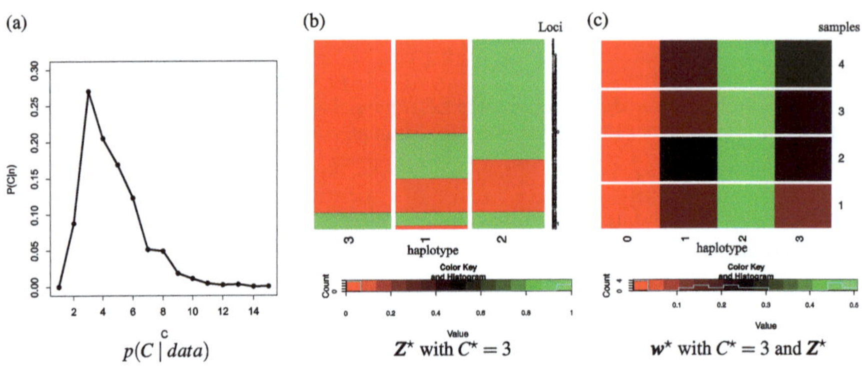

Fig. 8 Lung cancer data: the posterior distribution of C in (**a**), the heatmaps of $\boldsymbol{Z}^\star$ and $\boldsymbol{w}^\star$ with $C^\star = 3$ in (**b**) and (**c**), respectively. Note that for $c = 0$, $p_0^\star z_{t0}^\star$ is illustrated in the first column of panel (**c**)

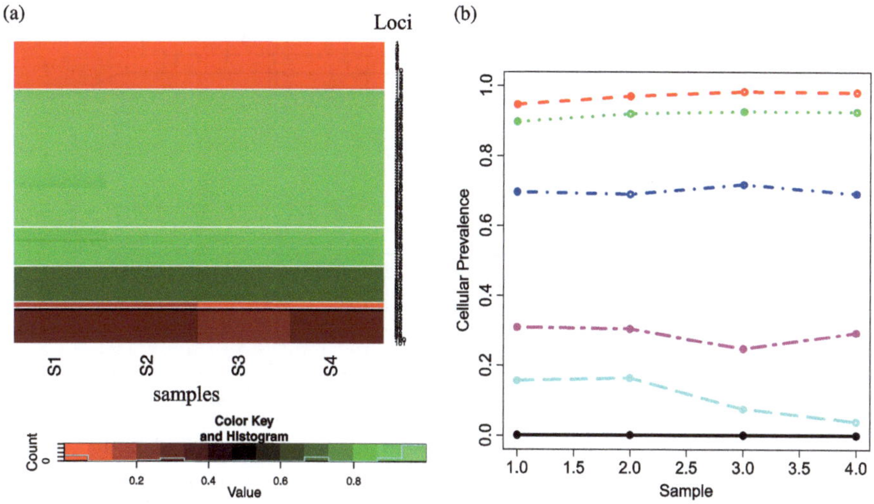

Fig. 9 Lung cancer data: estimated cellular prevalence of loci clusters over samples by PyClone. (**a**) Heatmap of cellular prevalence. (**b**) Mean prevalence for each cluster

3 Modeling Subclones Based on SNV and CNV

In [16] we build on the model of Sect. 2 to propose a Bayesian approach for joint modeling of CNVs and SNVs using deep DNA-Seq data. The extended model allows a subclone to have the copy number different from two. That is, it is assumed that subclonal CNVs as well as subclonal SNVs at the same loci are latent. The subclonal structure, as characterized by patterns of CNV and SNVs, is reconstructed to infer tumor heterogeneity using DNA-Seq data. The total number of reads and the number of reads with variant sequence in DNA-Seq data are used as data for CNVs and SNVs, respectively. TH is inferred as a decomposition of observed mutation frequencies into a mixture of latent subclones. The data are counts of aligned reads at each locus, as illustrated in Fig. 2. Figure 10 illustrates how TH is reflected in NGS data. In the illustration, a tumor sample has two hypothetical subclones that differ in CNVs and SNVs at the two shown loci. Suppose that the proportions of the two subclones in the sample are 0.75 and 0.25. Considering CNVs as shown in the figure, the expected copy numbers at the two loci become 2.75 and 1.75, respectively. This implies that 1.57 times as many reads are expected to be observed at locus 1 compared to locus 2 due to the CNVs. For locus 1, one allele in subclone 1 is mutated (G) and two alleles are not (A); in contrast both alleles in subclone 2 are not mutated (A). Therefore, at locus 1 the expected copy number with variant allele is $0.75(= 0.75 \times 1 + 0.25 \times 0)$, i.e., a weighted average across two subclones with weights being the relative proportions of the subclones. The expected variant allele fraction (VAF) is $0.27(= 0.75/2.75)$, which is the fraction of expected copy number with variant allele over the expected copy number. This implies that 27 % of short reads mapped to locus 1 may possess a variant sequence in DNA-Seq data.

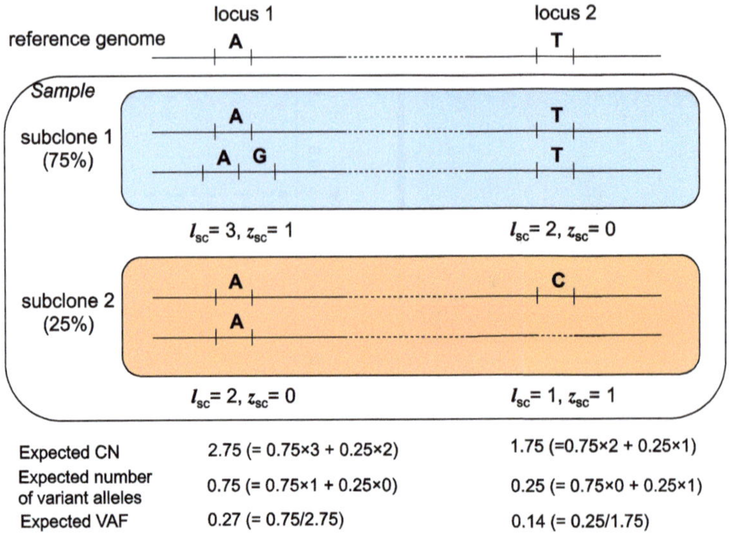

Fig. 10 A hypothetical example explaining how NGS data can be used for joint modeling of CNV and SNV. The figure shows that there are two subclones in a tumor sample with two loci: Subclone 1 has three copies at locus 1 and two copies at locus 2. Subclone 2 has two copies at locus 1 and one copy at locus 2. In addition, in subclone 1, among the three copies of locus 1, one copy possesses the mutated sequence and in subclone 2, one copy at locus 2 has the mutated sequence

In [15], we proposed a new Bayesian feature allocation model [1] to implement the ideas explained above using the observed NGS data. We first constructed an integer-valued matrix $\boldsymbol{L}$ to characterize subclonal copy numbers. Each column corresponds to a subclone and rows correspond to loci. Each column vector $\boldsymbol{\ell}_c = (\ell_{1c}, \ldots, \ell_{Sc})$ of integers is used to represent copy numbers at locus s for subclone c. For example, in Fig. 10, $\ell_{sc} = 3$ for $s = 1$ and $c = 1$ since subclone 1 has four alleles locus 1. As prior $p(\boldsymbol{L})$, we defined a finite version of a categorical Indian buffet process [26, 27]. Next, we introduced a second matrix $\boldsymbol{Z}$ with the same dimensions as $\boldsymbol{L}$ to record SNV's. Different from the previous approach, each column of $\boldsymbol{Z}$ represents the number of alleles with a variant sequence different from the reference sequence at the loci and is integer-valued. In particular, denoting by z_c the c-th column of $\boldsymbol{Z}$ conditional on $\boldsymbol{\ell}_c$, $z_c = (z_{1c}, \ldots, z_{Sc})$ represents the number of copies with a variant sequence at locus s, $s = 1, \ldots, S$ in subclone c. For example, in Fig. 10, $z_{sc} = 1$ for $s = 1$ and $c = 1$, indicating that one allele bears a variant sequence. The two random integer vectors, $\boldsymbol{\ell}_c$ and z_c describe a subclone and its genetic architecture at the corresponding loci. The remainder of this section describes the details of the model and a data analysis.

3.1 Models

3.1.1 Sampling Model

Recall that $\boldsymbol{N} = [N_{st}]$ and $\boldsymbol{n} = [n_{st}]$ denote the total number of reads and the number of reads that bear a mutated sequence, respectively, at locus s for tissue sample t, $s = 1, \ldots, S$ and $t = 1, \ldots, T$, from NSG experiments. Different from the approach in Sect. 2, we utilize N_{st} to model sample- and locus-specific copy numbers, denoted by M_{st} (which will later be decomposed similar to p_{st} in (2)). We assume a Poisson sampling model for N_{st},

$$N_{st} \mid \phi_t, M_{st} \overset{indep}{\sim} \text{Poi}(\phi_t M_{st}/2). \tag{5}$$

Here, ϕ_t adjusts differences in average numbers of reads among T samples at a locus with no CNV. The parameter ϕ_t can be interpreted as sequencing depth in sample t. Here, M_{st} is a sum of subclone specific copy numbers with weights being the proportion of subclone c in tissue sample t, w_{tc}. The construction of M_{st} based on subclonal copy number matrix $\boldsymbol{L}$ and subclone abundance matrix $\boldsymbol{w}$ will be discussed later in detail, as part of the prior construction. If there are no copy number variations in any subclone, then $M_{st} = 2$ and the Poisson mean becomes ϕ_t. Similar to (1), given N_{st} a binomial sampling model is assumed for n_{st};

$$n_{st} \mid N_{st}, p_{st} \overset{indep}{\sim} \text{Bin}(N_{st}, p_{st}). \tag{6}$$

Here p_{st} is the success probability of observing a read with a variant sequence at locus s in sample t. Similar to the previous development, we use subclonal SNV matrix $\boldsymbol{Z}$ to model p_{st}.

3.1.2 Construction of M_{st}

We assume the number of subclones in T samples, C is unknown. For any given C, the decomposition of M_{st} into subclonal CNVs, ℓ_{sc} with weights, w_{tc} is

$$M_{st} = \ell_{s0} w_{t0} + \sum_{c=1}^{C} w_{tc} \ell_{sc}, \tag{7}$$

where we have added the first term for a background subclone $c = 0$, to account for subclones that have negligible abundance in the sample, similar to ϵ_{t0} in (2). The abundance level of subclone c in sample t, w_{tc} is defined as the same as before. $\ell_{sc} \in \{0, 1, 2, \ldots, Q\}$ represent copy number at locus s in subclone c, where Q is a pre-specified maximum number of copies. The event $\ell_{sc} = 2$ means no copy number variant at locus s in subclone c and $\ell_{sc} \neq 2$ implies CNV, for example, $\ell_{sc} = 1$

indicates one copy loss and $\ell_{sc} = 3$ indicates one copy gain. We fix $\ell_{s0} = 2$, that is, we assume no CNV in the background subclone. ℓ_{sc}, $s = 1, \ldots, S$ and $c = 1, \ldots, C$ are collected in $S \times C$ integer matrix.

3.1.3 Prior on L

We now develop a prior distribution for a latent random matrix of copy numbers, $\boldsymbol{L} = [\ell_{sc}]$, where $\ell_{sc} \in \{0, 1, 2, \ldots, Q\}$ for $c = 1, \ldots, C$ and $s = 1, \ldots, S$. We first introduce a latent probability of having q copies in subclone c, $p(\ell_{sc} = q) = \pi_{cq}$. Assuming a priori independence among subclones, let $\boldsymbol{\pi}_c = (\pi_{c0}, \ldots, \pi_{cQ})$, $0 < \pi_{cq} < 1$ and $\sum_{q=0}^{Q} \pi_{cq} = 1$, $c = 1, \ldots, C$, i.i.d from a beta-Dirichlet distribution [12]:

$$\boldsymbol{\pi}_c \overset{iid}{\sim} \text{Be-Dir}(\alpha/C, \beta, \gamma_0, \gamma_1, \gamma_3, \ldots, \gamma_Q)$$

This implies that $p(\ell_{sc} \neq 2) = (1 - \pi_{c2})$ follows a beta distribution with parameters, α/C and β and conditional on $(1 - \pi_{c2})$, $\tilde{\boldsymbol{\pi}} = (\tilde{\pi}_{c0}, \tilde{\pi}_{c1}, \tilde{\pi}_{c3}, \ldots, \tilde{\pi}_{cQ})$, where $\tilde{\pi}_{cq} = \pi_{cq}/(1 - \pi_{c2})$ with $q \neq 2$, follows a Dirichlet distribution with parameters, $(\gamma_0, \gamma_1, \gamma_3, \ldots, \gamma_Q)$. Given C and $\boldsymbol{\pi}_c$, we let

$$p(\boldsymbol{L} \mid C, \boldsymbol{\pi}) = \prod_{s=1}^{S} \prod_{c=1}^{C} \prod_{q=0}^{Q} \pi_{cq}^{m_{cq}}$$

where the number of loci having q copies in subclone c, $m_{cq} = \sum_{s=1}^{S} I(\ell_{sc} = q)$. For $\beta = 1$, the marginal limiting distribution of $\boldsymbol{L}$ can be shown to define a categorical Indian buffet process (cIBP) as $C \to \infty$ [26, 27].

3.1.4 Construction of p_{st} and Prior $p(Z \mid L)$

For each locus s and subclone c, let $z_{sc} \in \{0, \ldots, \ell_{sc}\}$ denote the number of copies among the ℓ_{sc} copies that are bearing a variant sequence. Then the expected copy number with variant allele among the M_{st} copies can be expressed as $m_{st} = p_0 z_{s0} w_{t0} + \sum_{c=1}^{C} w_{tc} z_{sc}$. We add an additional term for a background subclone $c = 0$ similar to (7). The success probability in (6) is defined as

$$p_{st} = \frac{m_{st}}{M_{st}} = \frac{p_0 z_{s0} w_{t0} + \sum_{c=1}^{C} w_{tc} z_{sc}}{M_{st}}. \tag{8}$$

We fix $z_{s0} = 2$ for all s and add a global parameter p_0 to account for artifacts and experimental noise that would produce variant reads even if the subclones are not variant. Since p_0 does not depend on s or t, it can be estimated pooling data from all loci and samples and does not affect the identifiability of the model. We assume $p_0 \sim \text{Be}(a_{00}, b_{00})$ with $a_{00} \ll b_{00}$ to shrink p_0 to small values a priori. In words, p_{st}, the proportion of reads with SNV at locus s in sample t is the expected proportion of alleles having SNV. We continue the model construction with a prior $p(z_{sc} \mid \ell_{sc})$. Given ℓ_{sc}, we assume that z_{sc} is equally likely to be any integer in $\{0, \ldots, \ell_{sc}\}$. That is,

$$p(z_{sc} = z \mid \ell_{sc}) = \frac{1}{\ell_{sc} + 1}$$

and $z_{sc} = 0$ if $l_{sc} = 0$.

3.1.5 Priors for w, C and ϕ

We consider the same prior distributions for $\boldsymbol{w}_t$ and C in Sect. 3 as follows. The C subclones jointly defined in $\boldsymbol{L}$ and $\boldsymbol{Z}$ are common among all tumor samples, but their relative weights w_{tc} vary across tumor samples. we consider independent Dirichlet distributions for weights $\boldsymbol{w}_t$ in (7) and (8). That is, $\boldsymbol{w}_t \mid C \overset{iid}{\sim} \text{Dir}(d_0, d, \ldots, d)$ for $t = 1, \ldots, T$. Using $d_0 < d$ implies that the background subclone takes a smaller proportion in a sample. We also let the unknown number of latent subclones C follow a geometric distribution, $C \sim \text{Geom}(r)$ where $\text{E}(C) = 1/r$.

Lastly, we take account of different average read counts in T samples through ϕ_t. ϕ_t represent the expected read counts with two copies in sample t and assume $\phi_t \overset{indep}{\sim} \text{Gamma}(a_t, b_t)$ where $\text{E}(\phi_t) = a_t/b_t$. Recalling (5), N_{st} is determined by the average read count in sample t, ϕ_t and latent copy number at position s in sample t, M_{st}, in words.

The proposed model constructs C latent tumor subclones that are thought of composing the observed samples using the two latent matrices, $\boldsymbol{L}$ and $\boldsymbol{Z}$, conditional on C. Noting that $\boldsymbol{L}$ and $\boldsymbol{Z}$ are not directly observable, we use $\boldsymbol{n}$ and $\boldsymbol{N}$ to infer the latent structure including C. Joint inference on C, $\boldsymbol{L}$, $\boldsymbol{Z}$ and $\boldsymbol{w}_t$ explains tumor heterogeneity.

3.1.6 Posterior Simulation

The posterior simulation approach proposed in Sect. 2.1 can be extended for this generalized model with some minor modifications only. The unknown parameters are $\boldsymbol{x} = (\boldsymbol{L}, \boldsymbol{Z}, \boldsymbol{w}, \boldsymbol{\phi}, \boldsymbol{\pi}, p_0)$, where $\boldsymbol{w} = \{w_{tc}\}$ and $\boldsymbol{\pi} = \{\pi_{cq}\}$. Similar to the SNV only model, for fixed C, Gibbs sampling transition probabilities are used to update ℓ_{sc}, z_{sc}, π_{cq} and ϕ_t and Metropolis-Hastings transition probabilities are used to update $\boldsymbol{w}$ and p_0. Updating C is again implemented by the strategy of splitting the data into a small training set $(\boldsymbol{n}', \boldsymbol{N}')$ with $n'_{st} = b_{st} n_{st}$, $N'_{st} = b_{st} N_{st}$, and a test data set, $(\boldsymbol{n}'', \boldsymbol{N}'')$ with $n''_{st} = (1 - b_{st}) n_{st}$ etc, proposed in Sect. 2.1.

To summarize the joint posterior distribution, we first select MAP estimate of C, $C^{\star}$. Conditioning on $C^{\star}$, we find a posterior point estimate for $\boldsymbol{L}$, $\boldsymbol{L}^{\star}$ following [16]. Posterior point estimates $\boldsymbol{Z}^{\star}$, $\boldsymbol{w}^{\star}$ and $\boldsymbol{\pi}^{\star}$ are reported conditional on $C^{\star}$ and $\boldsymbol{L}^{\star}$. Finally, the posterior mean of $\boldsymbol{\phi}$ and p_0 are also reported conditional on $C^{\star}$.

3.2 *Lung Cancer Data*

The lung cancer dataset in Sect. 2.3 was re-analyzed in [15] by the model extended for CNV. The same bioinformatics pre-processing was conducted, resulting in having in the end $S = 101$ SNVs for the four intra-tumor samples ($T = 4$). Figure 11 shows the histograms of the total number of reads and the empirical read ratios, N_{st} and n_{st}/N_{st}.

To fit the proposed model, we fixed the hyperparameters as $r = 0.2$, $\alpha = 3$, $\gamma_q = 0.5$ for $q = 0, 1, 3(= Q)$, $d_0 = 0.5$, $d = 1$, $a_{00} = 0.3$ and $b_{00} = 5$. For the prior of ϕ_t, we let $b = 10$ and specified a by setting the median of the observed N_{st} to be the prior mean. For each value of C, we initialized $\boldsymbol{Z}$ using the observed sample proportions and $\boldsymbol{L}$ using the initial $\boldsymbol{Z}$. We generated initial values for $\boldsymbol{\theta}_{tc}$ and p_0 by prior draws. We generated $b_{st} \overset{iid}{\sim} \text{Be}(30, 970)$ to construct the training set and ran the MCMC simulation over 18,000 iterations, discarding the first 8000 iterations as initial burn-in.

Figure 12 summarizes posterior inference under the proposed model. Panel (a) shows $C^{\star} = 2$, i.e., two estimated subclones. Using posterior samples with $C = C^{\star}$, we computed $\hat{N}_{st}$ and $\hat{p}_{st}$ and compared them to the observed data. The differences are centered at 0, implying a good fit to the data. Conditional on $C^{\star} = 2$, we found $\boldsymbol{L}^{\star}$, $\boldsymbol{Z}^{\star}$ and $\boldsymbol{w}^{\star}$. The loci in $\boldsymbol{L}^{\star}$ and $\boldsymbol{Z}^{\star}$ are re-arranged in the same order for better illustration. From Fig. 11a we notice that many positions have large numbers of reads, over 200 reads. This is reflected in $\boldsymbol{L}^{\star}$ which estimates three copies at many

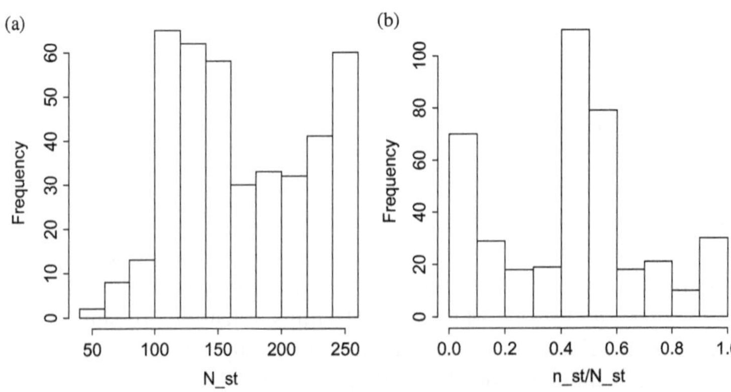

Fig. 11 Lung cancer data. (**a**) Histogram of N_{st}. (**b**) Histogram of n_{st}/N_{st}

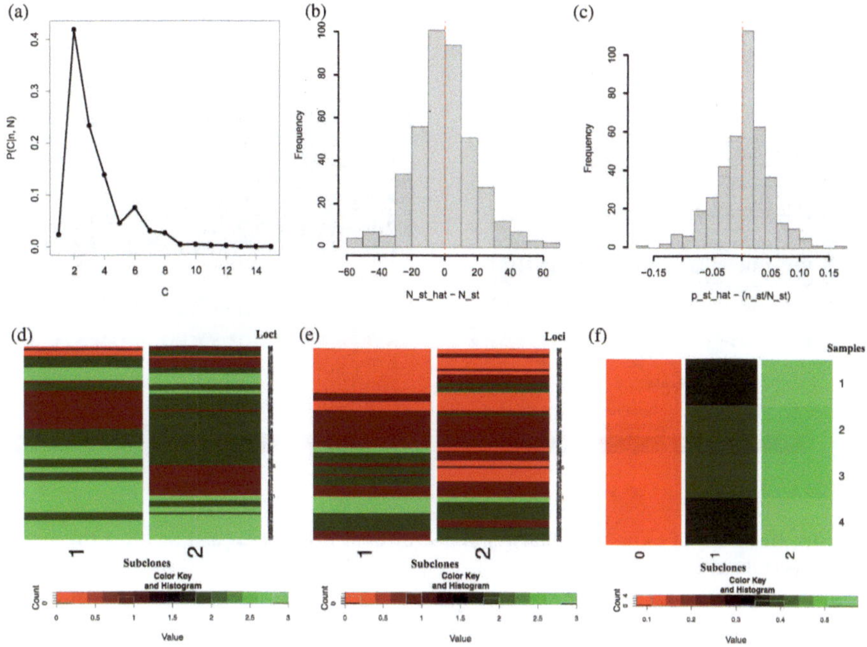

Fig. 12 Posterior inference for the lung cancer dataset. (**a**) $p(C \mid \boldsymbol{n}, N)$. (**b**) $\hat{N}_{st} - N_{st}$. (**c**) $\hat{p}_{st} - (n_{st}/N_{st})$. (**d**) $\boldsymbol{L}^{\star}$. (**e**) $\boldsymbol{Z}^{\star}$. (**f**) $\boldsymbol{w}^{\star}$

positions. The estimated weights $\boldsymbol{w}^{\star}$ in Fig. 12f show a great similarity across the four samples. This may be due to the fact that the four samples were dissected from close-by spatial locations in the tumor. Also, this is similar to what we found in Sect. 2.3.

Again, for comparison we implemented PyClone [24] for the lung cancer data. Different from the analysis by PyClone in Sect. 2.3, PyClone was set to consider copy number changes. We let the normal copy number, the minor parental copy number and the major parental copy number be 2, 0 and 3, respectively, at each locus. PyClone considers copy number changes and estimates the variant allelic prevalence (fraction of clonal population having a mutation) at a locus in a sample. The interpretation of variant allelic prevalences, referred to as "cellular prevalences" in PyClone, is similar to that of p_{st} in the proposed model. The posterior estimates of prevalence and the estimated clustering of the loci are shown in Fig. 13a. The clustering identified five clusters of the loci. The mean prevalences within a locus cluster are similar across samples, which is similar to $\boldsymbol{w}^{\star}$ in Fig. 12f. Panel (b) of Fig. 13 is a heatmap of fractions of reads bearing mutation for each locus and sample. Again, PyClone provides a reasonable estimate of a loci clustering based on the empirical fractions, but does not provide an inference on subclonal populations.

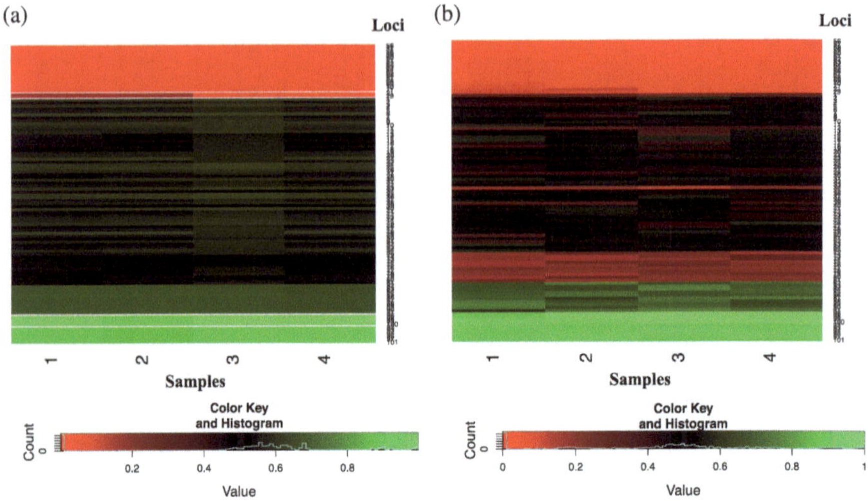

Fig. 13 Heatmaps of estimated cellular prevalences from PyClone (**a**) and (n_{st}/N_{st}) (**b**) for the lung cancer dataset

4 Conclusion

We presented the two Bayesian feature allocation models for TH developed in [16] and [15]. The proposed approaches infer the exact DNA sequences of each haplotype or subclone. They yield inference on the number and proportions of haplotypes or subclones in the sample. The inference produced by the developed methods will significantly impact downstream treatment of individual tumors, ultimately allowing personalized prognosis. For example, tumor samples with large proportions of cells bearing somatic mutations on tumor suppressor genes should be treated differently from those that have no or a small proportion of such cells. In addition, metastatic or recurrent tumors may possess very different compositions of cellular genomes and should be treated differently. Inference on TH can be exploited for improved treatment strategies for relapsed cancer patients, and can facilitate a significantly improvement in cancer treatment in practice.

A number of extensions are possible for the present model. For example, additional sources of information on CNVs such as a SNP array can be incorporated by extending the proposed model when such information is available, leading to improved inference on TH including $\boldsymbol{L}$. Another meaningful extension that we can consider is to cluster patients on the basis of the imputed TH, that is, we link a random partition and a feature allocation model. This extension may help clinicians assign different treatment strategies, and be the basis of adaptive clinical trial designs.

Acknowledgements Yuan Ji and Peter Müller's research is partially supported by NIH R01 CA132897.

References

1. Broderick, T., Jordan, M.I., Pitman, J., et al.: Cluster and feature modeling from combinatorial stochastic processes. Stat. Sci. **28**(3), 289–312 (2013)
2. Broderick, T., Pitman, J., Jordan, M.I.: Feature allocations, probability functions, and paintboxes. Bayesian Anal. **8**, 801–836 (2013)
3. Casella, G., Moreno, E.: Objective Bayesian variable selection. J. Am. Stat. Assoc. **101**(473), 157–167 (2006)
4. Church, D.M., Schneider, V.A., Graves, T., Auger, K., Cunningham, F., Bouk, N., Chen, H.C., Agarwala, R., McLaren, W.M., Ritchie, G.R., et al.: Modernizing reference genome assemblies. PLoS Biol. **9**(7), e1001091 (2011)
5. Gerlinger, M., Rowan, A., Horswell, S., Larkin, J., Endesfelder, D., Gronroos, E., Martinez, P., Matthews, N., Stewart, A., Tarpey, P., Varela, I., Phillimore, B., Begum, S., McDonald, N., Butler, A., Jones, D., Raine, K., Latimer, C., Santos, C., Nohadani, M., Eklund, A., Spencer-Dene, B., Clark, G., Pickering, L., Stamp, G., Gore, M., Szallasi, Z., Downward, J., Futreal, P., Swanton, C.: Intratumor heterogeneity and branched evolution revealed by multiregion sequencing. N. Engl. J. Med. **366**(10), 883–892 (2012)
6. Green, P.J.: Reversible jump Markov chain Monte Carlo computation and Bayesian model determination. Biometrika **82**(4), 711–732 (1995)
7. Griffiths, T.L., Ghahramani, Z.: Infinite latent feature models and the Indian buffet process. In: Neural Information Processing Systems, pp. 475–482. MIT Press, Cambridge (2005)
8. Griffiths, T.L., Ghahramani, Z.: The Indian buffet process: an introduction and review. J. Mach. Learn. Res. **12**, 1185–1224 (2011)
9. Jiao, W., Vembu, S., Deshwar, A., Stein, L., Morris, Q.: Inferring clonal evolution of tumors from single nucleotide somatic mutations. BMC Bioinf. **15**(1), 35 (2014). doi:10.1186/1471-2105-15-35. http://www.biomedcentral.com/1471-2105/15/35
10. Kanehisa, M., Goto, S., Furumichi, M., Tanabe, M., Hirakawa, M.: KEGG for representation and analysis of molecular networks involving diseases and drugs. Nucleic Acids Res. **38**(Suppl. 1), D355–D360 (2010)
11. Keats, J.J., Chesi, M., Egan, J.B., Garbitt, V.M., Palmer, S.E., Braggio, E., Van Wier, S., Blackburn, P.R., Baker, A.S., Dispenzieri, A., et al.: Clonal competition with alternating dominance in multiple myeloma. Blood **120**(5), 1067–1076 (2012)
12. Kim, Y., James, L., Weissbach, R.: Bayesian analysis of multistate event history data: beta-Dirichlet process prior. Biometrika **99**(1), 127–140 (2012)
13. Landau, D., Carter, S., Stojanov, P., McKenna, A., Stevenson, K., Lawrence, M., Sougnez, C., Stewart, C., Sivachenko, A., Wang, L., Wan, Y., Zhang, W., Shukla, S., Vartanov, A., Fernandes, S., Saksena, G., Cibulskis, K., Tesar, B., Gabriel, S., Hacohen, N., Meyerson, M., Lander, E., Neuberg, D., Brown, J., Getz, G., Wu, C.: Evolution and impact of subclonal mutations in chronic lymphocytic leukemia. Cell **152**(4), 714–726 (2013)
14. Lee, A.J., Endesfelder, D., Rowan, A.J., Walther, A., Birkbak, N.J., Futreal, P.A., Downward, J., Szallasi, Z., Tomlinson, I.P., Howell, M., et al.: Chromosomal instability confers intrinsic multidrug resistance. Cancer Res. **71**(5), 1858–1870 (2011)
15. Lee, J., Müller, P., Sengupta, S., Gulukota, K., Ji, Y.: Bayesian inference for tumor subclones accounting for sequencing and structural variants. Technical report, Applied Mathematics and Statistics, University of California Santa Cruz (2014)
16. Lee, J., Müller, P., Gulukota, K., Ji, Y.: A Bayesian feature allocation model for tumor heterogeneity. Ann. Appl. Stat. **9**, 621–639 (2015)

17. Li, H., Durbin, R.: Fast and accurate short read alignment with Burrows–Wheeler transform. Bioinformatics **25**(14), 1754–1760 (2009)
18. Marusyk, A., Polyak, K.: Tumor heterogeneity: causes and consequences. Biochim. Biophys. Acta **1085**(1), 105–117 (2010)
19. McKenna, A., Hanna, M., Banks, E., Sivachenko, A., Cibulskis, K., Kernytsky, A., Garimella, K., Altshuler, D., Gabriel, S., Daly, M., et al.: The genome analysis toolkit: a mapreduce framework for analyzing next-generation DNA sequencing data. Genome Res. **20**(9), 1297–1303 (2010)
20. Miller, C.A., White, B.S., Dees, N.D., Griffith, M., Welch, J.S., Griffith, O.L., Vij, R., Tomasson, M.H., Graubert, T.A., Walter, M.J., et al.: Sciclone: inferring clonal architecture and tracking the spatial and temporal patterns of tumor evolution. PLoS Comput. Biol. **10**(8), e1003665 (2014)
21. Navin, N., Krasnitz, A., Rodgers, L., Cook, K., Meth, J., Kendall, J., Riggs, M., Eberling, Y., Troge, J., Grubor, V., et al.: Inferring tumor progression from genomic heterogeneity. Genome Res. **20**(1), 68–80 (2010)
22. Oesper, L., Mahmoody, A., Raphael, B.J.: Theta: inferring intra-tumor heterogeneity from high-throughput dna sequencing data. Genome Biol. **14**(7), R80 (2013)
23. O'Hagan, A.: Fractional Bayes factors for model comparison. J. R. Stat. Soc. B **57**, 99–138 (1995)
24. Roth, A., Khattra, J., Yap, D., Wan, A., Laks, E., Biele, J., Ha, G., Aparicio, S., Bouchard-Côté, A., Shah, S.P.: Pyclone: statistical inference of clonal population structure in cancer. Nat. Methods. **11**, 396–398 (2014)
25. Russnes, H.G., Navin, N., Hicks, J., Borresen-Dale, A.L.: Insight into the heterogeneity of breast cancer through next-generation sequencing. J. Clin. Invest. **121**(10), 3810–3818 (2011)
26. Sengupta, S.: Two models involving Bayesian nonparametric techniques. Ph.D thesis, University of Florida (2013)
27. Sengupta, S., Guluokta, K., Lee, J., Müller, P., Ji, Y.: Bayclone: Bayesian nonparametric inference of tumor subclones using ngs data. In: Proceedings of the Pacific Symposium on Biocomputing (PSB), 467–78 (2015)
28. Strino, F., Parisi, F., Micsinai, M., Kluger, Y.: Trap: a tree approach for fingerprinting subclonal tumor composition. Nucleic Acids Res. **41**(17), e165 (2013). doi:10.1093/nar/gkt641. http://nar.oxfordjournals.org/content/41/17/e165.abstract
29. Teh, Y.W., Görür, D., Ghahramani, Z.: Stick-breaking construction for the Indian buffet process. In: Proceedings of the International Conference on Artificial Intelligence and Statistics, vol. 11 (2007)
30. Xu, Y., Mueller, P., Yuan, Y., Gulukota, K., Ji, Y.: MAD Bayes for tumor heterogeneity feature allocation with non-normal sampling. J. Am. Stat. Assoc. **110**, 503–514 (2015)
31. Zare, H., Wang, J., Hu, A., Weber, K., Smith, J., Nickerson, D., Song, C., Witten, D., Blau, C.A., Noble, W.S.: Inferring clonal composition from multiple sections of a breast cancer. PLoS Comput. Biol. **10**(7), e1003703 (2014)

Bayesian Penalty Mixing: The Case of a Non-separable Penalty

Veronika Ročková and Edward I. George

Abstract Separable penalties for sparse vector recovery are plentiful throughout statistical methodology and theory. Here, we confine attention to the problem of estimating sparse high-dimensional normal means. Separable penalized likelihood estimators are known to have a Bayesian interpretation as posterior modes under independent product priors. Such estimators can achieve rate-minimax performance when the correct level of sparsity is known. A fully Bayes approach, on the other hand, mixes the product priors over a shared complexity parameter. These constructions can yield a self-adaptive posterior that achieves rate-minimax performance when the sparsity level is unknown. Such optimality has also been established for posterior mean functionals. However, less is known about posterior modes in these setups. Ultimately, the mixing priors render the coordinates dependent through a penalty that is no longer separable. By tying the coordinates together, the hope is to gain adaptivity and achieve automatic hyperparameter tuning. Here, we study two examples of fully Bayes penalties: the fully Bayes LASSO and the fully Bayes Spike-and-Slab LASSO of Ročková and George (The Spike-and-Slab LASSO, Submitted). We discuss discrepancies and highlight the benefits of the two-group prior variant. We develop an Appell function apparatus for coping with adaptive selection thresholds. We show that the fully Bayes treatment of a complexity parameter is tantamount to oracle hyperparameter choice for sparse normal mean estimation.

1 Introduction

1.1 Separable Versus Non-separable

Separable penalty functions are limited by their inability to adapt to common features across model parameters because they treat these parameters independently. Non-separable penalties, on the other hand, can harvest structural knowledge such

V. Ročková (✉) • E.I. George
Statistics Department, The Wharton School of the University of Pennsylvania, Philadelphia, PA 19104, USA
e-mail: vrockova@wharton.upenn.edu; edgeorge@wharton.upenn.edu

A. Frigessi et al. (eds.), *Statistical Analysis for High-Dimensional Data*, Abel Symposia 11, DOI 10.1007/978-3-319-27099-9_11

as groupings, networks or temporal orderings, to induce similarity across related components. The Fused LASSO [27], the group LASSO [18], OSCAR [2] are just a few prominent examples, which exploit structural similarities among parameters. Our interest in non-separable penalties here is fundamentally different. We want to explore the degree of adaptivity to unknown sparsity levels that can be achieved with exchangeable non-separable penalties when estimating sparse signals. To this end, we take a fully Bayesian perspective on penalized likelihood estimation of sparse normal means.

We consider the classic problem of estimating a mean vector from a single multivariate observation. With $\boldsymbol{y} = (y_1, \ldots, y_n)'$ that arises from

$$y_i = \beta_{0i} + \varepsilon_i, \quad \text{where} \quad \varepsilon_i \overset{iid}{\sim} \mathcal{N}(0, 1), \quad i = 1, \ldots, n, \tag{1}$$

independently, the goal is to estimate $\boldsymbol{\beta}_0 = (\beta_{01}, \ldots, \beta_{0n})'$ under squared error loss, assuming that $\boldsymbol{\beta}_0$ is possibly sparse. Throughout the paper, sparsity is understood as a requirement that $p_n = o(n)$ as $n \to \infty$, where $p_n = \|\boldsymbol{\beta}_0\|_0$. The quality of recovery of $\boldsymbol{\beta}_0$ is often assessed relative to the benchmark minimax risk $2p_n \log(n/p_n)(1 + o(1))$ [7] and the "near-minimax" risk $2p_n \log n(1 + o(1))$, a perspective adopted here.

By regularizing towards sparsity, superbly behaving estimators can be obtained through maximization of the penalized likelihood

$$\widehat{\boldsymbol{\beta}} = \arg\max_{\boldsymbol{\beta} \in \mathbb{R}^n} \left\{ -\frac{1}{2} \sum_{i=1}^{n} (y_i - \beta_i)^2 + Pen_\lambda(\boldsymbol{\beta}) \right\}, \tag{2}$$

where $Pen_\lambda(\boldsymbol{\beta})$ is a regularizing penalty and $\lambda > 0$ is a user-specified penalty parameter. The known equivalence between penalized likelihood estimators and Bayesian posterior modes is obtained by associating a penalty function with a (possibly improper) prior $\pi(\boldsymbol{\beta} \mid \lambda)$ via $Pen_\lambda(\boldsymbol{\beta}) = \log \pi(\boldsymbol{\beta} \mid \lambda)$. Particularly appealing have been penalties that are separable in the sense: $Pen_\lambda(\boldsymbol{\beta}) = \sum_{i=1}^{n} pen_\lambda(\beta_i)$. These correspond to independent product priors $\pi(\boldsymbol{\beta} \mid \lambda) = \prod_{i=1}^{n} \pi(\beta_i \mid \lambda)$. Familiar examples of separable penalties include the ℓ_0 variable selection penalty $-\sum \lambda \delta_0(\beta_i)$, its closest concave relative the ℓ_1 LASSO penalty $-\sum \lambda |\beta_i|$ [26] and the plentiful LASSO variants [31, 32]. Recently there has been a surge of interest in separable penalties that are non-concave (SCAD of Fan and Li [8], MC+ of Zhang [29], log penalty of Friedman [10]). Such penalties eliminate modeling bias and can achieve more refined recovery rates [28].

Separable penalized likelihood estimators can achieve the minimax risk (up to a constant) with a suitable choice of λ that typically depends on p_n. Removing the need to assume that p_n is known, adaptive estimators can be obtained with empirical Bayes and fully Bayes approaches. The latter is of interest to us here.

To move beyond the independent product priors that give rise to separable penalties, more flexible penalty functions can be obtained from fully Bayes hierarchical prior constructions. Such priors are obtained by mixing over a shared parameter,

$$\pi(\boldsymbol{\beta}) = \int \prod_{i=1}^{n} \pi(\beta_i \mid \eta)\pi(\eta) \mathrm{d}\,\eta, \tag{3}$$

where $\pi(\eta)$ is a prior distribution. The coefficients $\beta_1, \ldots, \beta_n$ are now conditionally independent given η. Appropriately formulated, such exchangeable priors can be used to create multivariate estimators that "borrow strength" across the components of $\boldsymbol{\beta}$.

Such estimators have a long tradition. Perhaps the best known examples are the variety of posterior mean Stein estimators that can be motivated with hierarchical mixtures of normal priors. For example, the construction (3) with $\pi(\beta_i \mid \eta) = N(0, \eta)$ and uniform $\pi(\eta)$ over $(0, \infty)$, yields the harmonic prior $\pi_H(\boldsymbol{\beta}) = \left(\sum_i \beta_i^2\right)^{-n-2}$ under which the components of $\boldsymbol{\beta}$ are no longer independent. With this prior, the formal Bayes Stein estimator $\widehat{\boldsymbol{\beta}}^H$ is known to be minimax in the classical sense of having expected squared error loss less than the minimax value n, for all $\boldsymbol{\beta}$ whenever $n \geq 3$ [25]. It is also known to be admissible [3]. To appreciate the adaptive shrinkage behavior of $\widehat{\boldsymbol{\beta}}^H$, note that a large fixed value of η would cause the posterior mean to shrink very little, whereas a very small η would cause the posterior mean to shrink dramatically. By introducing a prior on η, $\widehat{\boldsymbol{\beta}}^H$ adaptively shrinks more towards 0 when smaller values of η (and $\sum_i \beta_i^2$) are supported by the data through the posterior. Further elaborations of (3) can be used to obtain generalized Stein estimators that adaptively exploit ensemble structure among the components of $\boldsymbol{\beta}$. For example, a location mixture of normals for each component of $\boldsymbol{\beta}$, namely $\pi(\beta_i \mid \eta_1, \ldots, \eta_K) = \sum_{k=1}^{K} w_k N(u_{ik}, \eta_k)$ with independent uniform priors on the η_k, leads to a minimax multiple shrinkage estimator that adaptively shrinks towards the prior mean best supported by the data [11, 12]. There are many possibilities for the construction of such estimators, which offer substantial risk reduction in the vicinity of their shrinkage targets.

The hierarchical normal priors for posterior mean Stein estimation could also be used to generate non-separable penalty functions $\log \pi(\boldsymbol{\beta})$ to obtain posterior mode estimators. Sometimes these modal estimators will be the same as the mean estimators, as occurs under the harmonic prior, but in general they will differ. In any case, the classical minimax guarantee offered by Stein estimators is less important in sparse settings where $p_n = o(n)$, as protection against all $\boldsymbol{\beta}$ is no longer needed. Instead, one can focus on obtaining risk reduction in the narrower region of interest where p_n is small. By using posterior mode estimators that adaptively threshold irrelevant coefficients in such regions, one can aim for the asymptotic minimax value $2p_n \log(n/p_n)$, a vast improvement over n.

1.2 Bayesian Penalty Mixing

As opposed to the simple addition of penalty terms that typically occurs with separable penalties, prior constructions such as (3) exemplify another route for penalty construction. This general approach, which we call Bayesian penalty mixing, is a strategy that combines penalty functions via mixtures of their underlying prior distributions. More precisely, let $Pen(\boldsymbol{\beta} \mid \eta) = \log \pi(\boldsymbol{\beta} \mid \eta)$ be a set of penalties corresponding to a set of priors $\pi(\boldsymbol{\beta} \mid \eta)$ indexed by η. Bayesian penalty mixing entails the creation of a penalty

$$Pen(\boldsymbol{\beta}) = \log \pi(\boldsymbol{\beta}) = \log \int \pi(\boldsymbol{\beta} \mid \eta)\pi(\eta)\, d\eta$$

induced by mixing the underlying priors over $\pi(\eta)$. Note that this mixing occurs in the space of priors rather than the space of penalties.

As is well-known, the derivatives of $Pen(\boldsymbol{\beta})$ and $Pen(\boldsymbol{\beta} \mid \eta)$ play a crucial role as the "bias terms" of the penalized likelihood solution $\widehat{\boldsymbol{\beta}}$ to (2), [8]. The adaptive potential of Bayesian penalty mixing is reflected in the relationship between these derivatives given by the following fundamental identity

$$\frac{\partial Pen(\boldsymbol{\beta})}{\partial|\beta_i|} = \int \frac{\partial Pen(\boldsymbol{\beta} \mid \eta)}{\partial|\beta_i|}\pi(\eta \mid \boldsymbol{\beta})\, \mathrm{d}\,\eta \tag{4}$$

which follows from

$$\frac{\partial \log \pi(\boldsymbol{\beta})}{\partial|\beta_i|} = \frac{1}{\pi(\boldsymbol{\beta})} \int \frac{\partial \pi(\boldsymbol{\beta} \mid \eta)}{\partial|\beta_i|}\pi(\eta)\mathrm{d}\,\eta = \int \frac{\partial \log \pi(\boldsymbol{\beta} \mid \eta)}{\partial|\beta_i|}\pi(\eta \mid \boldsymbol{\beta})\mathrm{d}\,\eta.$$

Thus the bias induced by $Pen(\boldsymbol{\beta})$ will be an adaptive convex combination of the biases induced by each of the combined penalties $Pen(\boldsymbol{\beta} \mid \eta)$. More weight is put on shrinkage terms that are better supported by $\pi(\eta \mid \boldsymbol{\beta})$. In this way, $Pen(\boldsymbol{\beta})$ automatically emphasizes those shrinkage terms which are better suited for each $\boldsymbol{\beta}$.

The principal thrust of this paper is to demonstrate the potential of Bayesian penalty mixing through three examples:

- A fully Bayes LASSO penalty obtained by mixing LASSO penalties *across* coordinates, (Sect. 2).
- A Spike-and-Slab LASSO penalty obtained by mixing pairs of LASSO penalties *within* coordinates, (Sect. 3).
- A fully Bayes Spike-and-Slab LASSO penalty obtained by mixing LASSO penalties both *within and across* coordinates, (Sect. 4).

These Spike-and-Slab LASSO examples complement the developments of Ročková [21], who introduced Spike-and-Slab LASSO priors, and Ročková and George [23, 24], who further developed and applied these priors for variable selection.

In each of these three examples, we pay particular attention to the ability of the modal estimator to adapt to the unknown sparsity level (a property known to hold for a posterior mean in similar spike-and-slab setups). Our exploration concludes with a very important finding. By mixing within coordinates and then adding a prior distribution over a complexity parameter, one achieves a level of adaptivity that is tantamount to an oracle hyperparameter choice. Our analysis constitutes an initial step towards the general development of more elaborate hierarchical penalty constructions for asymptotically minimax penalized likelihood estimation with unknown p_n.

In Sect. 2, we study the fully Bayes variant of the LASSO. Sections 3 and 4 review the Spike-and-Slab LASSO and its fully Bayes variant. Section 5 then develops an Appell function apparatus to deal with expectations under a certain class of generalized beta distributions. Section 6 shows the adaptability of the fully Bayes Spike-and-Slab LASSO in sparse normal means. Section 7 concludes with a discussion of future directions.

The following notation will be used throughout. For sequences a_n and b_n, $a_n \sim b_n$ means $a_n/b_n \to c$ for some $c > 0$, $a_n \succeq b_n$ means $b_n = \mathcal{O}(a_n)$, $a_n \succ b_n$ means $b_n = o(a_n)$. We will denote by $|\cdot|$ the ℓ_1 norm.

2 Fully Bayes LASSO

The ℓ_1 penalty $Pen_\lambda(\boldsymbol{\beta}) = -\lambda|\boldsymbol{\beta}|$, arguably the most prominent separable regularizer, gives rise to the LASSO estimator $\widehat{\boldsymbol{\beta}}^L$ in (2). With the universal threshold choice $\lambda \sim \sqrt{2\log n}$, the LASSO estimator enjoys oracle properties [6] and achieves a near-minimax risk rate when $p_n = o(n)$. In practice, however, the parameter λ is often chosen by performance based criteria such as cross-validation, generalized cross-validation or ideas based on Stein's unbiased estimate of risk [26]. Park and Casella [19] offer Bayesian alternatives to choosing λ: an empirical Bayes strategy through marginal maximum likelihood and a fully Bayes solution with an appropriate prior distribution $\pi(\lambda)$. All of these approaches use the data to inform the penalty hyperparameter, thereby potentially boosting performance. Whereas Park and Casella [19] used fully Bayes for posterior median estimation via MCMC, here we investigate the implications for direct penalized likelihood estimation.

For any given prior distribution $\pi(\lambda)$, a fully-Bayes-LASSO penalty is defined as

$$Pen_{FL}(\boldsymbol{\beta}) = \log \int_0^\infty \left(\frac{\lambda}{2}\right)^n \mathrm{e}^{-\lambda|\boldsymbol{\beta}|} \mathrm{d}\,\pi(\lambda). \tag{5}$$

Except for trivial point-mass priors $\pi(\lambda)$, (5) is a non-separable penalty. The well-known closed-form solution for the LASSO estimator, which treats λ as fixed, writes $\widehat{\boldsymbol{\beta}}^L = (\widehat{\beta}_1^L, \ldots, \widehat{\beta}_n^L)'$ as

$$\widehat{\beta}_i^L = (|y_i| - \lambda)_+ \mathrm{sign}(y_i). \tag{6}$$

This follows from the KKT conditions, using the fact that $-\lambda$ is the derivative of the LASSO penalty. With the fully-Bayes-LASSO penalty, the derivative is instead

$$\frac{\partial Pen_{FL}(\boldsymbol{\beta})}{\partial|\beta_i|} = -\frac{\int_0^\infty \lambda \left(\frac{\lambda}{2}\right)^n \mathrm{e}^{-\lambda|\boldsymbol{\beta}|}\mathrm{d}\,\pi(\lambda)}{\int_0^\infty \left(\frac{\lambda}{2}\right)^n \mathrm{e}^{-\lambda|\boldsymbol{\beta}|}\mathrm{d}\,\pi(\lambda)} = -\mathsf{E}\,[\lambda \mid \boldsymbol{\beta}],$$

a special case of (4). Thereby, the fully-Bayes-LASSO estimator $\widehat{\boldsymbol{\beta}}^{FL} = (\widehat{\beta}_1^{FL},\ldots,\widehat{\beta}_n^{FL})'$ satisfies

$$\widehat{\beta}_i^{FL} = \left[|y_i| - \mathsf{E}\left(\lambda \mid \widehat{\boldsymbol{\beta}}^{FL}\right)\right]_+ \mathrm{sign}(y_i). \tag{7}$$

Here, the shrinkage term is adaptive, depending on the data through $\widehat{\boldsymbol{\beta}}^{FL}$. Interestingly, the fully Bayes approach is seen to manifest itself through the plug-in choice $\mathsf{E}\,[\lambda \mid \widehat{\boldsymbol{\beta}}^{FL}]$ in empirical Bayes-like fashion. Note, however, that $\widehat{\boldsymbol{\beta}}^{FL}$ is contained on both sides of (7), in contrast with approaches which insert a single derived estimate for λ. With the fully Bayes plug-in, the amount of shrinkage reflects the size of $|\widehat{\boldsymbol{\beta}}^{FL}|$, as will be seen below.

It can be shown[1] that the risk of the LASSO estimator $\widehat{\boldsymbol{\beta}}^L$ satisfies

$$\mathsf{E}_{\boldsymbol{\beta}_0}||\widehat{\boldsymbol{\beta}}^L - \boldsymbol{\beta}_0||^2 \le p_n(2 + 4\lambda^2) + (n - p_n)4\lambda\phi(\lambda), \tag{8}$$

when $||\boldsymbol{\beta}_0||_0 = p_n$. In order to obtain the near-minimax rate, one would need to select $\lambda \sim \sqrt{2\log n}$ so that $\mathsf{E}_{\boldsymbol{\beta}_0}||\widehat{\boldsymbol{\beta}}^L - \boldsymbol{\beta}_0||^2 \preceq p_n\lambda^2 = 2p_n\log n$.

Analogously, it can be shown that the fully-Bayes-LASSO estimator satisfies

$$\mathsf{E}_{\boldsymbol{\beta}_0}||\widehat{\boldsymbol{\beta}}^{FL} - \boldsymbol{\beta}_0||^2 \le p_n(2 + 4\mathsf{E}_{\boldsymbol{\beta}_0}\widehat{\lambda}^2) + (n - p_n)4\mathsf{E}_{\boldsymbol{\beta}_0}\widehat{\lambda}\phi(\widehat{\lambda}),$$

where $\widehat{\lambda} = \mathsf{E}\left(\lambda \mid \widehat{\boldsymbol{\beta}}^{FL}\right)$. One would hope that the fully Bayes variant will self-adapt, yielding ideally $\mathsf{E}_{\boldsymbol{\beta}_0}\widehat{\lambda} \sim \sqrt{2\log n}$, the desired LASSO tuning. To get a sense of this possibility, let's take a closer look at $\widehat{\lambda}$.

For the purpose of illustration, consider the conjugate class[2] of priors $\pi(\lambda) = \frac{b^a}{\Gamma(a)}\lambda^{a-1}\mathrm{e}^{-b\lambda}\mathbb{I}(\lambda > 0)$, so that

$$\pi(\boldsymbol{\beta}) = \frac{b^a}{2^n\Gamma(a)}\int_0^\infty \lambda^{n+a-1}\mathrm{e}^{-\lambda(|\boldsymbol{\beta}|+b)}\mathrm{d}\,\lambda = \frac{b^a\Gamma(n+a)}{2^n\Gamma(a)(|\boldsymbol{\beta}|+b)^{n+a}}.$$

---

[1]Following the proving technique of Ročková [21], Remark 5.1. This upper bound is useful for illustration and can be sharpened.

[2]Park and Casella [19] use a gamma prior on λ^2 for the ease of MCMC implementation.

This yields

$$\widehat{\lambda} = \mathsf{E}[\lambda \mid \widehat{\boldsymbol{\beta}}^{FL}] = \frac{n+a}{|\widehat{\boldsymbol{\beta}}^{FL}| + b}. \tag{9}$$

Thus $\widehat{\lambda}$ is an adaptive threshold that depends not only on the sparsity of $\widehat{\boldsymbol{\beta}}^{FL}$, but also on the size of the nonzero coefficients. The dependence on $|\widehat{\boldsymbol{\beta}}^{FL}|$, and hence on $|\boldsymbol{\beta}_0|$, makes it impossible to tune a and b so that $\mathsf{E}_{\boldsymbol{\beta}_0}\widehat{\lambda} \sim \sqrt{2\log n}$. Thus, there seems to be a disconnect between the universal LASSO tuning for near-minimax rates, and the fully Bayes LASSO approach.

Moreover, note that in (7), all coordinates are shrunk by the same amount. As opposed to the classical LASSO, the adaptive weight here depends on the size of the coefficients $\widehat{\boldsymbol{\beta}}$. With just one tuning-parameter, despite its adaptivity, the penalty will fail to shrink globally and act locally [20]. As a locally adaptive extension of the LASSO prior, Griffin and Brown [14] propose individual penalties λ_i for each coordinate, where $\lambda_i \sim \pi(\lambda)$. Each λ_i is a realization from a mixing distribution. Marginally, such strategies induce sharply peaked separable penalties.

Although the fully Bayes treatment of the LASSO offers the possibility for self-tuning, the penalty $\mathsf{E}\,(\lambda \mid \widehat{\boldsymbol{\beta}}^{FL})$ cannot both circumvent the bias issue and adapt to sparsity at the same time. For this, it is imperative that each coefficient is given a unique opportunity to escape the overall shrinkage effect. This is achieved with global/local shrinkage priors and two-group spike-and-slab priors. In the sequel, we explore the two group mixture prior formulations for penalty creation. Instead of mixing across coordinates immediately, we begin by mixing within coordinates.

3 Spike-and-Slab LASSO

Penalty mixing within coordinates provides an opportunity to enhance the performance of penalized likelihood estimators (2) by combining the benefits of single penalties. For instance, the elastic net [32] blends the LASSO and the ridge, inducing a grouping effect in estimation while maintaining the ability to threshold. Other combinations of convex and concave penalties have been proposed to achieve good subset recovery and bias elimination [9]. In these two cases, the mixing operates at the penalty level through the linear superposition of penalty terms.

In sharp contrast, Bayesian penalty mixing, which operates at the prior level, is inherently nonlinear and probabilistic. Such Bayesian penalty mixing arises naturally in the context of spike-and-slab mixture formulations for Bayesian variable selection. In particular, let us turn to the recently proposed Spike-and-Slab LASSO (SSL) prior of Ročková [21]. Viewed as a continuous relaxation of the point mass mixture prior (Castillo and van der Vaart [5]), the SSL prior deploys a two-point mixture of a Laplace spike distribution $\pi(\beta \mid \lambda_0) = \frac{\lambda_0}{2}\mathrm{e}^{-|\beta|\lambda_0}$ and a Laplace slab

$\pi(\beta \mid \lambda_1) = \frac{\lambda_1}{2} e^{-|\beta|\lambda_1}$, i.e.

$$\pi(\boldsymbol{\beta} \mid \theta, \lambda_1, \lambda_0) = \prod_{i=1}^{n} [\theta \pi(\beta_i \mid \lambda_1) + (1 - \theta)\pi(\beta_i \mid \lambda_0)],$$

where $\theta \in (0, 1)$ is a mixing weight. It is assumed $\lambda_0 >> \lambda_1 > 0$. Note that the SSL prior reduces to a single Laplace (LASSO) prior when $\lambda_0 = \lambda_1$, and converges to a point mass spike-and-slab mixture as $\lambda_0 \to \infty$. Here we have three parameters $(\lambda_1, \lambda_0, \theta)$, where $0 < \lambda_1 < 1$ is a small fixed constant treated as known (made precise by the theoretical study of Ročková [21]) and λ_0 and θ are the two parameters subject to tuning. In what follows, we suppress λ_1 from the conditioning.

Tailored for Bayesian variable selection [21, 22, 24], each β_i is thought of as arriving from the diffuse slab distribution $\pi(\beta_i \mid \lambda_1)$, with probability $\theta \in (0, 1)$, or from the sharply peaked spike distribution $\pi(\beta_i \mid \lambda_0)$. In the context of Bayesian regression analysis, selection with a spike-and-slab prior has traditionally entailed a decision to include the ith regressor only when the "posterior probability that β_i came from $\pi(\beta_i \mid \lambda_1)$" is high. However, when approached from a penalized likelihood perspective, the selection strategy is very different.

In the context of penalized likelihood estimation, variable selection capitalizes on a penalty of the form

$$Pen_{SL}(\boldsymbol{\beta} \mid \theta, \lambda_0) = \sum_{i=1}^{n} \log[\theta \pi(\beta_i \mid \lambda_1) + (1 - \theta)\pi(\beta_i \mid \lambda_0)]. \tag{10}$$

The penalty (10) stands out from classical penalty functions as nonlinear in both $|\beta_i|$ and $(\lambda_1, \lambda_0, \theta)$. The benefits of using this rather complex nonlinear functional are revealed by its implicit shrinkage term, the derivative. As a special case of (4), we obtain

$$\frac{\partial Pen_{SL}(\boldsymbol{\beta} \mid \theta, \lambda_0)}{\partial |\beta_i|} = -\lambda_1 p_\theta^\star(\beta_i) - \lambda_0[1 - p_\theta^\star(\beta_i)] \equiv -\lambda_\theta^\star(\beta_i), \tag{11}$$

where

$$p_\theta^\star(\beta_i) = \frac{\theta \pi(\beta_i \mid \lambda_1)}{\theta \pi(\beta_i \mid \lambda_1) + (1 - \theta)\pi(\beta_i \mid \lambda_0)} = \frac{1}{1 + \frac{1-\theta}{\theta}\frac{\lambda_0}{\lambda_1} e^{-|\beta_i|(\lambda_0 - \lambda_1)}} \tag{12}$$

is the conditional probability that β_i came from $\pi(\beta_i \mid \lambda_1)$ having seen β_i. Thus, the spike-and-slab LASSO shrinkage term $\lambda_\theta^\star(\beta_i)$ mixes the two LASSO shrinkage terms (λ_1, λ_0) and does so adaptively. Ideally, one would like to use $\lambda_1 < 1$ when $|\beta_i|$ is large, and $\lambda_0 >> 1$ when $|\beta_i|$ is small. This is essentially effectuated with the adaptive exponential weight $0 < p_\theta^\star(\beta_i) < 1$, which gears $\lambda_\theta^\star(\beta_i)$ towards λ_0, when $|\beta_i|$ is small, and towards λ_1 when $|\beta_i|$ is large.

The first order KKT conditions immediately yield a necessary characterization of the global mode $\widehat{\boldsymbol{\beta}}^{SL}$, where the coordinate estimators must satisfy

$$\widehat{\beta}_i^{SL} = \left[|y_i| - \lambda_\theta^\star(\widehat{\beta}_i^{SL})\right]_+ \operatorname{sign}(y_i),\ i = 1, \ldots, n. \tag{13}$$

The form (13) resembles the LASSO estimator (6). However, here the SSL penalty term $\lambda_\theta^\star(\widehat{\beta}_i^{SL})$ is not constant, but rather depends on the data through $\widehat{\beta}_i^{SL}$. As with the adaptive LASSO, [31], each coefficient has its own penalty, which serves as a basis for "differential" shrinkage. Adaptive in this way, the SSL estimator deploys a large penalty (close to λ_0) to threshold small estimates, and a small penalty (close to λ_1) to hold large estimates steady with only slight bias. This is very much in contrast to a single LASSO estimator which shrinks all estimates equally with a constant penalty.

To further eliminate local modal solutions, the necessary characterization (13) can be sharpened [21], where $\widehat{\boldsymbol{\beta}}^{SL}$ can be shown to be sandwiched between soft and hard thresholding operators. When λ_0 is large enough, the coordinate estimates must satisfy

$$\widehat{\beta}_i^{SL} = \left[|y_i| - \lambda_\theta^\star(\widehat{\beta}_i^{SL})\right] \operatorname{sign}(y_i)\, \mathrm{I}(|y_i| > \Delta),\ i = 1, \ldots, n, \tag{14}$$

where

$$\Delta \sim \sqrt{2\log[1/p_\theta^\star(0)]} + \lambda_1, \tag{15}$$

when $\lambda_1 \le \mathrm{e}^{-2}$ and $\lambda_0 \ge 1/\theta + 3$, and $0 < \theta \le 0.5$. Thus, letting λ_0 increase with the sample size, the asymptotic risk of $\widehat{\boldsymbol{\beta}}^{SL}$ is ultimately governed by the threshold Δ through a functional

$$1/p_\theta^\star(0) = 1 + \frac{\lambda_0}{\lambda_1}\frac{(1-\theta)}{\theta}. \tag{16}$$

It follows from the proof of Theorem 5.1 of [21] that

$$\mathsf{E}_{\boldsymbol{\beta}_0}||\widehat{\boldsymbol{\beta}}^{SL} - \boldsymbol{\beta}_0||^2 \preceq p_n\Delta^2 + (n - p_n)\Delta\phi(\Delta). \tag{17}$$

This upper bound is similar to (8), where Δ now plays the role of selection threshold. The rate-minimax performance of the global posterior mode $\widehat{\boldsymbol{\beta}}^{SL}$ will be then achieved when $1/p_\theta^\star(0) \sim (n/p_n)^\alpha$ for some $\alpha > 0$. This will occur, for instance, when $\lambda_1 < \mathrm{e}^{-2}$, $\theta \sim p_n/n$ and $\lambda_0 \sim 1/\theta$. Under this "oracle" choice, the threshold Δ is of the optimal order $\sqrt{2\log[n/p_n]}$, yielding (Corollary 5.1 of Ročková [21])

$$\sup_{\boldsymbol{\beta}_0 \in l_0[p_n;n]} \mathsf{E}_{\boldsymbol{\beta}_0}||\widehat{\boldsymbol{\beta}}^{SL} - \boldsymbol{\beta}_0||^2 \sim p_n \log(n/p_n).$$

Moreover, with this parameter choice, the entire posterior distribution $\pi(\boldsymbol{\beta} \mid \boldsymbol{y})$ concentrates around the true vector $\boldsymbol{\beta}_0$ at the minimax rate (Corollary 6.1 of Ročková [21]). Namely,

$$\sup_{\boldsymbol{\beta}_0 \in l_0[p_n;n]} \mathsf{E}_{\boldsymbol{\beta}_0} \mathsf{P}(\boldsymbol{\beta} \in \mathbb{R}^n : ||\boldsymbol{\beta} - \boldsymbol{\beta}_0||^2 > M p_n \log[n/p_n] \,|\, \boldsymbol{y}^{(n)}) \to 0 \tag{18}$$

for a suitably large constant $M > 0$. This property fails to hold for a single LASSO Laplace prior (Castillo et al. [4]), despite the optimality of the LASSO mode.

Nevertheless, the oracle parameter setup will be unavailable when p_n is unknown, as will typically be the case in practice. To get around this problem, one could consider an empirical Bayes plug-in choice for θ and λ_0 (along the lines of Johnstone and Silverman [16]). However, here we explore a fully Bayes approach which places a prior distribution on θ. The hope is that by treating θ as unknown in this way, we can mimic the performance obtained by the oracle choice.

It is important to note that the spike penalty λ_0 also requires proper tuning. Here, we focus exclusively on adapting θ, assuming that λ_0 satisfies $\lambda_0/\lambda_1 \sim n^\alpha$ for $\alpha > 0$). This scenario is instructive for understanding the basic mechanisms underlying the adaptivity of fully Bayes penalty mixing. It is also a fundamental first step towards fully adaptive procedures, obtained by inducing a prior on λ_0. We discuss some of these alternatives at the end of Sect. 6.

4 Fully Bayes Spike-and-Slab LASSO

In Sect. 2, we considered a fully Bayes treatment of the original LASSO, mixing its single penalty parameter over a prior distribution. This mixing produces a data-dependent penalty, which ties the coordinates together. In Sect. 3, we considered a very different approach, mixing penalties within coordinates over a spike-and-slab prior, keeping the value of the shared hyperparameter θ fixed. This mixing treated each coefficient uniquely, preventing the borrowing of strength across coordinates. We now proceed to combine these two perspectives, by mixing the spike-and-slab prior over a prior distribution on θ. This will allow the coordinates to share a global hyperparameter, while the spike-and-slab prior allows each coefficient to be treated locally.

Adaptive mixing of spike-and-slab penalties across the coordinates of β_i can be achieved with a suitable prior $\pi(\theta)$ [24]. The prior mixing proportion θ plays the role of a complexity parameter, determining the sparsity of the solution. In the absence of knowledge about p_n, setting θ fixed to a constant may diminish performance by over/underestimating the dimensionality. The hope is that by introducing $\pi(\theta)$, the penalty can adapt to the sparsity level and help yield oracle-like performance automatically, avoiding the need for setting θ close to p_n/n.

With a prior on θ, the coordinates in $\boldsymbol{\beta}$ are now marginally dependent, yielding

$$\pi(\boldsymbol{\beta}) = \int_0^1 \prod_{i=1}^n [\theta\pi(\beta_i \mid \lambda_1) + (1-\theta)\pi(\beta_i \mid \lambda_0)]\, d\,\pi(\theta) \tag{19}$$

which will be non-separable for all but trivial choices of $\pi(\theta)$. Generally, the integral above does not have a closed form solution, complicating the tractability of the penalty $Pen(\boldsymbol{\beta}) = \log \pi(\boldsymbol{\beta})$. Fortunately, a revealing and simple form can still be found for its derivative.

With θ fixed, a simple necessary characterization of the global mode was obtained in (14). Following the development in Ročková and George [24], we can still obtain a similar simple characterization under the dependent prior $\pi(\boldsymbol{\beta})$. As another special case of (4), we have

$$\begin{aligned}\frac{\partial \log \pi(\boldsymbol{\beta})}{\partial|\beta_i|} &= \frac{1}{\pi(\boldsymbol{\beta})}\int_0^1 \frac{\partial \pi(\boldsymbol{\beta} \mid \theta)}{\partial|\beta_i|}\pi(\theta)\mathrm{d}\,\theta = \int_0^1 \frac{\partial \log \pi(\boldsymbol{\beta} \mid \theta)}{\partial|\beta_i|}\pi(\theta \mid \boldsymbol{\beta})\mathrm{d}\,\theta \\ &= -\lambda_1 \int_0^1 p_\theta^\star(\beta_i)\pi(\theta \mid \boldsymbol{\beta})\mathrm{d}\,\theta - \lambda_0\left[1 - \int_0^1 p_\theta^\star(\beta_i)\pi(\theta \mid \boldsymbol{\beta})\mathrm{d}\,\theta\right].\end{aligned} \tag{20}$$

The difference between (11) and (20) is illuminating. Instead of the "fixed-θ" mixing probability $p_\theta^\star(\beta_i)$ in (11), (20) employs an aggregated mixing probability $\int_0^1 p_\theta^\star(\beta_i)\pi(\theta \mid \boldsymbol{\beta})\mathrm{d}\,\theta$ that averages $p_\theta^\star(\beta_i)$ over $\pi(\theta \mid \boldsymbol{\beta})$. The implicit bias term (20) reveals the mechanism underlying the adaptivity. By averaging over the conditional distribution $\pi(\theta \mid \boldsymbol{\beta})$, the penalty is given an opportunity to learn about the level of sparsity of $\boldsymbol{\beta}$.

Going further, substantial insight and simplification is provided by the following surprising identity from Ročková and George [24]

$$p_{\theta_i}^\star(\beta_i) \equiv \int_0^1 p_\theta^\star(\beta_i)\pi(\theta \mid \boldsymbol{\beta})\mathrm{d}\,\theta, \quad \theta_i \equiv E[\theta \mid \boldsymbol{\beta}_{\setminus i}]. \tag{21}$$

Here $\boldsymbol{\beta}_{\setminus i}$ denotes the sub-vector of $\boldsymbol{\beta}$ containing all but the ith entry. Even though $p_\theta^\star(\beta_i)$ is a nonlinear function of θ, its average value over $\pi(\theta \mid \boldsymbol{\beta})$ is obtained by simply substituting $\theta_i \equiv E[\theta \mid \boldsymbol{\beta}_{\setminus i}]$ for θ to obtain $p_{\theta_i}^\star(\beta_i)$. With the representation (21), the implicit bias term (20) is of the simple form

$$\frac{\partial \log \pi(\boldsymbol{\beta})}{\partial|\beta_i|} = \lambda_1 p_{\theta_i}^\star(\beta_i) + \lambda_0\left[1 - p_{\theta_i}^\star(\beta_i)\right] \equiv \lambda_{\theta_i}^\star(\beta_i), \tag{22}$$

which similarly comes from $\lambda_\theta^\star(\beta_i)$ in (11) by simple substitution of θ_i for θ.

A direct analogue of (14) is now readily available. The coordinates of the global modal estimator $\widehat{\boldsymbol{\beta}}^{FSL}$ under the fully Bayes non-separable SSL penalty will jointly satisfy

$$\widehat{\beta}_i^{FSL} = \left[|y_i| - \lambda^{\star}_{\hat{\theta}_i}(\widehat{\beta}_i^{FSL})\right]_+ \operatorname{sign}(y_i)\, \mathrm{I}(|y_i| > \Delta_i), \tag{23}$$

where $\widehat{\theta}_i \equiv \mathsf{E}\,[\theta \mid \widehat{\boldsymbol{\beta}}_{\setminus i}^{FSL}]$, and

$$\Delta_i \sim \sqrt{2\log[1/p^{\star}_{\hat{\theta}_i}(0)]} + \lambda_1. \tag{24}$$

Compared to Eq. (14), each coordinate in (23) now has a penalty $\lambda^{\star}_{\hat{\theta}_i}(\widehat{\beta}_i^{FSL})$ which depends on all the coordinates through $\widehat{\beta}_i$ and $\widehat{\theta}_i$, not just the ith. This dependency originates from the mixing distribution $\pi(\theta \mid \widehat{\boldsymbol{\beta}}^{FSL})$, used to obtain the "average" inclusion probability (21). The fewer zeros in $\widehat{\boldsymbol{\beta}}^{FSL}$, the less concentrated this distribution will be around the origin, thereby leading to a larger value of $\widehat{\theta}_i$.

Another essential difference between (14) and (23), is the replacement of Δ by the adaptive thresholds Δ_i. In the separable case, we have a single threshold for which

$$(\Delta - \lambda_1)^2 \sim 2\,\log\left[1 + \frac{\lambda_0}{\lambda_1}\frac{1-\theta}{\theta}\right]. \tag{25}$$

With θ fixed to a constant, (25) deploys *prior odds* of non-entering the model $(1-\theta)/\theta$. Substituting $\widehat{\theta}_i$ for θ, we have

$$(\Delta_i - \lambda_1)^2 \sim 2\,\log\left[1 + \frac{\lambda_0}{\lambda_1}\frac{1-\mathsf{E}\,(\theta \mid \widehat{\boldsymbol{\beta}}_{\setminus i}^{FSL})}{\mathsf{E}\,(\theta \mid \widehat{\boldsymbol{\beta}}_{\setminus i}^{FSL})}\right] \tag{26}$$

which shows how very different the non-separable formulation is from the separable one. By treating θ as random, (26) uses the "*posterior odds*" $\frac{[1-\mathsf{E}\,(\theta \mid \widehat{\boldsymbol{\beta}}_{\setminus i}^{FSL})]}{\mathsf{E}\,(\theta \mid \widehat{\boldsymbol{\beta}}_{\setminus i}^{FSL})}$. Through $\widehat{\boldsymbol{\beta}}$, the data inform θ about the sparsity level through the proportion of its nonzero entries. This observation is fundamental to understanding the mechanism through which the fully Bayes formulation transmits information into the posterior mode.

5 Bounds and Rates for the Fully Bayes Selection Thresholds

The selection thresholds Δ_i are indispensable to describing the properties of the global mode estimator. For this purpose, Ročková and George [24] present bounds for the quantity $\mathsf{E}\,[\theta \mid \widehat{\boldsymbol{\beta}}_{\setminus i}]$, and thereby also Δ_i when $\theta \sim \mathscr{B}(a,b)$. Note that the posterior expectations $\mathsf{E}\,(\theta \mid \widehat{\boldsymbol{\beta}}_{\setminus i})$ will be very similar for each $i = 1,\ldots,n$, when n is sufficiently large. Thus, despite Δ_i's that are coordinate-specific, they will not be dramatically different. For a relatively uninformative choice of $\pi(\theta)$, one would expect $\mathsf{E}\,(\theta \mid \widehat{\boldsymbol{\beta}}_{\setminus i})$ to be close to $\widehat{p}^i/n$, where $\widehat{p}^i = \|\widehat{\boldsymbol{\beta}}_{\setminus i}\|_0$.

Let us assume that it is the first $\widehat{p}$ entries in $\widehat{\boldsymbol{\beta}}$ that are nonzero. Under $\theta \sim \mathscr{B}(a,b)$, the density of the conditional distribution $\pi(\theta \mid \widehat{\boldsymbol{\beta}})$ is given by

$$\pi(\theta \mid \widehat{\boldsymbol{\beta}}) \propto \theta^{a-1}(1-\theta)^{b-1}(1-\theta z)^{n-\widehat{p}}\prod_{j=1}^{\widehat{p}}(1-\theta x_j), \tag{27}$$

where $z = 1 - \frac{\lambda_1}{\lambda_0}$, $x_j = \left(1 - \frac{\lambda_1}{\lambda_0}\mathrm{e}^{|\widehat{\beta}_j|(\lambda_0-\lambda_1)}\right)$. This distribution turns out to be a generalization of the Gauss hypergeometric distribution [1, 15]. The normalizing constant writes as an Euler integral representation of the hypergeometric function of several variables [13]. Consequently, the expectation can be written as

$$\mathsf{E}\,[\theta \mid \widehat{\boldsymbol{\beta}}] = \frac{\int_0^1 \theta^{a}(1-\theta)^{b-1}\,(1-\theta z)^{n-\widehat{p}}\prod_{j=1}^{\widehat{p}}\left(1-\theta x_j\right)\mathrm{d}\,\theta}{\int_0^1 \theta^{a-1}(1-\theta)^{b-1}\,(1-\theta z)^{n-\widehat{p}}\prod_{j=1}^{\widehat{p}}\left(1-\theta x_j\right)\mathrm{d}\,\theta}. \tag{28}$$

Ročková and George [24] suggest approximating (28) by

$$\frac{\mathscr{B}(a+1,b)}{\mathscr{B}(a,b)}\frac{F_1(a+1,\widehat{p}-n,-\widehat{p},a+b+1;z,x)}{F_1(a,\widehat{p}-n,-\widehat{p},a+b;z,x)}, \tag{29}$$

for some suitable x, where

$$F_1(a',b',c',d';z,x) = \frac{1}{\mathscr{B}(d'-a',a')}\int_0^1 \theta^{a'-1}(1-\theta)^{d'-a'-1}(1-\theta z)^{-b'}(1-\theta x)^{-c'}\,\mathrm{d}\,\theta$$

is the Appell F1 function. To obtain suitable lower and upper bounds for $\mathsf{E}\,[\theta \mid \widehat{\boldsymbol{\beta}}]$, we begin with the following lemma which establishes that the ratio (29) is monotone in x and z.

Lemma 1 (Monotonicity Ratio of Appell F1 Functions) *Assume $\delta > 0$. Then the function*

$$f_\delta(a',b',c',d';z,x) = \frac{F_1(a'+\delta,b',c',d'+\delta;z,-x)}{F_1(a',b',c',d';z,-x)} \tag{30}$$

is monotone increasing when $c' < 0$ and monotone decreasing when $c' > 0$ for $x > -1$.

Proof Denote by $A_\delta = \frac{1}{\mathscr{B}(d'-a',a'+\delta)}$. Then

$$f_\delta(a',b',c',d';z,x) = \frac{A_\delta\int_0^1 \theta^{a'+\delta-1}(1+\theta x)^{-c'}g(a',d',b',z;\theta)\mathrm{d}\,\theta}{A_0\int_0^1 \theta^{a'-1}(1+\theta x)^{-c'}g(a',d',b',z;\theta)\mathrm{d}\,\theta}, \tag{31}$$

where $g(a', d', b', z; \theta) = (1-\theta)^{d'-a'-1}(1-\theta z)^{-b'}$. By differentiating ratio (31) with respect to x, the function $f_\delta(a', b', c', d'; z, x)$ is monotone increasing for $c' < 0$ (and monotone decreasing for $c' > 0$) if

$$\int_0^1 q(\theta)p(\theta)\mathrm{d}\theta \int_0^1 h(\theta)p(\theta)\mathrm{d}\theta < \int_0^1 q(\theta)h(\theta)p(\theta)\mathrm{d}\theta \int_0^1 p(\theta)\mathrm{d}\theta, \tag{32}$$

where

$$p(\theta) = \theta^{a'-1}(1+\theta x)^{-c'} g(a', d', b', z; \theta)$$

$$q(\theta) = \theta^{\delta}, \quad h(\theta) = \frac{\theta}{1+\theta x}$$

The inequality (32) follows from Chebyshev's integral inequality, because the function $p(\theta)$ is positive and both $q(\theta)$ and $h(\theta)$ are monotone increasing on $(0, \theta)$ for $x > -1$.

Remark 1 Lemma 1 is a generalization of Lemma 1.1 of Karp and Sitnik [17], who showed the monotonicity of ratios of Gauss Hypergeometric functions (a special case of the Appell F1 functions) with shifted hyperparameters. Their result is obtained as a special case when either $b' = 0$ or $c' = 0$. Lemma 1 can also be formulated in terms of z, where the ratio will be monotone increasing in z when $b' < 0$ and decreasing when $b' > 0$.

The next lemma will be a stepping stone for deriving the upper bound on the selection threshold.

Lemma 2 *Assume* $\delta > 0$ *and let* $f_\delta(a', b', c', d'; z, x)$ *be as in* (30). *Assume* $c' < 0$ *and* $0 < z < 1$. *Then we have*

$$\lim_{x\to\infty} f_\delta(a', b', c', d'; z, x) < \frac{\mathscr{B}(d'-a', a')}{\mathscr{B}(d'-a', a'+\delta)} \frac{\mathscr{B}(d'-a', a'+\delta-c')}{\mathscr{B}(d'-a', a'-c')}. \tag{33}$$

Proof Let A_δ be as in the proof of Lemma 1. Repeatedly applying l'Hospital's rule (with respect to x), we obtain for $c' < 0$

$$\lim_{x\to\infty} f_\delta(a', b', c', d'; z, x) = \frac{A_\delta}{A_0} \frac{\int_0^1 \theta^{a'+\delta-c'-1}(1-\theta)^{d'-a'-1}[1-\theta z]^{-b'}\mathrm{d}\theta}{\int_0^1 \theta^{a'-c'-1}(1-\theta)^{d'-a'-1}[1-\theta z]^{-b'}\mathrm{d}\theta} \tag{34}$$

$$= \frac{A_\delta}{A_0} \frac{\mathscr{B}(d'-a', a'+\delta-c')}{\mathscr{B}(d'-a', a'-c')} \frac{F_1(a'+\delta-c', b', 0, d'+\delta; z, 1)}{F_1(a'-c', b', 0, d'; z, 1)} \tag{35}$$

Note that $F_1(a', b', 0, d'; z, 1) = F_2^1(b', a', d'; z)$, where F_2 is the Gauss hypergeometric function. We can apply Lemma 1.1 of Karp and Sitnik [17] or Lemma 1 to conclude that the ratio of two Gauss functions with shifted arguments is monotone decreasing in z. Since $0 < z < 1$, we have $\frac{F_1(a'+\delta-c',b',0,d'+\delta;z,1)}{F_1(a'-c',b',0,d';z,1)} < \frac{F_1(a'+\delta-c',b',0,d'+\delta;0,1)}{F_1(a'-c',b',0,d';0,1)} = 1$.

Having developed the apparatus of Appell F1 functions, we are ready to state and prove the following key lemma.

Lemma 3 *Assume $\pi(\theta \mid \widehat{\boldsymbol{\beta}})$ is distributed according to* (27)*. Let $\widehat{p} = \|\widehat{\boldsymbol{\beta}}\|_0$. Then*

$$C\,\frac{\widehat{p}+a}{b+a+n} < \mathsf{E}\,[\theta \mid \widehat{\boldsymbol{\beta}}] < \frac{\widehat{p}+a}{b+a+\widehat{p}},$$

where $0 < C < 1$. Moreover, when $a = 1, b = n$ and $(\lambda_0 - \lambda_1)^2\, n/\widehat{p}^2 \to \infty$, then $\lim_{n\to\infty} C = 1$.

Proof Let $x_j = \left(1 - \frac{\lambda_1}{\lambda_0} e^{|\widehat{\beta}_j|(\lambda_0-\lambda_1)}\right)$ and assume (without loss of generality) that $x_j = x$ for $1 \le j \le \widehat{p}$. Note that $x < 1$ and $x \to -\infty$ as $\lambda_0 \to \infty$. Applying Lemma 1 and Lemma 2 (with $\delta = 1$) , we obtain

$$\mathsf{E}\,[\theta \mid \widehat{\boldsymbol{\beta}}] = \frac{\mathscr{B}(a+1,b)}{\mathscr{B}(a,b)}\frac{F_1(a+1,\widehat{p}-n,-\widehat{p},a+b+1;z,x)}{F_1(a,\widehat{p}-n,-\widehat{p},a+b;z,x)} \tag{36}$$

$$< \frac{\mathscr{B}(\widehat{p}+a+1,b)}{\mathscr{B}(\widehat{p}+a,b)} = \frac{\widehat{p}+a}{\widehat{p}+a+b}. \tag{37}$$

Next, we can write

$$\mathsf{E}\,[\theta \mid \widehat{\boldsymbol{\beta}}] > \frac{\int_0^1 \theta^{\widehat{p}+a}(1-\theta)^b(1-\theta z)^{n-\widehat{p}}\mathrm{d}\,\theta}{\int_0^1 \theta^{\widehat{p}+a-1}(1-\theta)^b(1-\theta z)^{n-\widehat{p}}\mathrm{d}\,\theta}\times$$
$$\frac{\int_0^1 \theta^{\widehat{p}+a-1}(1-\theta)^b(1-\theta z)^{n-\widehat{p}}\mathrm{d}\,\theta}{\int_0^1 \theta^{\widehat{p}+a-1}(1-\theta)^b(1-\theta z)^{n-\widehat{p}}(1+\frac{1-\theta}{\theta}\frac{\lambda_0}{\lambda_1}e^{-|\beta_i|(\lambda_0-\lambda_1)})^{\widehat{p}}\mathrm{d}\,\theta},$$

where we used the fact that $1/p^\star_\theta(\beta_i) = 1 + \frac{1-\theta}{\theta}\frac{\lambda_0}{\lambda_1}e^{-|\beta_i|(\lambda_0-\lambda_1)]} > 1$. Denote by $R(z)$ the first term in the product above and by C the second term. Then

$$R(z) = \frac{\mathscr{B}(\widehat{p}+a+1,b)}{\mathscr{B}(\widehat{p}+a,b)}\frac{F_1(\widehat{p}+a+1,0,\widehat{p}-n,\widehat{p}+a+b+1;0,z)}{F_1(\widehat{p}+a,0,\widehat{p}-n,\widehat{p}+a+b;0,z)}$$

$$> R(1) = \frac{\widehat{p}+a}{b+a+n}, \tag{38}$$

where we applied Lemma 1.

Next, we show that $C \to 1$ as $\lambda_0 \to \infty$. First, we denote by $\tilde{\pi}(\theta) \propto \theta^{a+\widehat{p}-1}(1-\theta)^{b-1}(1-\theta z)^{n-\widehat{p}}(1+\frac{1-\theta}{\theta}\frac{\lambda_0}{\lambda_1}e^{-|\beta_i|(\lambda_0-\lambda_1)})^{\widehat{p}}$, the density of a generalized

Gauss hypergeometric distribution, and by $\mathsf{E}_{\widetilde{\pi}}[\cdot]$ its expectation operator. Then

$$C = \mathsf{E}_{\widetilde{\pi}}\left\{\left[1 + \frac{1-\theta}{\theta}\frac{\lambda_0}{\lambda_1}\mathrm{e}^{-|\widehat{\beta}_i|(\lambda_0-\lambda_1)}\right]^{-\widehat{p}}\right\}.$$

We now use the fact that nonzero values $\widehat{\beta}_i$ are larger than a certain threshold, $p^\star_{\theta_i}(\widehat{\beta}_i) > 0.5(1+\sqrt{1-4/(\lambda_0-\lambda_1)^2}$, [21]. This can be equivalently written as

$$\frac{\lambda_0}{\lambda_1}\mathrm{e}^{-|\widehat{\beta}_i|(\lambda_0-\lambda_1)} < \frac{\mathsf{E}\,[\theta \mid \widehat{\boldsymbol{\beta}}_{\setminus i}]}{1-\mathsf{E}\,[\theta \mid \widehat{\boldsymbol{\beta}}_{\setminus i}]}\frac{1}{(\lambda_0-\lambda_1)^2/2-1} < \frac{\widehat{p}+a}{b-1}\frac{1}{(\lambda_0-\lambda_1)^2/2-1}.$$

In the second inequality above, we applied the upper bound (36). Next,

$$1 > \left[1 + \frac{1-\theta}{\theta}\frac{\lambda_0}{\lambda_1}\mathrm{e}^{-|\widehat{\beta}_i|(\lambda_0-\lambda_1)}\right]^{-\widehat{p}} > \mathrm{e}^{-\frac{1-\theta}{\theta}\frac{\widehat{p}+a}{b-1}\frac{\widehat{p}}{(\lambda_0-\lambda_1)^2/2-1}} \equiv g(\theta)$$

Assuming $(\lambda_0-\lambda_1)^2\, n/\widehat{p}^2 \to \infty$ as $n \to \infty$ and $b = n, a = 1$, we have $\lim_{n\to\infty} g(\theta) = 1\, \forall \theta \in (0,1)$ and $\lim_{n\to\infty} C = 1$, by the bounded convergence theorem.

The arguments apply also when $x_i \neq x_j, 1 \leq i,j \leq \widehat{p}_n$, yielding ultimately the same upper/lower bounds.

Lemma 3 has important implications for the tuning of a and b. With $a = 1$ and $b = n$, we obtain $\mathsf{E}\,[\theta \mid \widehat{\boldsymbol{\beta}}] \sim \frac{\widehat{p}}{n}$, which is the actual proportion of nonzero coefficients in $\widehat{\boldsymbol{\beta}}$. Using Lemma 3, we obtain that with $a = 1$ and $b = n$, the posterior odds satisfy

$$\frac{n+\widehat{p}+1}{\widehat{p}+1} - 1 < \frac{1-\mathsf{E}\,[\theta \mid \widehat{\boldsymbol{\beta}}]}{\mathsf{E}\,[\theta \mid \widehat{\boldsymbol{\beta}}]} < \frac{2n+1}{\widehat{p}+1} - 1. \tag{39}$$

These posterior odds play a key role in determining the selection thresholds Δ_i, which in turn drive the risk of the global mode estimator.

6 Risk Properties of the Global Mode

Now consider the fully-Bayes SSL estimator $\widehat{\boldsymbol{\beta}}^{FSL}$, and again assume that it is the first p entries in $\boldsymbol{\beta}_0$ that are nonzero. Adapting the proof of Theorem 5.1 of Ročková [21], we obtain

$$\mathsf{E}_{\boldsymbol{\beta}_0}||\widehat{\boldsymbol{\beta}}^{FSL} - \boldsymbol{\beta}_0||^2 \preceq \sum_{i=1}^{p_n} \mathsf{E}_{\boldsymbol{\beta}_0}\Delta_i^2 + \sum_{i=p_n+1}^{n} \mathsf{E}_{\boldsymbol{\beta}_0}\Delta_i\phi(\Delta_i). \tag{40}$$

With $a = 1$ and $b = n$, using (39) we obtain

$$\mathsf{E}_{\boldsymbol{\beta}_0}||\widehat{\boldsymbol{\beta}}^{FSL} - \boldsymbol{\beta}_0||^2 \preceq p_n \,\mathsf{E}_{\boldsymbol{\beta}_0} \log\left[1 + \frac{\lambda_0}{\lambda_1}\frac{n}{\widehat{p}+1}\right]. \tag{41}$$

It is worthwhile to compare (41) with the upper risk bound (17) obtained for the non-adaptive estimator. Here, we have a different selection threshold for each coordinate and deploy an expected value of these thresholds under $\pi(\boldsymbol{Y} \mid \boldsymbol{\beta}_0)$. In the absence of knowledge of p_n, the automatic choice $\lambda_0/\lambda_1 = n^\alpha$, for $\alpha > 0$, and $\theta = 1/n$ yielded $\Delta \sim \sqrt{2\log(1 + n^{\alpha+1})}$ in the non-adaptive case. Here, by adapting the parameter θ, we obtain an improvement, where $\Delta_i \sim \sqrt{2\log(1 + n^{\alpha+1}/\widehat{p})}$. In either case, with $\lambda_0/\lambda_1 = n^\alpha$ one achieves the near-minimax risk rate $\sqrt{2\log n}$. However, in the adaptive case we have obtained a sharper upper bound.

Whereas the fully Bayes LASSO selection threshold $\mathsf{E}[\lambda \mid \widehat{\boldsymbol{\beta}}^L]$ could not be scaled as $\sqrt{2\log n}$, here the adaptive thresholds Δ_i are themselves logarithms and scale as $\sqrt{2\log n}$ under a suitable beta prior $\mathscr{B}(1, n)$. Thus, with the spike-and-slab LASSO, there is no longer a disconnect between the fully Bayes and universal hyperparameter tuning.

6.1 Adapting to the Dimensionality

The purpose of this section is to demonstrate the ability of the "posterior odds" $[1 - \mathsf{E}(\theta \mid \widehat{\boldsymbol{\beta}}_{\setminus i})]/\mathsf{E}(\theta \mid \widehat{\boldsymbol{\beta}}_{\setminus i})$ to adapt to the true unknown sparsity level p_n. For $\theta \sim \mathscr{B}(1, n)$, the asymptotic rate of the odds ratio (39) is governed by $n/\widehat{p}$. Our goal in this section is to show that these odds are of the optimal order n/p_n with large probability. The following lemma will be instrumental in the result to follow.

Lemma 4 *We have*

$$\log\left[\frac{\pi(\boldsymbol{\beta}_0)}{\pi(\widehat{\boldsymbol{\beta}})}\right] > -\lambda_1|\widehat{\boldsymbol{\beta}} - \boldsymbol{\beta}_0| + (\widehat{p} - p_n)\log\left[\frac{\lambda_0}{\lambda_1}\frac{b+k+a}{\widehat{p}+a}\right] + \log C,$$

where $k = \widehat{p}\,\mathrm{I}(\widehat{p} < p_n) + n\,\mathrm{I}(\widehat{p} > p_n)$ *and* C *was defined in the proof of Lemma 3.*

Proof We can write

$$\log\left[\frac{\pi(\boldsymbol{\beta}_0)}{\pi(\widehat{\boldsymbol{\beta}})}\right] > -\lambda_1|\widehat{\boldsymbol{\beta}} - \boldsymbol{\beta}_0| + (\widehat{p} - p_n)\log\left(\frac{\lambda_0}{\lambda_1}\right) + \log\left[\frac{N(z)}{D(z)}\right] + \log C \tag{42}$$

where $z = (1 - \frac{\lambda_1}{\lambda_0})$ and

$$N(z) \equiv \int_0^1 \theta^{p_n+a-1}(1-\theta)^{b-1}(1-\theta z)^{n-p_n} d\,\theta, \tag{43}$$

$$D(z) \equiv \int_0^1 \theta^{\widehat{p}+a-1}(1-\theta)^{b-1}(1-\theta z)^{n-\widehat{p}} d\,\theta. \tag{44}$$

Denote by $R(z) = \frac{\mathscr{B}(\hat{p}_n+a,b)}{\mathscr{B}(p_n+a,b)} \frac{N(z)}{D(z)}$. First, assume $p_n = \widehat{p} + \delta$ for some $\delta > 0$. We can write

$$R(z) = \frac{F_1(\widehat{p}+a+\delta, 0, \widehat{p}-n+\delta, b+\widehat{p}+a+\delta; 0, z)}{F_1(\widehat{p}+a, 0, \widehat{p}-n, b+\widehat{p}+a; 0, z)}. \tag{45}$$

As in Lemma 1, we can show (using similar arguments) that $R(z)$ is monotone decreasing in z and thus can be lower-bounded by $R(1)$. Therefore

$$\frac{N(z)}{D(z)} > \frac{\mathscr{B}(p_n+a, b+n-p_n)}{\mathscr{B}(\widehat{p}+a, b+n-\widehat{p})} > \left(\frac{b+n+a}{\widehat{p}+a}\right)^{\widehat{p}-p_n}. \tag{46}$$

Now assume $\widehat{p} = p_n + \delta$ for some $\delta > 0$. Using again the monotonicity argument, we find that $1/R(z)$ can be upper-bounded by $1/R(0)$. This yields

$$\frac{N(z)}{D(z)} > \frac{\mathscr{B}(p_n+a, b)}{\mathscr{B}(\widehat{p}+a, b)} > \left(\frac{b+\widehat{p}+a}{\widehat{p}+a}\right)^{\widehat{p}-p_n}.$$

In the following theorem we show that, with high probability, $\widehat{p}$ has the same order as p_n, assuming that the signal is strong enough. Namely, we provide a non-asymptotic upper and lower bound for $\widehat{p}$, focusing on a set $\tau_0 = \{\boldsymbol{Y} : ||\boldsymbol{Y} - \boldsymbol{\beta}_0||_\infty \leq \bar{\lambda}\}$, where $\bar{\lambda} = 2\sqrt{\log n}$. The complement of this set has a small probability, i.e. $\mathsf{P}(\tau_0^c) \leq \frac{2}{n}$ (Castillo et al. [4], Lemma 2).

Theorem 1 *Assume $\lambda_0/\lambda_1 = n^\alpha$ where $\alpha > 0$ and $\lambda_1 < \bar{\lambda}$. Assume $|\beta_{0i}| \geq b_0$, when $\beta_{0i} \neq 0$, where $b_0 > C_1\sqrt{p_n \log n}$ for some $C_1 > 0$. Then with probability at least $1 - \frac{2}{n}$, we have*

$$p_n \leq \widehat{p} \leq 2p_n + 1. \tag{47}$$

Proof Denote by $Q(\boldsymbol{\beta}) = -\frac{1}{2}||\boldsymbol{Y}-\boldsymbol{\beta}||^2 + \log \pi(\boldsymbol{\beta})$, where $\pi(\boldsymbol{\beta})$ is the non-separable prior (19). Using the global optimality $0 \geq Q(\boldsymbol{\beta}^0) - Q(\widehat{\boldsymbol{\beta}})$, we can write

$$0 \geq ||\widehat{\boldsymbol{\beta}} - \boldsymbol{\beta}^0||^2 - 2\boldsymbol{\varepsilon}'(\widehat{\boldsymbol{\beta}} - \boldsymbol{\beta}^0) + 2\,\log\left(\frac{\pi(\boldsymbol{\beta}_0)}{\pi(\widehat{\boldsymbol{\beta}})}\right) \tag{48}$$

Now, we condition on the set τ_0 and use the Hölder inequality $|\boldsymbol{\alpha}'\boldsymbol{\beta}| \leq |\boldsymbol{\alpha}|_\infty |\boldsymbol{\beta}|$ to find that

$$0 \geq ||\widehat{\boldsymbol{\beta}} - \boldsymbol{\beta}^0||^2 - 2\,\bar{\lambda}|\widehat{\boldsymbol{\beta}} - \boldsymbol{\beta}_0| + 2\,\log\left(\frac{\pi(\boldsymbol{\beta}_0)}{\pi(\widehat{\boldsymbol{\beta}})}\right). \tag{49}$$

Denote by $\boldsymbol{\delta} = \widehat{\boldsymbol{\beta}} - \boldsymbol{\beta}_0$. Using the fact $|\boldsymbol{\delta}| \leq ||\boldsymbol{\delta}||\,||\boldsymbol{\delta}||_0^{1/2}$, we have

$$0 \geq ||\boldsymbol{\delta}||^2 - 2\,\bar{\lambda}||\boldsymbol{\delta}||\,||\boldsymbol{\delta}||_0^{1/2} + 2\,\log\left(\frac{\pi(\boldsymbol{\beta}_0)}{\pi(\widehat{\boldsymbol{\beta}})}\right). \tag{50}$$

We will first show the upper bound $\widehat{p} \leq C_2 p_n$ for some $C_2 > 1$. To this end, we assume $\widehat{p} > p_n$. Using the lower-bound of the log-prior ratio in Lemma 4 we have

$$\log\left[\frac{\pi(\boldsymbol{\beta}_0)}{\pi(\widehat{\boldsymbol{\beta}})}\right] \geq -\lambda_1|\boldsymbol{\beta}_0 - \widehat{\boldsymbol{\beta}}_0| + (\widehat{p} - p_n)\log\left(\frac{\lambda_0}{\lambda_1}\frac{b+n+a}{\widehat{p}+a}\right) + 2\log C.$$

To continue with (50), we can write

$$\left[||\boldsymbol{\delta}|| - (\bar{\lambda}+\lambda_1)||\boldsymbol{\delta}||_0^{1/2}\right]^2 + 2\,(\widehat{p}-p_n)\log\left(\frac{\lambda_0}{\lambda_1}\frac{b+n+a}{\widehat{p}+a}\right) \leq (\bar{\lambda}+\lambda_1)^2||\boldsymbol{\delta}||_0 + 2\log 1/C. \tag{51}$$

With (51) and using the fact $||\boldsymbol{\delta}||_0 \leq \widehat{p} + p_n$, we obtain

$$2\,(\widehat{p} - p_n)\log\left(\frac{\lambda_0}{\lambda_1}\frac{b+n+a}{\widehat{p}+a}\right) \leq (\bar{\lambda}+\lambda_1)^2(\widehat{p}+p_n) + 2\log 1/C$$

which is equivalent to writing

$$\widehat{p} \leq p_n\left(1 + \frac{2(\bar{\lambda}+\lambda_1)^2}{2\log\left(\frac{\lambda_0}{\lambda_1}\frac{b+n+a}{\widehat{p_n}+a}\right) - (\bar{\lambda}+\lambda_1)^2}\right) + 2\log 1/C.$$

With $\lambda_1 < \bar{\lambda}$ and $\lambda_0/\lambda_1 = n^\alpha$ for sufficiently large $\alpha > 0$, we have $\log\left(\frac{\lambda_0}{\lambda_1}\frac{b+n+a}{\widehat{p}+a}\right) > (\bar{\lambda}+\lambda_1)^2$. Because $C \to 1$ under given assumptions, $\log 1/C < 1/2$ for n large enough. We obtain the upper bound in (47) with $C_2 = 2$.

What remains to be shown is $p_n \leq \widehat{p}$. We prove this statement by contradiction. Assume $\widehat{p} < p_n$ and let $0 < q = p_n - \widehat{p}$. To continue with (50), we use Lemma 4 to obtain

$$0 \geq ||\boldsymbol{\delta}||\left[||\boldsymbol{\delta}|| - 2\,(\bar{\lambda}+\lambda_1)||\boldsymbol{\delta}||_0^{1/2}\right] + 2(\widehat{p} - p_n)\log\left(\frac{\lambda_0}{\lambda_1}\frac{b+\widehat{p}+a}{\widehat{p}+a}\right) + 2\log C.$$

Because $||\boldsymbol{\delta}|| < p_n + \widehat{p} < (1 + C_2)p_n + 1$, this writes as

$$0 \geq ||\boldsymbol{\delta}|| \left[||\boldsymbol{\delta}|| - 2\,(\bar{\lambda} + \lambda_1)\sqrt{p_n(1 + C_2) + 1} \right] + 2(\widehat{p} - p_n) \log \left(\frac{\lambda_0}{\lambda_1} \frac{b + \widehat{p} + a}{\widehat{p} + a} \right) + 2 \log C. \quad (52)$$

Assuming the minimal-strength condition $|\beta_{0i}| > b_0$ when $\beta_{0i} \neq 0$, we can write

$$\frac{1}{2}||\boldsymbol{\delta}|| > \frac{1}{2}\sqrt{q}b_0 > C_1\sqrt{p_n \log n} > 2\,(\bar{\lambda} + \lambda_1)\sqrt{p_n(1 + C_1) + 1}$$

for suitably large C_1. Assuming $\lambda_0/\lambda_1 = n^\alpha$, (52) yields

$$\begin{aligned} 0 &\geq \frac{1}{2}||\boldsymbol{\delta}||^2 - 2q \log \left(\frac{\lambda_0}{\lambda_1} \frac{b + \widehat{p} + a}{\widehat{p} + a} \right) + 2 \log C \\ &> 2C_1^2\sqrt{p_n \log n} - 2q \log \left(\frac{\lambda_0}{\lambda_1} \frac{b + \widehat{p} + a}{\widehat{p} + a} \right) + 2 \log C > 0 \end{aligned}$$

for C_1 sufficiently large.

Remark 2 The minimal strength condition in Lemma 1 is a bit stronger than typical beta-min conditions in the LASSO literature. This stronger condition was used previously by Fan and Lv [9] and Zheng et al. [30] to show sign consistency of non-concave regularizers.

We conclude the paper with the following result which follows directly from Lemma 3 and Theorem 1.

Corollary 1 *Assume $\theta \sim \mathscr{B}(1, n)$. Under the same conditions as in Theorem 1, we obtain*

$$\frac{1 - \mathsf{E}\,[\theta \mid \widehat{\boldsymbol{\beta}}_{\setminus i}]}{\mathsf{E}\,[\theta \mid \widehat{\boldsymbol{\beta}}_{\setminus i}]} \sim n/p_n$$

and thus $(\Delta_i - \lambda_1)^2 \sim 2 \log \left(\frac{\lambda_0}{\lambda_1} \frac{n}{p_n} \right)$, with probability at least $1 - \frac{2}{n}$.

Corollary 1 conveys the very important conclusion that the portion of the selection threshold Δ_i involving θ is *self-adaptive*. In other words, the non-separable penalty obtained with the prior $\pi(\theta) = \mathscr{B}(1, n)$ removes the need for setting θ equal to the true proportion of true coefficients p_n/n, because it can adapt to the ambient dimensionality of the data. Thus, the fully Bayes treatment of θ here mimics oracle performance. This behavior was confirmed by simulations, where self-tuning θ with the fully Bayes formulation was tantamount to selecting θ by cross-validation.

Adapting θ is only halfway towards a fully automatic procedure that would adapt λ_0 and θ simultaneously, removing the need for assuming p_n is known. Observing that $(1-\theta)/\theta$ and λ_0 should be of the same order n/p_n, Ročková [21] proposed tying λ_0 and θ through $\lambda_0 \sim 1/\theta$ to borrow strength. This amounts to inducing a beta prime distribution on the spike penalty. Another potentially useful approach would be to treat θ and λ_0 independently by assigning two prior distributions. In any case, adapting λ_0 simultaneously with θ requires several nontrivial modifications of our approach and will be reported elsewhere.

7 Discussion

In this paper we demonstrated the potential of the fully Bayes approach for adaptive penalty creation. We compared two deployments of this strategy in terms of their ability to adapt to unknown sparsity: the fully Bayes LASSO and the fully Bayes Spike-and-Slab LASSO. In the first example, the fully Bayes adaptation could not overcome the restrictive form of the penalty. In the second example, however, the fully Bayes adaptation automatically performed universal hyperparameter tuning. For the Spike-and-Slab LASSO, treating a penalty hyperparameter as random with a prior was shown to be tantamount to an oracle choice of the hyperparameter. Thus, penalty functions arising from such fully Bayes prior constructions exert self-adapting ability. This adaptability is reminiscent of an empirical Bayes strategy, and constitutes an alternative to cross-validation and other calibration approaches.

Acknowledgements This work was supported by NSF grant DMS-1406563 and AHRQ grant R21-HS021854.

References

1. Armero, C., Bayarri, M.: Prior assessments in prediction in queues. The Stat. **45**, 139–153 (1994)
2. Bondell, H., Reich, B.: Simultaneous regression shrinkage, variable selection, and supervised clustering of predictors with OSCAR. Biometrics **64**, 115–123 (2008)
3. Brown, L.: Admissible estimators, recurrent diffusions, and insoluble boundary value problems. Ann. Math. Stat. **42**, 855–903 (1971)
4. Castillo, I., Schmidt-Hieber, J., van der Vaart, A.: Bayesian linear regression with sparse priors. Ann. Stat. **43**, 1986–2018 (2015)
5. Castillo, I., van der Vaart, A.: Needles and straw in a haystack: posterior concentration for possibly sparse sequences. Ann. Stat. **40**, 2069–2101 (2012)
6. Donoho, D., Johnstone, I.M.: Ideal spatial adaptation by wavelet shrinkage. Biometrika **81**, 425–455 (1994)
7. Donoho, D., Johnstone, I.M., Hoch, J.C., Stern, A.S.: Maximum entropy and the nearly black object. J. R. Stat. Soc. B **54**, 41–81 (1992)
8. Fan, J., Li, R.: Variable selection via nonconcave penalized likelihood and its oracle properties. J. Am. Stat. Assoc. **96**, 1348–1360 (2001)
9. Fan, Y., Lv, J.: Asymptotic properties for combined l1 and concave regularization. Biometrika **101**, 67–70 (2014)

10. Friedman, J.: Fast sparse regression and classification. Technical Report, Department of Statistics, Stanford University (2008)
11. George, E.I.: Combining minimax shrinkage estimators. J. Am. Stat. Assoc. **81**, 437–445 (1968a)
12. George, E.I.: Minimax multiple shrinkage estimation. Ann. Stat. **14**, 188–205 (1968b)
13. Gradshteyn, I., Ryzhik, E.: Table of Integrals Series and Products. Academic, New York (2000)
14. Griffin, J.E., Brown, P.J.: Bayesian hyper-LASSOS with non-convex penalization. Aust. N. Z. J. Stat. **53**, 423–442 (2012)
15. Ismail, M., Pitman, J.: Algebraic evaluations of some Euler integrals, duplication formulae for Appell's hypergeometric function f_1, and Brownian variations. Can. J. Math. **52**, 961–981 (2000)
16. Johnstone, I.M., Silverman, B.W.: Needles and straw in haystacks: empirical Bayes estimates of possibly sparse sequences. Ann. Stat. **32**, 1594–1649 (2004)
17. Karp, D., Sitnik, S.M.: Inequalities and monotonicity of ratios for generalized hypergeometric function. J. Approx. Theory **161**, 337–352 (2009)
18. Meier, L., Van de Geer, S., Bühlmann, P.: The group LASSO for logistic regression. J. R. Stat. Soc. B **70**, 53–71 (2008)
19. Park, T., Casella, G.: The Bayesian LASSO. J. Am. Stat. Assoc. **103**, 681–686 (2008)
20. Polson, N., Scott, J.: Shrink globally, act locally: sparse Bayesian regularization and prediction. Bayesian Stat. **9**, 501–539 (2010)
21. Ročková, V.: Bayesian estimation of sparse signals with a continuous spike-and-slab prior. In revision Annals of Statistics (2015)
22. Ročková, V., George, E.: EMVS: The EM approach to Bayesian variable selection. J. Am. Stat. Assoc. **109**, 828–846 (2014)
23. Ročková, V., George, E.: Fast Bayesian factor analysis via automatic rotations to sparsity. J. Am. Stat. Assoc., JASA (2015a, accepted for publication)
24. Ročková, V., George, E.: The Spike-and-Slab LASSO, JASA (2015b, Submitted)
25. Stein, C.: Estimation of the mean of a multivariate normal distribution. In: Hajek, J. (ed.) Prague Symposium on Asymptotic Statistics. Univerzita Karlova, Prague, Czech republic (1974)
26. Tibshirani, R.: Regression shrinkage and selection via the LASSO. J. R. Stat. Soc. B **58**, 267–288 (1994)
27. Tibshirani, R., Saunders, M., Rosset, S., Zhu, J., Knight, K.: Sparsity and smoothness via the fused LASSO. J. R. Stat. Soc. B **67**, 91–108 (2005)
28. Wang, Z., Liu, H., Zhang, T.: Optimal computational and statistical rates of convergence for sparse nonconvex learning problems. Ann. Stat. **42**, 2164–2201 (2014)
29. Zhang, C.H.: Nearly unbiased variable selection under minimax concave penalty. Ann. Stat. **38**, 894–942 (2010)
30. Zheng, Z., Fan, Y., Lv, J.: High dimensional thresholded regression and shrinkage effect. J. R. Stat. Soc. B **76**, 627–649 (2014)
31. Zou, H.: The adaptive LASSO and its oracle properties. J. Am. Stat. Assoc. **101**, 1418–1429 (2006)
32. Zou, H., Hastie, T.: Regularization and variable selection via the elastic net. J. R. Stat. Soc. B **67**, 301–320 (2005)

Confidence Intervals for Maximin Effects in Inhomogeneous Large-Scale Data

Dominik Rothenhäusler, Nicolai Meinshausen, and Peter Bühlmann

Abstract One challenge of large-scale data analysis is that the assumption of an identical distribution for all samples is often not realistic. An optimal linear regression might, for example, be markedly different for distinct groups of the data. Maximin effects have been proposed as a computationally attractive way to estimate effects that are common across all data without fitting a mixture distribution explicitly. So far just point estimators of the common maximin effects have been proposed in Meinshausen and Bühlmann (Ann Stat 43(4):1801–1830, 2015). Here we propose asymptotically valid confidence regions for these effects.

1 Introduction

Large-scale regression analysis often has to deal with inhomogeneous data in the sense that samples are not drawn independently from the same distribution. The optimal regression coefficient might for example be markedly different in distinct groups of the data or vary slowly over a chronological ordering of the samples. One option is then to either model the exact variation of the regression vector with a varying-coefficient model in the latter case [5, 7] or to fit a mixture distribution in the former [1, 6, 8]. For large-scale analysis with many groups of data samples or many predictor variables this approach might be too expensive computationally and also yield more information than necessary in settings where one is just interested in effects that are present in all sub-groups of data. A maximin effect was defined in [9] as the effect that is common to all sub-groups of data and a simple estimator based on subsampling of the data was proposed in [3]. However, the estimators for maximin effects proposed so far just yield point estimators but we are interested here in confidence intervals. While we are mostly dealing with low-dimensional data where the sample size exceeds the number of samples, the results could potentially be extended to high-dimensional regression using similar ideas as proposed for

D. Rothenhäusler (✉) • N. Meinshausen • P. Bühlmann
Seminar für Statistik, ETH Zürich, Rämistrasse 101, 8092 Zürich, Switzerland
e-mail: rothenhaeusler@stat.math.ethz.ch; meinshausen@stat.math.ethz.ch; buehlmann@stat.math.ethz.ch

A. Frigessi et al. (eds.), *Statistical Analysis for High-Dimensional Data*, Abel Symposia 11, DOI 10.1007/978-3-319-27099-9_12

example in [12] or [11] for the estimation of optimal linear regression effects for high-dimensional data.

1.1 Model and Notation

We first present a model for inhomogeneous data as considered in [9]. Specifically, we look at a special case where the data are split into several known groups $g = 1, \ldots, G$. In each group g, we assume a linear model of the form

$$Y_g = \mathbf{X}_g b_g^0 + \varepsilon_g, \tag{1}$$

where Y_g is a n-dimensional response vector of interest, b_g^0 a deterministic p-dimensional regression parameter vectors and $\mathbf{X}_g$ a $n \times p$-dimensional design matrix containing in the columns the n observations of p predictor variables. The noise contributions ε_g are assumed to be independent with distribution $\mathcal{N}_n(0, \sigma^2 \mathrm{Id}_n)$. We assume the sample size n to be identical in each group. Generalizations to varying-coefficient models [5, 7] are clearly possible but notationally more cumbersome. Inhomogeneity is caused by the different parameter vectors in the group. We define $\mathbf{X}$ as the row-wise concatenation of the design matrices $\mathbf{X}_1, \mathbf{X}_2, \ldots, \mathbf{X}_G$ and assume that the groups are known, that is we know which observations belong to the groups $g = 1, \ldots, G$, respectively. For the distribution of $\mathbf{X}_g$, $g = 1, \ldots, G$ we consider different scenarios.

1.1.1 Scenario 1

Random design. The observations of the predictor variables are independent samples of an unknown multivariate distribution F with finite fourth moments. We assume this distribution to be common across all groups $g = 1, \ldots, G$.

1.1.2 Scenario 2

Random design in each group. The observation in each group are independent samples of an unknown distribution F_g with finite fourth moments. Observations in different groups are independent. The distribution F_g may be different in different groups.

In the following if not mentioned otherwise we assume Scenario 1. The generalization to Scenario 2 is to a large extent only notational.

1.2 Aggregation

The question arises how the inhomogeneity of the optimal regression across groups is taken into account when trying to estimate the relationship between the predictor variables and the outcome of interest. Several known alternatives such as mixed effects models [10], mixture models [8] and clusterwise regression models [4] are possibilities and are useful especially in cases where the group structure is unknown. They are at the same time computationally quite demanding.

A computationally attractive alternative (especially for the discussed case of known groups but also more generally) is to estimate the optimal regression coefficient separately in each group, which are either known (as assumed in the following) or sampled in some appropriate form [9]. As estimates for the b_g^0 we use in the following standard least squares estimators

$$\hat{b}_g = \arg\min_{b \in \mathbb{R}^p} \|Y_g - \mathbf{X}_g b\|_2^2.$$

The restriction to this estimator is only for the purpose of simplicity. Regularization can be added if necessary but the essential issues are already visible for least-squares estimation.

Now a least-squares estimator is obtained in each group of data and the question is how these different estimators can be aggregated. The simplest and perhaps most widely-used aggregation scheme is bagging (bootstrap aggregation), as proposed by Breiman [2], where the aggregated estimator is given by

$$\textbf{Bagging}: \quad \hat{b} := \sum_g w_g \hat{b}_g, \qquad \text{where } w_g = \frac{1}{G} \;\; \forall g = 1, \ldots, G. \tag{2}$$

If the data from different groups originate from an independent sampling mechanism, the bagging is a useful aggregation scheme. In particular, computing the bagged estimator is computationally more attractive than computing a single least-squares estimator as it allows the data to be split up into distinct subsets and processed independently before the aggregation step. For inhomogeneous data, the variability of the estimates $\hat{b}_g$ for $g = 1, \ldots, G$ allows to gain some insight into the nature of the inhomogeneity. However, as argued in [3], averaging is the wrong aggregation mechanism for inhomogeneous data.

1.3 Maximin Effect and Magging

For inhomogeneous data, instead of looking for an estimator that works best on average, Meinshausen and Bühlmann [9] proposed to aim to maximize the minimum explained variance across several settings $g = 1, \ldots, G$. To be more precise, in our setting,

$$b_{\text{maximin}} := \arg\max_{b \in \mathbb{R}^p} \min_{g=1,\ldots,G} V(b, b_g^0),$$

where $V(b, b_g^0)$ is the explained variance in group g (with true regression vector b_g^0) when using a regression vector b. That is

$$\begin{aligned} V(b, b_g^0) &:= \mathbb{E}\|Y_g\|_2^2 - \mathbb{E}\|Y_g - X_g b\|_2^2 \\ &= 2b^t \Sigma^0 b_g^0 - b^t \Sigma^0 b, \end{aligned}$$

where $\Sigma^0 := \mathbb{E}\hat{\Sigma}$ with $\hat{\Sigma} := (nG)^{-1}\mathbf{X}^t\mathbf{X}$ is the sample covariance matrix. In words, the maximin effect is defined as the estimator that maximises the explained variance in the most adversarial scenario ("group"). In this sense, the maximin effect is the effect that is common among all groups in the data and ignores the effects that are present in some groups but not in others. It was shown in [9] that the definition above is equivalent to

$$b_{\text{maximin}} = \arg\min_{b \in \text{CVX}(B^0)} b^t \Sigma^0 b,$$

where $B^0 = (b_1^0, \ldots, b_G^0) \in \mathbb{R}^{p \times G}$ the matrix of the regression parameter vectors and $CVX(B^0)$ denotes the closed convex hull of the G vectors in B^0. The latter definition motivates **ma**ximin **agg**regat**ing**, or **magging** [3], which is the convex combination that minimizes the ℓ_2-norm of the fitted values:

$$\textbf{Magging: } \hat{b} := \sum_{g=1}^{G} \alpha_g \hat{b}_g, \qquad \text{where } \alpha := \arg\min_{\alpha \in C_G} \|\sum_{g=1}^{G} \alpha_g \mathbf{X}\hat{b}_g\|_2 \text{ and}$$

$$C_G := \{\alpha \in \mathbb{R}^G : \min_g \alpha_g \geq 0 \text{ and } \sum_g \alpha_g = 1\}$$

The magging regression vector is unique if $\mathbf{X}^t\mathbf{X}$ is positive definite. Otherwise, we can only identify the prediction effect $\mathbf{X}b_{\text{maximin}}$ and the solution above is meant to be any member of the feasible set of solutions. To compute the estimator, the dataset is split into several smaller datasets and we assume here that the split separates the data into already known groups. After computing estimators on all of these groups separately, possibly in parallel, magging can be used to find common effects of all datasets. This is in particular interesting if there is inhomogeneity in the data. For known groups, as in our setting, magging can be interpreted as the plug-in estimate of the maximin effect.

In the following we need additional notation. For $B := (b_1, \ldots, b_G) \in \mathbb{R}^{p\times G}$ and for $\Sigma \in \mathbb{R}^{p\times p}$ positive definite define

$$M_\Sigma(B) := \underset{b\in \mathrm{CVX}(B)}{\arg\min}\, b^t \Sigma b$$

We obtain the original definition of the magging estimator for $M_{\hat{\Sigma}}(\hat{B})$ with $\hat{B} = (\hat{b}_1, \ldots, \hat{b}_G)$ and the maximin effect with $M_{\Sigma^0}(B^0)$.

1.4 Novel Contribution and Organization of the Paper

So far only point estimators of maximin effects have been proposed in the literature. In Sect. 2 we discuss an asymptotic approach to construct confidence regions for the maximin effect. Specifically, we calculate the asymptotic distribution of $\sqrt{n}(M_{\hat{\Sigma}}(\hat{B}) - M_{\Sigma^0}(B^0))$ and derive corresponding asymptotically valid confidence regions. This gives us (asymptotically) tight confidence regions and will shed more light on the (asymptotic) nature of the fluctuations of the magging estimator. We evaluate the actual coverage of this approximation on simulated datasets in Sect. 3. The proofs of the corresponding theorems and an alternative non-asymptotic approach can be found in the Appendix. The advantages and disadvantages of the approaches are discussed in Sect. 4.

2 Confidence Intervals for Maximin Effects

In Scenario 1, the random design of the predictor variables is identical across all groups of data. For fixed G and $n \to \infty$, we can then use the delta method to derive the asymptotic distribution of the scaled difference between the true and estimated magging effects

$$\sqrt{n}(M_{\hat{\Sigma}}(\hat{B}) - M_{\Sigma^0}(B^0)).$$

This in turn allows to construct confidence intervals for the true maximin effects. Let $W(\hat{B}, \hat{\Sigma})$ be a consistent estimator of the (positive definite) variance of the Gaussian distribution

$$\lim_{n\to\infty} \sqrt{n}(M_{\hat{\Sigma}}(\hat{B}) - M_{\Sigma^0}(B^0)).$$

Let $\alpha > 0$. Choose τ as the $(1-\alpha)$-quantile of the χ^2_p-distribution. Define then a confidence region as

$$\mathbf{C}(\hat{\Sigma}, \hat{B}) := \{M \in \mathbb{R}^p : (M_{\hat{\Sigma}}(\hat{B}) - M)^t W(\hat{B}, \hat{\Sigma})^{-1}(M_{\hat{\Sigma}}(\hat{B}) - M) \le \frac{\tau}{n}\} \tag{3}$$

The definition of $W(\hat{B}, \hat{\Sigma})$ is deferred to the Appendix, section "Definitions and Formulas". We will show in the following that we obtain asymptotically valid confidence intervals with this approach. For simplicity, we work with Scenario 1 here and assume that the noise contributions ε_g in Eq. (1) are independent with distribution $\mathcal{N}_n(0, \sigma^2 \mathrm{Id}_n)$. Furthermore, each $\mathbf{X}_g \in \mathbb{R}^{n \times p}$ is assumed to have full rank, requiring $p \leq n$. Though the framework for the result is a Gaussian linear model, it can be easily extended to more general settings.

The following theorem describes the coverage properties of the confidence interval (3). In the following, for $x, y \in \mathbb{R}^p$ and $\Sigma \in \mathbb{R}^{p \times p}$ positive definite define $\langle x, y \rangle_\Sigma := x^t \Sigma y$.

Theorem 1 *Let Σ^0 be positive definite. Let $M_{\Sigma^0}(B^0) = \sum_{g=1}^G \alpha_g b_g^0$ with $\alpha_g \geq 0$, $\sum_{g=1}^G \alpha_g = 1$ and let this representation be unique. Let $|\{g : \alpha_g \neq 0\}| > 1$. Suppose that the hyperplane orthonormal to the maximin effect contains only "active" b_g^0, i.e. $\{b_g^0 : g = 1, \ldots, G\} \cap \{M \in \mathbb{R}^p : \langle M - M_{\Sigma^0}(B^0), M_{\Sigma^0}(B^0)\rangle_{\Sigma^0} = 0\} \subset \{b_g^0 : \alpha_g \neq 0\}$. Then*

$$\lim_{n \to \infty} \mathbb{P}[M_{\Sigma^0}(B^0) \in \mathbf{C}(\hat{\Sigma}, \hat{B})] = 1 - \alpha.$$

In other words, the set defined in (3) is an asymptotically valid confidence region for $M_{\Sigma^0}(B^0)$ under the made assumptions. If the true coefficients b_g^0 in each group are drawn from a multivariate density, then the assumptions are fulfilled with probability one.

The special case $|\{g : \alpha_g \neq 0\}| = 1$ is excluded, as the magging estimator is identical to a solution in one individual group in this case, which is equivalent to $M_{\hat{\Sigma}}(\hat{B}) = \hat{b}_g$ for a $g \in \{1, \ldots, G\}$, up to an asymptotically negligible set. This case is mainly excluded for notational reasons. The assumptions of Theorem 1 guarantee that the derivative of magging $M_\Sigma(B)$ exists and is continuous at B^0 and Σ^0. If the latter condition is violated, it is still possible to obtain asymptotic bounds in the more general setting, as $\lim_{n \to \infty} \sqrt{n}(M_{\hat{\Sigma}}(\hat{B}) - M_{\Sigma^0}(B^0))$ is still subgaussian. We explore the violation of these assumptions with simulation studies in the next section. The proof of Theorem 1 is an application of Slutsky's Theorem, combined with the following result about the asymptotic variance of the magging estimator.

Theorem 2 *Let the assumptions of Theorem 1 be true. Then, for $n \to \infty$,*

$$\sqrt{n}\left(M_{\hat{\Sigma}}(\hat{B}) - M_{\Sigma^0}(B^0)\right) \tag{4}$$

$$\rightharpoonup \mathcal{N}\left(0, \sigma^2 \sum_{g \in A(B^0, \Sigma^0)} \mathrm{D}_g^t M_{\Sigma^0}(B^0) \Sigma^{-1} \mathrm{D}_g M_{\Sigma^0}(B^0) + V(B^0_{A(B^0,\Sigma^0)}, \Sigma^0)\right).$$

Here, D_g denotes the differential in direction b_g. This derivative is calculated in the Appendix, see section "Definitions and Formulas". The set $A(B, \Sigma) \subset \{1, \ldots, G\}$ denotes indices g for which b_g has nonvanishing coefficient α_g in one of the convex combinations $M_\Sigma(B) = \sum_{g=1,\dots,G} \alpha_g b_g$ with $\alpha_g \geq 0$, $\sum_{g=1,\dots,G} \alpha_g = 1$. Note that by the assumptions of Theorem 1 this convex combination is unique for $M_{\Sigma^0}(B^0)$. The definition of $V(B_{A(B,\Sigma)}, \Sigma)$ is somewhat lengthy and can be found in the Appendix, section "Definitions and Formulas".

The first summand in the variance in formula (4) is due to fluctuations of the estimator of B^0, the second summand is due to fluctuations of the estimator of Σ^0. If Σ^0 is known in advance, we can use $\hat{\Sigma} := \Sigma^0$ and in the theorem above $V = 0$. Figure 1 is an illustration of Theorem 2.

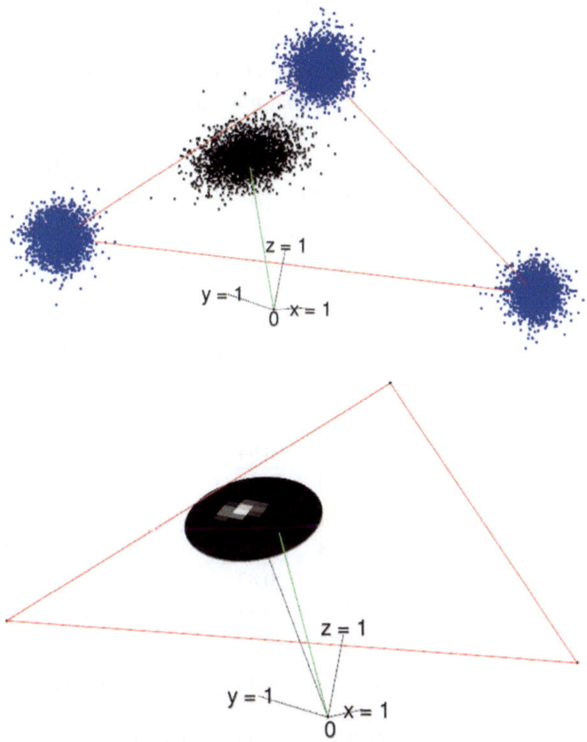

Fig. 1 An illustration of Theorems 1 and 2. On the *upper plot* the *blue dots* represent 3000 realizations of $\hat{b}_g$, $g = 1, 2, 3$ with dimension $p = 3$. The *black dots* are the corresponding magging estimates $M_{\hat{\Sigma}}(\hat{B})$. The *green line* indicates the true maximin effect $M_{\Sigma^0}(B^0)$. On the *lower plot*, the *black line* indicates one of the $M_{\hat{\Sigma}}(\hat{B})$ with the corresponding approximate 95 %-confidence region calculated with the terms of Eq. (3)

3 Numerical Examples

The aim of this section is to evaluate the actual coverage of the approximate confidence regions as defined above. We study several examples. They have in common that the entries in $\mathbf{X}$ are i.i.d. $\mathcal{N}(0,1)$. Furthermore the ε_g are i.i.d. $\mathcal{N}(0, \mathrm{Id}_n)$ and independent of $\mathbf{X}$. The tables show the coverage of the true maximin effect $M_{\Sigma^0}(B^0)$ by the proposed 95 % confidence regions. We calculate the confidence intervals only for $p < n$ scenarios as long as least squares estimators are used (Tables 1, 2, and 3), while the case of $p \geq n$ is covered in Tables 4 and 5 by the use of a ridge penalty. All simulations were run 1000 times.

In the setting of Table 1 all assumptions of Theorem 1 are satisfied. As expected, for large p the convergence of the actual coverage seems to be slower. Note that for validity of Theorem 1 it is not necessary that $p = G$, as we have asymptotically tight coverage for all $1 < G \leq p$.

In Tables 2 and 3 we explore the violation of one of the assumptions in Theorem 1. The maximin effect is $M_{\Sigma^0}(B^0) = (1, 0, 0 \ldots)$, and the convex combination $M_{\Sigma^0}(B^0) = \sum_{g=1}^{G} \alpha_g b_g^0$ with $\alpha_g \geq 0$, $\sum \alpha_g = 1$ is not unique. In both cases, this seems to lead to too conservative confidence regions. Generally, in these

Table 1 $b_g^0 = e_g$, $g = 1, \ldots, G = p$, where the e_g denote the vectors of the standard basis, 1000 iterations

	$n = 5$	10	15	100	200	500	1000	2000	4000
$p = 3$	0.70	0.78	0.82	0.92	0.94	0.95	0.94	0.94	0.95
5		0.69	0.76	0.90	0.93	0.95	0.94	0.95	0.95
10			0.62	0.84	0.88	0.94	0.95	0.96	0.94
15				0.78	0.85	0.93	0.92	0.95	0.95
20				0.72	0.83	0.90	0.91	0.95	0.94
40				0.54	0.63	0.79	0.88	0.91	0.94
80				0.57	0.38	0.50	0.74	0.85	0.92

The coverage can be seen to be approximately correct if n is sufficiently large

Table 2 $b_g^0 = e_1 + z_g e_2$, $g = 1, \ldots, G = p$, $z_g \sim \mathcal{N}(0, 1)$ independent

	$n = 5$	10	15	100	200	500	1000	2000	4000
$p = 3$	0.64	0.84	0.91	0.97	0.96	0.82	0.98	0.96	0.97
5		0.61	0.79	0.99	0.97	0.88	0.82	0.91	1.00
10			0.23	0.99	0.99	1.00	0.99	0.93	0.98
15				0.99	0.99	1.00	1.00	0.99	0.99
20				0.99	1.00	0.99	1.00	1.00	0.99
40				0.94	1.00	1.00	1.00	1.00	1.00
80				0.00	1.00	1.00	1.00	1.00	1.00

The assumptions are violated, yielding too conservative confidence intervals. The 0.00 at $n = 100$, $p = 80$ is due to a large bias of $M_{\hat{\Sigma}}(\hat{B})$ towards 0. For larger n, however, this bias quickly vanishes and we get the desired coverage (starting at approximately $n = 120$)

Table 3 $b_g^0 = e_1, g = 1, \ldots, G = [0.8p]$

	$n = 5$	10	15	100	200	500	1000	2000	4000
$p = 3$	0.76	0.87	0.90	0.99	0.99	0.99	1.00	1.00	1.00
5		0.65	0.78	1.00	1.00	1.00	1.00	1.00	1.00
10			0.33	1.00	1.00	1.00	1.00	1.00	1.00
15				0.99	1.00	1.00	1.00	1.00	1.00
20				0.99	1.00	1.00	1.00	1.00	1.00
40				0.93	1.00	1.00	1.00	1.00	1.00
80				0.00	1.00	1.00	1.00	1.00	1.00

The assumptions are again violated and coverage is too high. At $p = 80$ and $n = 100$ we observe the same effect as in Table 2. In this scenario the estimated confidence regions can become arbitrarily large. This stems from the fact that if some of the $\hat{b}_g$ corresponding to $A(\hat{B}, \hat{\Sigma})$ are very close, the estimated variance of magging may become large. In this setting a different approach, for example as discussed in section "Relaxation-Based Approach" in the Appendix makes more sense

Table 4 $b_g^0 = e_g, g = 1, \ldots, G = p$

	$n = 5$	10	15	100	200	500	1000	2000	4000
$p = 3$	0.71	0.77	0.84	0.92	0.94	0.96	0.95	0.94	0.93
5	0.74	0.69	0.76	0.90	0.94	0.94	0.95	0.95	0.95
10	0.55	0.70	0.60	0.86	0.88	0.93	0.94	0.94	0.95
15	0.52	0.53	0.70	0.77	0.86	0.91	0.94	0.95	0.95
20	0.53	0.48	0.52	0.73	0.81	0.89	0.93	0.92	0.94
40	0.40	0.47	0.37	0.52	0.62	0.81	0.87	0.90	0.94
80	0.20	0.40	0.37	0.56	0.38	0.52	0.72	0.84	0.90

The diagonal elements of $\hat{\Sigma}$ and $\hat{\Sigma}_g$ where increased by a value 10^{-4} in order to make them invertible and not too ill-conditioned for $n \leq p$. Again, coverage is approximately correct for n sufficiently large

Table 5 This table shows the average maximum eigenvalues of the estimated covariance matrix of $\sqrt{n}(M_{\Sigma^0}(B^0) - M_{\hat{\Sigma}}(\hat{B}))$, analogous to Table 4

	$n = 5$	10	15	100	200	500	1000	2000	4000
$p = 3$	41.70	2.97	1.59	0.59	0.53	0.49	0.47	0.47	0.46
5	831.50	13.52	4.83	0.42	0.34	0.30	0.28	0.26	0.26
10	6.56	1935.77	27.78	0.29	0.20	0.16	0.14	0.13	0.12
15	0.29	19.83	3844.87	0.26	0.16	0.12	0.10	0.09	0.08
20	0.08	4.25	41.04	0.29	0.15	0.09	0.08	0.07	0.06
40	0.01	0.04	4.61	2.71	0.16	0.07	0.05	0.04	0.03
80	0.00	0.00	0.01	205.85	1.09	0.06	0.03	0.02	0.02

settings the difficulty arises from the fact that the derivative of $M_\Sigma(B)$ does not exist at $M_{\Sigma^0}(B^0)$. As a result, the fluctuations of $\lim_n \sqrt{n}(M_{\Sigma^0}(B^0) - M_{\hat{\Sigma}}(\hat{B}))$—provided that this limit exists—are not necessarily Gaussian anymore.

In the last simulation, depicted in Table 4 the $\hat{b}_g$, $g = 1, \ldots, G$ were not calculated by ordinary least squares but ridge regression. The diagonal elements of $\hat{\Sigma}$ and $\hat{\Sigma}_g$ where increased by a value 10^{-4} in order to make them invertible and not too ill-conditioned for $n \le p$. Apart from that we used the same setting as in Table 1. As in Table 1, for large n the coverage seems to be (approximately) correct but severe undercoverage can still occur for $n \ll p$. In these high-dimensional settings, the tuning ridge parameter would need to be better adjusted for a useful balance between bias and variance and the bias of the ridge penalty would have to be adjusted for, something which is beyond the current scope. In Table 5 the corresponding maximum eigenvalues of the estimated variance of $\sqrt{n}(M_{\Sigma^0}(B^0) - M_{\hat{\Sigma}}(\hat{B}))$ were plotted, each entry being the average over all 1000 runs. We observe a spike for $p = n$. This peaking is similar to a related effect in ridge and lasso regression. Specifically, for fixed p and varying n, the norm of the regression estimate is growing as n is increased, reaching its peak at approximately $p = n$ while then decreasing again as the solution converges towards the true parameter as n grows very large.

4 Discussion

We derived the asymptotic distribution of the magging estimator and proposed asymptotically tight and valid confidence regions for the maximin effect. The corresponding theorems requires a rather weak assumption on the true regression coefficients $b_1^0, \ldots, b_G^0$. However, if this assumption is not satisfied, as studied in simulations, the resulting confidence regions seem to become too conservative. Especially when all of the "active" vectors $\{\hat{b}_g : g \in A(\hat{\Sigma}, \hat{B})\}$ are very close to each other, the proposed confidence regions tend to become large. Furthermore, in this scenario the magging estimator may suffer from a large bias. Then it may make more sense to use an approach based on relaxation. Such an approach is outlined in the Appendix in section "Relaxation-Based Approach" and it would also allow for non-asymptotic confidence intervals at the price of coverage probabilities well above the specified level. The proposed asymptotic confidence interval on the other hand is arguably more intuitive and yields in most scenarios tight bounds for large sample sizes.

Appendix

The structure is as follows: the first part is devoted to the most important definitions and explicit formulas which were omitted in the main section of the paper. The second part contains the proof of Theorem 2 and several lemmata. The third part contains the proof of Theorem 1. Finally, the last part contains a relaxation-based idea to construct confidence intervals for maximin effects.

Definitions and Formulas

Definition 1 ($A(B, \Sigma)$) The set $A(B, \Sigma) \subset \{1, \ldots, G\}$ denotes indices g for which b_g has nonvanishing coefficient α_g in one of the convex combinations $M_\Sigma(B) = \sum_{g=1,\ldots,G} \alpha_g b_g$ with $\alpha_g \geq 0$, $\sum_{g=1,\ldots,G} \alpha_g = 1$. Note that by the assumptions of Theorem 1 or Theorem 2 the α_g are unique for $M_{\Sigma^0}(B^0)$.

Definition 2 ($W(B, \Sigma)$) $W(\hat{B}, \hat{\Sigma})$ is a consistent estimator of the variance of $\lim_n \sqrt{n}(M_{\hat{\Sigma}}(\hat{B}) - M_{\Sigma^0}(B^0))$, see proof of Theorem 2.

$$W(B, \Sigma) = \sigma^2 \sum_{g \in A(B,\Sigma)} \mathrm{D}_g^t M_\Sigma(B_{A(B,\Sigma)}) \Sigma^{-1} \mathrm{D}_g M_\Sigma(B_{A(B,\Sigma)}) + V(B_{A(B,\Sigma)}, \Sigma)$$

Definitions and explicit formulas of these terms can be found below. We estimate Σ^0 by $\hat{\Sigma} = \frac{1}{nG}\mathbf{X}^t\mathbf{X}$. $\mathrm{D}_g^t M_\Sigma(B)$ denotes the derivative of $M_\Sigma(B)$ with respect to b_g.

Explicit Formula for $V(\hat{B}_{A(\hat{B},\hat{\Sigma})}, \hat{\Sigma})$

(Compare with Lemma 5)

Consistent estimator of the additional variance of $\lim_n \sqrt{n}(M_{\hat{\Sigma}}(\hat{B}) - M_{\Sigma^0}(B^0))$ "caused" by not knowing Σ^0, see proof of Theorem 2 and Lemma 5.

$$V(\hat{B}_{A(\hat{B},\hat{\Sigma})}, \hat{\Sigma}) = \hat{D}(\hat{D}^t \hat{\Sigma} \hat{D})^{-1} \hat{D}^t \hat{C} \hat{D} (\hat{D}^t \hat{\Sigma} \hat{D})^{-1} \hat{D}^t,$$

where $\hat{C}$ is the empirical covariance matrix of the p-dimensional vectors $\frac{1}{\sqrt{G}} \mathbf{X}_{k\cdot}^t \mathbf{X}_{k\cdot} M_{\hat{\Sigma}}(\hat{B})$, $k = 1, \ldots, (nG)$. Furthermore, with $\tilde{B} = \hat{B}_{A(\hat{B},\hat{\Sigma})}$, $G' = |A(\hat{B}, \hat{\Sigma})|$:

$$\hat{D} := (\tilde{b}_2, \ldots, \tilde{b}_{G'}) - (\tilde{b}_1, \ldots, \tilde{b}_1).$$

Explicit Formula for $\mathrm{D}_g M_{\hat{\Sigma}}(\hat{B}_{A(\hat{\Sigma},\hat{B})})$

(Compare with Lemma 1)

Let us again write $\tilde{B} = \hat{B}_{A(\hat{B},\hat{\Sigma})}$, $G' = |A(\hat{B}, \hat{\Sigma})|$,

$$\mathrm{D}_g M_{\hat{\Sigma}}(\hat{B}_{A(\hat{\Sigma},\hat{B})}) = - \frac{\|M_{\hat{\Sigma}}(\tilde{B})\|_{\hat{\Sigma}}}{\|(\mathrm{Id} - \widehat{\mathrm{PA}}^{(g)})\tilde{b}_g\|_{\hat{\Sigma}}} \frac{(\mathrm{Id} - \widehat{\mathrm{PA}}^{(g)})\tilde{b}_g}{\|(\mathrm{Id} - \widehat{\mathrm{PA}}^{(g)})\tilde{b}_g\|_{\hat{\Sigma}}} \frac{M_{\hat{\Sigma}}(\tilde{B})^t}{\|M_{\hat{\Sigma}}(\tilde{B})\|_{\hat{\Sigma}}} \hat{\Sigma}$$
$$+ \frac{\|(\mathrm{Id} - \widehat{\mathrm{PA}}^{(g)}) M_{\hat{\Sigma}}(\tilde{B})\|_{\hat{\Sigma}}}{\|(\mathrm{Id} - \widehat{\mathrm{PA}}^{(g)})\tilde{b}_g\|_{\hat{\Sigma}}} \hat{\Pi}_{\tilde{B}}.$$

Here, $\widehat{\mathrm{PA}}^{(g)}$ denotes the affine projection on the smallest affine space containing $\tilde{b}_1, \ldots, \tilde{b}_{g-1}, \tilde{b}_{g+1}, \ldots, \tilde{b}_{G'}$. Let $\Pi_{\tilde{B}} \in \mathbb{R}^{p\times p}$ denote the projection on $\langle \tilde{b}_2 - \tilde{b}_1, \ldots, \tilde{b}_{G'} - \tilde{b}_1\rangle^{\perp}$. These geometric definitions are meant with respect to the scalar product $\langle x, y\rangle_{\hat{\Sigma}} = x^t \hat{\Sigma} y$.

Proof of Theorem 2

Proof The proof is based on the delta method. As $\hat{B} \rightharpoonup B^0$ and $\hat{\Sigma} \rightharpoonup \Sigma^0$, by Lemma 2, $A(B^0, \Sigma^0) = A(\hat{B}, \hat{\Sigma})$ up to an asymptotically negligible set. Hence $M_{\Sigma^0}(B^0) = M_{\Sigma^0}(B^0_{A(B^0,\Sigma^0)})$ and $M_{\hat{\Sigma}}(\hat{B}) = M_{\hat{\Sigma}}(\hat{B}_{A(B^0,\Sigma^0)})$ up to an asymptotically negligible set. So without loss of generality let us assume (without changing the definition of $\hat{\Sigma}$) that $A(B^0, \Sigma^0) = A(\hat{B}, \hat{\Sigma}) = \{1, \ldots, G\}$, and hence $B^0 = B^0_{A(B^0,\Sigma^0)}$, $\hat{B} = \hat{B}_{A(\hat{B},\hat{\Sigma})}$. By Lemmas 1 and 3, $M_{\Sigma}(B)$ is continuously differentiable in a neighborhood of B^0 and Σ^0. Using Taylor in a neighborhood of B^0 and Σ^0 we can write

$$\begin{aligned}
\sqrt{n}\left(M_{\hat{\Sigma}}(\hat{B}) - M_{\Sigma^0}(B^0)\right) &= \mathrm{D}_B M_{\Xi}(\xi)\sqrt{n}(\hat{B} - B^0)\\
&\quad + \mathrm{D}_\Sigma M_{\Xi}(\xi)\sqrt{n}(\hat{\Sigma} - \Sigma^0) + o_{\mathbb{P}}(1)\\
&= (\mathrm{D}_B M_{\Xi}(\xi) - \mathrm{D}_B M_{\Sigma^0}(B^0))\sqrt{n}(\hat{B} - B^0)\\
&\quad + (\mathrm{D}_\Sigma M_{\Xi}(\xi) - \mathrm{D}_\Sigma M_{\Sigma^0}(B^0))\sqrt{n}(\hat{\Sigma} - \Sigma^0)\\
&\quad + \mathrm{D}_B M_{\Sigma^0}(B^0)\sqrt{n}(\hat{B} - B^0)\\
&\quad + \mathrm{D}_\Sigma M_{\Sigma^0}(B^0)\sqrt{n}(\hat{\Sigma} - \Sigma^0) + o_{\mathbb{P}}(1),
\end{aligned}$$

with $\xi = \gamma B^0 + (1-\gamma)\hat{B}$ and $\Xi = \gamma\Sigma^0 + (1-\gamma)\hat{\Sigma}$ for some random variable $\gamma \in [0, 1]$. We now want to show that the first and second term are negligible, and calculate the asymptotic Gaussian distributions of the last two terms. Furthermore we want to show that the last two terms are asymptotically independent. This guarantees that the variance of $\lim_n \sqrt{n}\left(M_{\hat{\Sigma}}(\hat{B}) - M_{\Sigma^0}(B^0)\right)$ is the sum of the variances of the two asymptotic Gaussian distributions.

Hence, to prove (4) it suffices to show:

(1) $\mathrm{D}_B M_{\Xi}(\xi) - \mathrm{D}_B M_{\Sigma^0}(B^0) = o_{\mathbb{P}}(1)$
(2) $\mathrm{D}_\Sigma M_{\Xi}(\xi) - \mathrm{D}_\Sigma M_{\Sigma^0}(B^0) = o_{\mathbb{P}}(1)$
(3) $\sqrt{n}(\hat{b}_g - b^0_g) \rightharpoonup \mathcal{N}(0, \sigma^2(\Sigma^0)^{-1})$ for $g = 1, \ldots, G$.
(4) $\mathrm{D}_B M_{\Sigma^0}(B^0)\sqrt{n}(\hat{B} - B^0) \rightharpoonup \mathcal{N}\left(0, \sigma^2 \sum_{g\in A(B^0,\Sigma^0)} \mathrm{D}^t_g M_{\Sigma^0}(B^0)(\Sigma^0)^{-1}\, \mathrm{D}_g M_{\Sigma^0}(B^0)\right)$

(5) $\mathrm{D}_\Sigma M_{\Sigma^0}(B^0)\sqrt{n}(\hat{\Sigma}-\Sigma^0) \rightharpoonup \mathcal{N}(0, V(B^0, \Sigma^0))$
(6) For $\delta_n := \sqrt{n}(\hat{B}-B^0)$ and $\Delta_n := \sqrt{n}(\hat{\Sigma}-\Sigma^0)$ we have $(\delta_n, \Delta_n) \rightharpoonup (\delta, \Delta)$ with δ_g, $g = 1, \dots, G$ and Δ independent.

Part (1) and (2): By Lemmas 1 and 3 the derivatives are continuous at B^0 and Σ^0 and $\hat{\Sigma} \to \Sigma^0$, $\hat{B} \to B^0$ in probability (which implies $\xi \to B^0$ and $\Xi \to \Sigma^0$ in probability).

Part (3): This is immediate, as under the chosen model, conditioned on $\mathbf{X}$,

$$\hat{b}_g \sim \mathcal{N}(b_g, \sigma^2(\mathbf{X}_g^t\mathbf{X}_g)^{-1})$$

and $\frac{1}{n}\mathbf{X}_g^t\mathbf{X}_g \to \Sigma$ in probability.

Part (4): Part (3) and a linear transformation.

Part (5): We defer this part to Lemma 5.

Part (6): We saw the convergence of δ_n in part (3). The convergence of Δ_n is deferred to Lemma 4. In the following we use the notation $\delta = (\delta_1, \dots, \delta_G)$ and $\delta_n = (\delta_{n,1}, \dots, \delta_{n,G})$. For the asymptotic independence of part (6). we have to show that for any bounded continuous function g,

$$\mathbb{E}g(\delta_n, \Delta_n) \to \int\int g(\delta, \Delta)\frac{(\det\Sigma^0)^{G/2}}{(2\pi\sigma^2)^{G/2}}\prod_{g=1}^{G}\exp\left(-\delta_g^t\frac{\Sigma^0}{2\sigma^2}\delta_g\right)d\delta_1\cdots d\delta_G\mathbb{P}[d\Delta].$$

In the following equation the inner integral is bounded by 2, and for $n \to \infty$, $\frac{1}{n}\mathbf{X}_g^t\mathbf{X}_g \to \Sigma^0$ in probability. Hence, by dominated convergence on the inner and outer integral,

$$\int\int\Bigg|\prod_{g=1}^{G}\frac{\sqrt{\det\frac{1}{n}\mathbf{X}_g^t\mathbf{X}_g}}{(2\pi\sigma^2)^{1/2}}\exp\left(-\delta_{n,g}^t\frac{\mathbf{X}_g^t\mathbf{X}_g}{2n\sigma^2}\delta_{n,g}\right)$$
$$-\prod_{g=1}^{G}\frac{\sqrt{\det\Sigma^0}}{(2\pi\sigma^2)^{1/2}}\exp\left(-\delta_{n,g}^t\frac{\Sigma^0}{2\sigma^2}\delta_{n,g}\right)\Bigg|d\delta_{n,1}\cdots d\delta_{n,G}\mathbb{P}[d\Delta_n] \to 0.$$

Using this,

$$\limsup_{n\to\infty}|\mathbb{E}g(\delta_n, \Delta_n) - g(\delta, \Delta_n)| = 0,$$

where δ is independent of Δ_n, $\delta_g \sim \mathcal{N}(0, \sigma^2(\Sigma^0)^{-1})$ i.i.d.. Finally, with Δ independent of δ, $\Delta \sim \lim_n \sqrt{n}(\hat{\Sigma}-\Sigma^0)$,

$$\limsup_{n\to\infty}|\mathbb{E}g(\delta_n, \Delta_n) - \mathbb{E}g(\delta, \Delta)|$$
$$= \limsup_{n\to\infty}|\mathbb{E}g(\delta, \Delta_n) - \mathbb{E}g(\delta, \Delta)|$$

$$= \limsup_{n\to\infty} \left| \int \mathbb{E}[(g(\delta, \Delta_n) - g(\delta, \Delta))|\delta] \frac{(\det \Sigma^0)^{G/2}}{(2\pi\sigma^2)^{G/2}} \prod_{g=1}^{G} \exp\left(-\delta_g^t \frac{\Sigma^0}{2\sigma^2} \delta_g\right) d\delta_1 \cdots d\delta_G \right|$$

$$= 0.$$

In the second line we used Eq. (4), in the last line we used dominated convergence and $\Delta_n \rightharpoonup \Delta$. This concludes the proof.

Let $\Sigma \in \mathbb{R}^{p\times p}$ be symmetric positive definite. In the following, we work in the Hilbert space $(\mathbb{R}^p, \langle\cdot,\cdot\rangle_\Sigma)$, where for $x, y \in \mathbb{R}^p$,

$$\langle x, y\rangle_\Sigma := x^t \Sigma y,$$

and induced norm

$$\|x\|_\Sigma = \sqrt{x^t \Sigma x}.$$

This means that projections and orthogonality etc. are always meant with respect to this space. Let PA denote the affine projection on the smallest affine space containing $b_1, \ldots, b_G$. Let $\mathrm{PA}^{(g)}$ denote the affine projection on the smallest affine space containing $b_1, \ldots, b_{g-1}, b_{g+1}, \ldots, b_G$. Note that for $g = 1$ this space can be expressed as $b_2 + \langle b_3 - b_2, \ldots, b_G - b_2\rangle$. Let $\Pi_B \in \mathbb{R}^{p\times p}$ denote the projection on $\langle b_2 - b_1, \ldots, b_G - b_1\rangle^\perp$.

Lemma 1 *If $M_\Sigma(B) = \alpha_1 b_1 + \ldots + \alpha_G b_G$ with $0 < \alpha_g < 1$ for $g = 1, \ldots, G > 1$ and this representation is unique (i.e. $B = (b_1, \ldots, b_G)$ has full rank), then M_Σ is continuously differentiable in a neighborhood of B with*

$$\mathrm{D}_{g,v} M_\Sigma(B) = -\frac{\|M_\Sigma(B)\|_\Sigma}{\|(Id - PA^{(g)})b_g\|_\Sigma} \langle \frac{M_\Sigma(B)}{\|M_\Sigma(B)\|_\Sigma}, v\rangle_\Sigma \frac{(Id - PA^{(g)})b_g}{\|(Id - PA^{(g)})b_g\|_\Sigma} + \frac{\|(Id - PA^{(g)})M_\Sigma(B)\|_\Sigma}{\|(Id - PA^{(g)})b_g\|_\Sigma} \Pi_B v. \quad (5)$$

Here, $\mathrm{D}_{g,v} M_\Sigma(B)$ denotes the differential with respect to the variable b_g in direction v.

Remark 1 In the proof of Theorem 2, we could assume that without loss of generality $\{1, \ldots, G\} = A(B, \Sigma)$, i.e. $B = B_{A(B,\Sigma)}$. We saw that in a neighborhood of B and Σ, magging depends only on $B_{A(B,\Sigma)}$. Hence, for using the formula of $\mathrm{D}_g M_\Sigma(B)$ in the context of Theorems 1 and 2, replace in the definition B by $B_{A(B,\Sigma)}$. The derivatives with respect to b_g, $g \in \{1, \ldots, G\} - A(B, \Sigma)$ are zero.

Proof Without loss of generality, let us assume that $g = 1$. We will show that the partial derivatives exist and are continuous.

Let $\Delta_1 \in \langle b_2 - b_1, \dots, b_G - b_1\rangle^{\perp}$ and $\Delta_2 \in \langle b_2 - b_1, \dots, b_G - b_1\rangle$ and define $\tilde{B} := (b_1 + \Delta_1 + \Delta_2, b_2, \dots, b_G)$. First, we want to show that, if $\|\Delta_1 + \Delta_2\|_\Sigma$ small,

$$M_\Sigma(\tilde{B}) = \mathrm{PA}^{(1)} M_\Sigma(B) - \frac{\langle \mathrm{PA}^{(1)} M_\Sigma(B), (\mathrm{Id} - \mathrm{PA}^{(1)})\tilde{b}_1\rangle_\Sigma}{\|(\mathrm{Id} - \mathrm{PA}^{(1)})\tilde{b}_1\|_\Sigma^2}(\mathrm{Id} - \mathrm{PA}^{(1)})\tilde{b}_1. \tag{6}$$

Let us denote the r.h.s. by $\xi(\tilde{B})$. We have to show:

1. $\xi(\tilde{B}) \perp (\mathrm{Id} - \mathrm{PA}^{(1)})\tilde{b}_1$
2. $\xi(\tilde{B}) \perp \langle b_3 - b_2, \dots, b_G - b_2\rangle$
3. $\xi(\tilde{B}) \in \mathrm{CVX}(\tilde{B})$, the convex hull generated by the columns of $\tilde{B}$.

Note that 1. and 2. guarantee that the r.h.s. in (6) is perpendicular to the linear space generated by the columns of $\tilde{B}$.

1. is trivial. 2. By definition, $(\mathrm{Id} - \mathrm{PA}^{(1)})\tilde{b}_1 \perp \langle b_3 - b_2, \dots, b_G - b_2\rangle$. $\mathrm{PA}^{(1)} M_\Sigma(B) \perp \langle b_3 - b_2, \dots, b_G - b_2\rangle$ as we can decompose into $\mathrm{PA}^{(1)} M_\Sigma(B) = M_\Sigma(B) - (\mathrm{Id} - \mathrm{PA}^{(1)}) M_\Sigma(B)$, which are both, by definition, perpendicular to $\langle b_3 - b_2, \dots, b_G - b_2\rangle$.

Now let us show 3.: $M_\Sigma(B) = \sum_{g=1}^G \alpha_g b_g$ for some $0 < \alpha_g$ and $\sum_{g=1}^G \alpha_g = 1$, i.e. $(B^t B)^{-1} B^t M_\Sigma(B) = (B_{\restriction \langle b_1, \dots, b_G\rangle})^{-1} M_\Sigma(B) = \alpha$. Similarly, as $\xi(\tilde{B})$ lies on the affine space generated by $\tilde{b}_1, \dots, \tilde{b}_G$, we have $\xi(\tilde{B}) = \sum_{g=1}^G \tilde{\alpha}_g \tilde{b}_g$ with $\sum_{g=1}^G \tilde{\alpha}_g = 1$. For small $\|\Delta_1 + \Delta_2\|_\Sigma$, $\tilde{B}$ has full rank and as $\xi(\tilde{B}) \to M_\Sigma(B)$,

$$\lim_{\Delta \to 0} (\tilde{B}_{\restriction \langle \tilde{b}_1, \dots, \tilde{b}_G\rangle})^{-1} \xi(\tilde{B}) = \lim_{\Delta \to 0} (\tilde{B}^t \tilde{B})^{-1} \tilde{B}^t \xi(\tilde{B}) = \alpha.$$

Hence, for small $\|\Delta_1 + \Delta_2\|_\Sigma$, $\tilde{\alpha}_g > 0$ and $\sum_{g=1}^G \tilde{\alpha}_g = 1$, hence $\xi(\tilde{B}) \in \mathrm{CVX}(\tilde{B})$ and thus $M_\Sigma(\tilde{B}) = \xi(\tilde{B})$. This concludes the proof of (6).

Note that, as $\Delta_1 \perp \langle b_2 - b_1, \dots, b_G - b_1\rangle = \langle b_1 - b_2, b_3 - b_2, \dots, b_G - b_2\rangle$,

$$\begin{aligned}
(\mathrm{Id} - \mathrm{PA}^{(1)})\tilde{b}_1 &= \tilde{b}_1 - \operatorname*{arg\,min}_{\gamma \in b_2 + \langle b_3 - b_2, \dots, b_G - b_2\rangle} \|\gamma - b_1 - \Delta_1 - \Delta_2\|_\Sigma^2 \\
&= \tilde{b}_1 - \operatorname*{arg\,min}_{\gamma \in b_2 + \langle b_3 - b_2, \dots, b_G - b_2\rangle} \|\gamma - b_1 - \Delta_2\|_\Sigma^2 + \|\Delta_1\|_\Sigma^2 \\
&= \Delta_1 + (\mathrm{Id} - \mathrm{PA}^{(1)})(b_1 + \Delta_2).
\end{aligned} \tag{7}$$

$(\mathrm{Id} - \mathrm{PA}^{(1)})(b_1 + \Delta_2)$ and $(\mathrm{Id} - \mathrm{PA}^{(1)})b_1$ are linearly dependent. To see this, observe that both lie in the one-dimensional space $\langle b_2 - b_1, \dots, b_G - b_1\rangle \cap \langle b_3 - b_2, \dots, b_G - b_2\rangle^{\perp}$. This implies that

$$\begin{aligned}
&\frac{\langle \mathrm{PA}^{(1)} M_\Sigma(B), (\mathrm{Id} - \mathrm{PA}^{(1)})(b_1 + \Delta_2)\rangle_\Sigma}{\|(\mathrm{Id} - \mathrm{PA}^{(1)})(b_1 + \Delta_2)\|_\Sigma^2}(\mathrm{Id} - \mathrm{PA}^{(1)})(b_1 + \Delta_2) \\
&= \frac{\langle \mathrm{PA}^{(1)} M_\Sigma(B), (\mathrm{Id} - \mathrm{PA}^{(1)})b_1\rangle_\Sigma}{\|(\mathrm{Id} - \mathrm{PA}^{(1)})b_1\|_\Sigma^2}(\mathrm{Id} - \mathrm{PA}^{(1)})b_1
\end{aligned} \tag{8}$$

Now we can put these pieces together: In the first step we use (6) and (7), in the second we use $\Delta_1 \in \langle b_2 - b_1, \ldots, b_G - b_1 \rangle^{\perp}$.

$$M_\Sigma(\tilde{B}) = \mathrm{PA}^{(1)} M_\Sigma(B) - \frac{\langle \mathrm{PA}^{(1)} M_\Sigma(B), \Delta_1 + (\mathrm{Id} - \mathrm{PA}^{(1)})(b_1 + \Delta_2) \rangle_\Sigma}{\| \Delta_1 + (\mathrm{Id} - \mathrm{PA}^{(1)})(b_1 + \Delta_2) \|_\Sigma^2}$$
$$(\Delta_1 + (\mathrm{Id} - \mathrm{PA}^{(1)})(b_1 + \Delta_2))$$
$$= \mathrm{PA}^{(1)} M_\Sigma(B) - \frac{\langle \mathrm{PA}^{(1)} M_\Sigma(B), \Delta_1 + (\mathrm{Id} - \mathrm{PA}^{(1)})(b_1 + \Delta_2) \rangle_\Sigma}{\| \Delta_1 \|^2 + \| (\mathrm{Id} - \mathrm{PA}^{(1)})(b_1 + \Delta_2) \|_\Sigma^2}$$
$$(\Delta_1 + (\mathrm{Id} - \mathrm{PA}^{(1)})(b_1 + \Delta_2)).$$

In the first step we do an expansion of the equation above and in the second, we use (8) and $(\mathrm{Id} - \mathrm{PA}^{(1)})(b_1 + \Delta_2) = (\mathrm{Id} - \mathrm{PA}^{(1)}) b_1 + \mathcal{O}(\|\Delta_2\|_\Sigma)$:

$$M_\Sigma(\tilde{B})$$
$$= \mathrm{PA}^{(1)} M_\Sigma(B) - \frac{\langle \mathrm{PA}^{(1)} M_\Sigma(B), (\mathrm{Id} - \mathrm{PA}^{(1)})(b_1 + \Delta_2) \rangle_\Sigma}{\| (\mathrm{Id} - \mathrm{PA}^{(1)})(b_1 + \Delta_2) \|_\Sigma^2} (\mathrm{Id} - \mathrm{PA}^{(1)})(b_1 + \Delta_2)$$
$$- \frac{\langle \mathrm{PA}^{(1)} M_\Sigma(B), \Delta_1 \rangle_\Sigma}{\| (\mathrm{Id} - \mathrm{PA}^{(1)})(b_1 + \Delta_2) \|_\Sigma^2} (\mathrm{Id} - \mathrm{PA}^{(1)})(b_1 + \Delta_2)$$
$$- \frac{\langle \mathrm{PA}^{(1)} M_\Sigma(B), (\mathrm{Id} - \mathrm{PA}^{(1)})(b_1 + \Delta_2) \rangle_\Sigma}{\| (\mathrm{Id} - \mathrm{PA}^{(1)})(b_1 + \Delta_2) \|_\Sigma^2} \Delta_1 + \mathcal{O}(\|\Delta_1\|_\Sigma^2 + \|\Delta_2\|_\Sigma^2))$$
$$= \mathrm{PA}^{(1)} M_\Sigma(B) - \frac{\langle \mathrm{PA}^{(1)} M_\Sigma(B), (\mathrm{Id} - \mathrm{PA}^{(1)}) b_1 \rangle_\Sigma}{\| (\mathrm{Id} - \mathrm{PA}^{(1)}) b_1 \|_\Sigma^2} (\mathrm{Id} - \mathrm{PA}^{(1)}) b_1$$
$$- \frac{\langle \mathrm{PA}^{(1)} M_\Sigma(B), \Delta_1 \rangle_\Sigma}{\| (\mathrm{Id} - \mathrm{PA}^{(1)}) b_1 \|_\Sigma^2} (\mathrm{Id} - \mathrm{PA}^{(1)}) b_1$$
$$- \frac{\langle \mathrm{PA}^{(1)} M_\Sigma(B), (\mathrm{Id} - \mathrm{PA}^{(1)}) b_1 \rangle_\Sigma}{\| (\mathrm{Id} - \mathrm{PA}^{(1)}) b_1 \|_\Sigma^2} \Delta_1 + \mathcal{O}(\|\Delta_1\|_\Sigma^2 + \|\Delta_2\|_\Sigma^2)).$$

From this and (6) we obtain

$$M_\Sigma(\tilde{B}) - M_\Sigma(B)$$
$$= - \frac{\langle \mathrm{PA}^{(1)} M_\Sigma(B), \Delta_1 \rangle_\Sigma}{\| (\mathrm{Id} - \mathrm{PA}^{(1)}) b_1 \|_\Sigma^2} (\mathrm{Id} - \mathrm{PA}^{(1)}) b_1$$
$$- \frac{\langle \mathrm{PA}^{(1)} M_\Sigma(B), (\mathrm{Id} - \mathrm{PA}^{(1)}) b_1 \rangle_\Sigma}{\| (\mathrm{Id} - \mathrm{PA}^{(1)}) b_1 \|_\Sigma^2} \Delta_1 + \mathcal{O}(\|\Delta_1\|_\Sigma^2 + \|\Delta_2\|_\Sigma^2)).$$

Now let us write $\Delta_1 + \Delta_2 = \gamma v$, $\Delta_1 = \gamma(M_\Sigma(B)/\|M_\Sigma(B)\|_\Sigma + \mu v_\perp)$ with $v_\perp \perp M_\Sigma(B)$ and $v_\perp \perp \langle b_2 - b_1, \ldots, b_G - b_1\rangle$. By noting that

$$\begin{aligned}\langle \mathrm{PA}^{(1)} M_\Sigma(B), \Delta_1\rangle_\Sigma &= \langle M_\Sigma(B) + (\mathrm{PA}^{(1)} - \mathrm{Id})M_\Sigma(B), \gamma\frac{M_\Sigma(B)}{\|M_\Sigma(B)\|_\Sigma} + \mu v_\perp)\rangle_\Sigma \\ &= \gamma\|M_\Sigma(B)\|_\Sigma \\ &= \gamma\langle\frac{M_\Sigma(B)}{\|M_\Sigma(B)\|_\Sigma}, v\rangle_\Sigma \|M_\Sigma(B)\|_\Sigma,\end{aligned}$$

and, as $(\mathrm{Id} - \mathrm{PA}^{(1)})M_\Sigma(B)$ and $(\mathrm{Id} - \mathrm{PA}^{(1)})b_1$ are linearly dependent (both lie in the one-dimensional space $\langle b_2 - b_1, \ldots, b_G - b_1\rangle \cap \langle b_3 - b_2, \ldots, b_G - b_2\rangle^\perp$),

$$\begin{aligned}-\langle \mathrm{PA}^{(1)} M_\Sigma(B), (\mathrm{Id} - \mathrm{PA}^{(1)})b_1\rangle_\Sigma &= \langle(\mathrm{Id} - \mathrm{PA}^{(1)})M_\Sigma(B), (\mathrm{Id} - \mathrm{PA}^{(1)})b_1\rangle_\Sigma \\ &= \|(\mathrm{Id} - \mathrm{PA}^{(1)})M_\Sigma(B)\|_\Sigma \|(\mathrm{Id} - \mathrm{PA}^{(1)})b_1\|_\Sigma.\end{aligned}$$

We obtain:

$$\begin{aligned}&M_\Sigma(\tilde{B}) - M_\Sigma(B) \\ &= -\gamma\frac{\|M_\Sigma(B)\|_\Sigma}{\|(\mathrm{Id} - \mathrm{PA}^{(1)})b_1\|_\Sigma^2}\langle\frac{M_\Sigma(B)}{\|M_\Sigma(B)\|_\Sigma}, v\rangle_\Sigma(\mathrm{Id} - \mathrm{PA}^{(1)})b_1 \\ &\quad - \gamma\frac{\|(\mathrm{Id} - \mathrm{PA}^{(1)})M_\Sigma(B)\|_\Sigma\|(\mathrm{Id} - \mathrm{PA}^{(1)})b_1\|_\Sigma}{\|(\mathrm{Id} - \mathrm{PA}^{(1)})b_1\|_\Sigma^2}\Pi_B v + \mathcal{O}(\|\Delta_1\|_\Sigma^2 + \|\Delta_2\|_\Sigma^2)).\end{aligned}$$

Hence the directional derivative exists and is equal to (5). The assertion follows by existence and continuity of the directional derivatives in a neighborhood of B.

Lemma 2 *Let Σ^0 be positive definite. $M_\Sigma(B)$ is continuous in B and Σ in a neighborhood of Σ^0. Furthermore, under the assumptions of Theorem 1 (or Theorem 2), in a neighborhood of B^0 and Σ^0, $A(B, \Sigma)$ is constant.*

Proof First, let us prove that magging is continuous. Proof by contradiction: Assume there exist sequences $B_k \to B$, $\Sigma_k \to \Sigma$ positive definite such that $M_{\Sigma_k}(B_k) \not\to M_\Sigma(B)$. Without loss of generality, as Σ is invertible, $M_{\Sigma_k}(B_k)$ converges, too. By definition of $M_{\Sigma_k}(B_k)$ we have

$$\|M_{\Sigma_k}(B_k)\|_{\Sigma_k} \le \|\Pi_{B_k} M_\Sigma(B)\|_{\Sigma_k},$$

where Π_{B_k} denotes the projection (in $\langle\cdot,\cdot\rangle$) on the convex set $\mathrm{CVX}(B_k)$. By continuity,

$$\|\lim_k M_{\Sigma_k}(B_k)\|_\Sigma \le \|M_\Sigma(B)\|_\Sigma.$$

We have $M_{\Sigma_k}(B_k) \in \mathrm{CVX}(B_k)$ and hence by continuity $\lim_k M_{\Sigma_k}(B_k) \in \mathrm{CVX}(B)$. As magging is unique ($\Sigma$ is positive definite), this yields a contradiction.

Consider b_g^0 with $g \in A(B^0, \Sigma^0)$. By the assumptions of Theorem 1, $M_{\Sigma^0}(B^0) = \sum_{i \in A(B^0,\Sigma^0)} \alpha_i b_i^0$ with $0 < \alpha_i < 1$. Hence for small $\gamma \in \mathbb{R}$, $(1-\gamma)M_{\Sigma^0}(B^0) + \gamma b_g^0 \in \mathrm{CVX}(B^0)$ and by definition of magging

$$\|M_{\Sigma^0}(B^0)\|_{\Sigma^0} \leq \|(1-\gamma)M_{\Sigma^0}(B^0) + \gamma b_g^0\|_{\Sigma^0} \tag{9}$$

Using this inequality for small $\gamma > 0$ and small $\gamma < 0$ we obtain $\langle M_{\Sigma^0}(B^0), b_g^0 - M_{\Sigma^0}(B^0)\rangle = 0$. Hence, for all $g \in A(B^0, \Sigma^0)$, $M_{\Sigma^0}(B^0)$ is perpendicular (with respect to $\langle\cdot,\cdot\rangle_{\Sigma^0}$) to $b_g^0 - M_{\Sigma^0}(B^0)$. Hence $A(B^0, \Sigma^0) \subset M_{\Sigma^0}(B^0) + M_{\Sigma^0}(B^0)^{\perp}$.

Furthermore, by assumptions of Theorem 1, if $g \notin A(B^0, \Sigma^0)$ we have $b_g^0 \notin M_{\Sigma^0}(B^0) + M_{\Sigma^0}(B^0)^{\perp}$. By continuity, for $B = (b_1, \ldots, b_G)$ close to B^0 and Σ close to Σ^0 (in $\|\cdot\|_2$) we have $b_g \notin M_{\Sigma}(B) + M_{\Sigma}(B)^{\perp}$. By an analogous argument as in Eq. (9), $g \notin A(B, \Sigma)$. This proves $A(B^0, \Sigma^0) \subset A(B, \Sigma)$.

It remains to show $A(B, \Sigma) \subset A(B^0, \Sigma^0)$: For notational simplicity let us assume $A(B^0, \Sigma^0) = \{1, \ldots, G\}$. For B close to B^0 and Σ close to Σ^0, $M_{\Sigma}(B) = B\tilde{\alpha}$ with $\sum_{i=1}^{G} \tilde{\alpha}_i = 1$, $0 \leq \tilde{\alpha}_i \leq 1$. We want to show that for B close to B^0 and Σ close to Σ^0 (in $\|\cdot\|_2$), $0 < \tilde{\alpha}_i < 1$.

To this end, note that by the assumptions of Theorem 1 we have that $B^0_{A(B^0,\Sigma^0)}$ (here without loss of generality: B^0) has full rank, hence for B close to B^0 and Σ close to Σ^0, $(B^tB)^{-1} B^t M_{\Sigma}(B) = \tilde{\alpha}$ with $\tilde{\alpha}_i \geq 0$, $\sum_i \tilde{\alpha}_i = 1$. Furthermore,

$$\lim_{B \to B^0, \Sigma \to \Sigma^0} (B^tB)^{-1} B^t M_{\Sigma}(B) = \left((B^0)^t B^0\right)^{-1} (B^0)^t M_{\Sigma^0}(B^0) = \alpha.$$

Hence for B close to B^0 and Σ close to Σ^0 (in $\|\cdot\|_2$)), $0 < \tilde{\alpha}_i < 1$. This concludes the proof.

Lemma 3 *Let $G > 2$. Let $M_{\Sigma}(B) = \alpha_1 b_1 + \ldots + \alpha_G b_G$ with unique $0 < \alpha_g < 1$ satisfying $\sum_{g=1}^{G} \alpha_g = 1$. Then the mapping*

$$\{\textit{positive definite matrices in } \mathbb{R}^{p\times p}\} \to \mathbb{R}^p$$
$$\Sigma \mapsto M_{\Sigma}(B)$$

is continuously differentiable at B, Σ. Let Δ be a symmetric matrix. The differential in direction Δ is

$$\mathrm{D}_{\Sigma} M_{\Sigma}(B)\Delta = -D(D^t \Sigma D)^{-1} D^t \Delta M_{\Sigma}(B),$$

where

$$D := (b_2, \ldots, b_G) - (b_1, \ldots, b_1).$$

Proof By elementary analysis, it suffices to show that the directional derivatives exist in a neighborhood and that they are continuous.

For a small symmetric perturbation $\lambda\Delta$, by continuity of magging (Lemma 2), $M_{\Sigma+\lambda\Delta}(B)$ has to satisfy

$$M_{\Sigma+\lambda\Delta}(B) = M_{\Sigma}(B) + D\gamma$$

for some (small) vector $\gamma \in \mathbb{R}^{G-1}$. By definition of magging, and as $0 < \alpha_g < 1$ we have $\|M_{\Sigma+\lambda\Delta}(B)\|_{\Sigma+\lambda\Delta} \leq \|M_{\Sigma+\lambda\Delta}(B) + D\gamma'\|_{\Sigma+\lambda\Delta}$ for all small vectors $\gamma' \in \mathbb{R}^{G-1}$. Hence,

$$M_{\Sigma+\lambda\Delta}(B)^t(\Sigma + \lambda\Delta)D = 0. \tag{10}$$

Putting these two conditions together, we get

$$(M_{\Sigma}(B) + D\gamma)^t(\Sigma + \lambda\Delta)D = 0.$$

Furthermore, analogously as in Eq. (10) we obtain

$$M_{\Sigma}(B)^t\Sigma D = 0.$$

By combining the last two equations,

$$\gamma^t D^t(\Sigma + \lambda\Delta)D = -M_{\Sigma}(B)^t\lambda\Delta D.$$

As $D^t(\Sigma + \lambda\Delta)D$ is invertible (D has full rank as B has full rank. B has full rank as the α_g are unique),

$$\gamma^t = -M_{\Sigma}(B)^t\lambda\Delta D(D^t(\Sigma + \lambda\Delta)D)^{-1},$$
$$D\gamma = -D(D^t(\Sigma + \lambda\Delta)D)^{-1}D^t\lambda\Delta M_{\Sigma}(B).$$

Dividing by λ and letting $\lambda \to 0$ gives the desired result.

Lemma 4 *Let $\mathbf{X}_{k\cdot} \sim F$, $k = 1, \ldots, nG$ denote the i.i.d. rows of $\mathbf{X}$. Let $\mathbb{E}[\|\mathbf{X}_{1\cdot}^t\mathbf{X}_{1\cdot}\|_2^2] < \infty$ and $\Sigma^0 = \mathbb{E}[\mathbf{X}_{1\cdot}^t\mathbf{X}_{1\cdot}]$ positive definite. Then, for $n \to \infty$,*

$$\frac{1}{G\sqrt{n}}\sum_{k=1}^{nG}\left(\mathbf{X}_{k\cdot}^t\mathbf{X}_{k\cdot} - \Sigma^0\right) \rightharpoonup \Delta$$

where the symmetric matrix Δ has centered multivariate normal distributed entries under and on the diagonal with covariance

$$c_{ijkl} := Covar(\Delta_{ij}, \Delta_{kl}) = \frac{1}{G}\mathbb{E}[(\mathbf{X}_{1i}\mathbf{X}_{1j} - \mathbb{E}[\mathbf{X}_{1i}\mathbf{X}_{1j}])(\mathbf{X}_{1k}\mathbf{X}_{1l} - \mathbb{E}[\mathbf{X}_{1k}\mathbf{X}_{1l}])].$$

Proof *Apply the CLT.*

In the following Lemma, we want to calculate the distribution of

$$-D(D^t \Sigma D)^{-1} D^t \Delta M_\Sigma(B).$$

Lemma 5 *Let us use setting of Lemma 3 and 4.*

$$\mathrm{D}_\Sigma M_\Sigma(B)\sqrt{n}(\hat{\Sigma} - \Sigma) \rightharpoonup \mathcal{N}(0, V(B, \Sigma))$$

with

$$V(B, \Sigma) = D(D^t \Sigma D)^{-1} D^t C D(D^t \Sigma D)^{-1} D^t,$$

where

$$C_{ij} = \sum_{k,l=1}^{p} M_\Sigma(B)_k M_\Sigma(B)_l c_{iklj},$$

is the covariance matrix of $\Delta M_\Sigma(B)$ *and*

$$D := (b_2, \ldots, b_G) - (b_1, \ldots, b_1).$$

Remark 2 In the proof of Theorem 2, we could assume that without loss of generality $\{1, \ldots, G\} = A(B, \Sigma)$, i.e. $B = B_{A(B,\Sigma)}$. For using the definition of V in the context of Theorems 1 and 2, replace in the definition B by $B_{A(B,\Sigma)}$. The G in the definition of C stays the same, i.e. it is still the total number of groups.

Proof With Lemmas 3 and 4 it suffices to calculate the distribution of

$$-D(D^t \Sigma D)^{-1} D^t \Delta M_\Sigma(B),$$

i.e. the nontrivial part is to calculate the distribution of $\Delta M_\Sigma(B)$. We know it is Gaussian and centered, hence it suffices to determine the covariance matrix:

$$\begin{aligned}
\mathbb{E}\left(\Delta M_\Sigma(B) M_\Sigma(B)^t \Delta\right)_{ij} &= \mathbb{E} \sum_{k,l=1}^{p} \Delta_{ik} (M_\Sigma(B) M_\Sigma(B)^t)_{kl} \Delta_{lj} \\
&= \sum_{k,l=1}^{p} M_\Sigma(B)_k M_\Sigma(B)_l \mathbb{E} \Delta_{ik} \Delta_{lj} \\
&= \sum_{k,l=1}^{p} M_\Sigma(B)_k M_\Sigma(B)_l c_{iklj}.
\end{aligned}$$

In the last line we used Lemma 4. This concludes the proof.

Proof of Theorem 1

Proof First, note that by Lemma 1, $W(\Sigma^0, B^0)$ is invertible. Using Lemma 2, in a neighborhood of B^0 and Σ^0 the set-valued function $A(B, \Sigma)$ is constant. Hence, by Lemma 1 and Lemma 3, the derivatives of $M_\Sigma(B) = M_\Sigma(B_{A(B,\Sigma)})$ are continuous at B^0 and Σ^0. Furthermore, $V(B_{A(B,\Sigma)}, \Sigma)$ is continuous in C and in B and Σ at B^0 and Σ^0. All together, $W(\Sigma, B)$ is continuous at B^0 and Σ^0 in all its variables. By the definition of C in Lemma 5 and the definition of $\hat{C}$ in section "Definitions and Formulas" in this Appendix, $\hat{C} \to C$.

Hence, $W(\hat{\Sigma}, \hat{B}) \to W(\Sigma^0, B^0)$ in probability and we obtain that $W(\hat{B}, \hat{\Sigma})^{-1} \to W(B^0, \Sigma^0)^{-1}$ in probability. By Theorem 2 and Slutsky's Theorem we obtain

$$\sqrt{n}(M_{\hat{\Sigma}}(\hat{B}) - M_{\Sigma^0}(B^0))^t W(\hat{B}, \hat{\Sigma})^{-1} \sqrt{n}(M_{\hat{\Sigma}}(\hat{B}) - M_{\Sigma^0}(B^0)) \rightharpoonup \chi^2(p)$$

for $n \to \infty$. Hence

$$\begin{aligned} &\mathbb{P}[M_{\Sigma^0}(B^0) \in \mathbf{C}(\hat{\Sigma}, \hat{B})] \\ =&\mathbb{P}[(M_{\hat{\Sigma}}(\hat{B}) - M_{\Sigma^0}(B^0))^t W(\hat{B}, \hat{\Sigma})^{-1} (M_{\hat{\Sigma}}(\hat{B}) - M_{\Sigma^0}(B^0)) \leq \frac{\tau}{n}] \\ \to& 1 - \alpha \end{aligned}$$

for $n \to \infty$. This concludes the proof.

Relaxation-Based Approach

A simple approach is as follows: For given $\alpha > 0$, take random sets $\mathcal{R}_B$, $\mathcal{R}_\Sigma$ such that

$$\mathbb{P}[\Sigma^0 \in \mathcal{R}_\Sigma, B^0 \in \mathcal{R}_B] \geq 1 - \alpha,$$

where $B^0 = (b_1^0, \ldots, b_G^0)$ is the matrix of regression coefficients in all G groups. A generic approach is to choose a confidence region for Σ^0 on the confidence level $1-\alpha/2$ and confidence regions for b_g^0 on the confidence level $1-\alpha/(2G)$. However, this approach can easily be improved by taking larger regions around $\hat{b}_g$ that are far away from zero (thus have negligible influence on $M_{\hat{\Sigma}}(\hat{B})$) and smaller regions around $\hat{b}_g$ that are close to zero. Then calculate

$$\mathcal{R} = \{M_{\tilde{\Sigma}}(\tilde{B}) : \tilde{\Sigma} \in \mathcal{R}_\Sigma, \tilde{B} \in \mathcal{R}_B\} \subset \mathbb{R}^p,$$

which is a $1 - \alpha$ confidence region for the maximin effect. However, direct computation of this confidence region is computationally cumbersome.

For known Σ^0 the idea can be relaxed to the following scheme:

For $m \in \mathbb{R}^p$ and $\Sigma \in \mathbb{R}^{p \times p}$ positive definite let us define $\|m\|_\Sigma := \sqrt{m^T \Sigma m}$. Note that this defines a norm on $\mathbb{R}^p$. Now,

$$\begin{aligned}
\|M_{\Sigma^0}(B')\|_{\Sigma^0} &= \min_{\gamma \geq 0, \sum_{g=1}^G \gamma_g = 1} \|B'\gamma\|_{\Sigma^0} \\
&= \min_{\gamma \geq 0, \sum_{g=1}^G \gamma_g = 1} \|B'\gamma\|_{\Sigma^0} - \|B\gamma\|_{\Sigma^0} + \|B\gamma\|_{\Sigma^0} \\
&\leq \sup_{\gamma \geq 0, \sum_{g=1}^G \gamma_g = 1} |\|B'\gamma\|_{\Sigma^0} - \|B\gamma\|_{\Sigma^0}| + \min_{\gamma \geq 0, \sum_{g=1}^G \gamma_g = 1} \|B\gamma\|_{\Sigma^0} \\
&\leq \sup_{\gamma \geq 0, \sum_{g=1}^G \gamma_g = 1} \|(B' - B)\gamma\|_{\Sigma^0} + \min_{\gamma \geq 0, \sum_{g=1}^G \gamma_g = 1} \|B\gamma\|_{\Sigma^0}
\end{aligned}$$

and hence

$$\begin{aligned}
\|M_{\Sigma^0}(B')\|_{\Sigma^0} &\leq \sup_{\gamma \geq 0, \sum_{g=1}^G \gamma_g = 1} \sum_{g=1}^G \gamma_g \|b'_g - b_g\|_{\Sigma^0} + \min_{\gamma \geq 0, \sum_{g=1}^G \gamma_g = 1} \|B\gamma\|_{\Sigma^0} \\
&= \max_{g=1,\ldots,G} \|b'_g - b_g\|_{\Sigma^0} + \min_{\gamma \geq 0, \sum_{g=1}^G \gamma_g = 1} \|B\gamma\|_{\Sigma^0} \\
&= \max_{g=1,\ldots,G} \|b'_g - b_g\|_{\Sigma^0} + \|M_\Sigma(B)\|_{\Sigma^0}
\end{aligned}$$

By symmetry,

$$|\|M_{\Sigma^0}(B')\|_{\Sigma^0} - \|M_{\Sigma^0}(B)\|_{\Sigma^0}| \leq \max_{g=1,\ldots,G} \|b'_g - b_g\|_{\Sigma^0}. \tag{11}$$

We can now choose a covering of the confidence region $\mathscr{R}_B$ with $B^{(k)} \in \mathscr{R}_B, k = 1, \ldots, K$ such that balls $\mathscr{B}_{\epsilon_k}(B^{(k)})$ with radius ϵ_k around $B^{(k)}$ cover $\mathscr{R}_B$ with respect to the maximum norm $\|B\|_{\max} := \max_g \|b_g\|_{\Sigma^0}$.

A confidence region of the maximin effect can then be constructed as

$$\tilde{\mathscr{R}} = \bigcup_{k=1,\ldots,K} \{M : |\|M\|_{\Sigma^0} - \|M_{\Sigma^0}(B^{(k)})\|_{\Sigma^0}| \leq \epsilon_k\} \cap \mathrm{CVX}\left(\mathscr{B}_{\epsilon_k}(B^{(k)})\right).$$

This confidence region is valid: For all $M_{\Sigma^0}(B') \in \mathscr{R}_B$ there exists $k \in \{1, \ldots, K\}$ such that $\|B' - B^{(k)}\|_{\max} \leq \epsilon_k$. By Eq. (11), $|\|M_{\Sigma^0}(B')\|_{\Sigma^0} - \|M_{\Sigma^0}(B^{(k)})\|_{\Sigma^0}| \leq \epsilon_k$, hence $M_{\Sigma^0}(B') \in \tilde{\mathscr{R}}_B$. This implies $\mathscr{R}_B \subset \tilde{\mathscr{R}}_B$;

$$\mathbb{P}[M_{\Sigma^0}(B^0) \in \tilde{\mathscr{R}}] \geq \mathbb{P}[M_{\Sigma^0}(B^0) \in \mathscr{R}] \geq \mathbb{P}[B^0 \in \mathscr{R}_B] \geq 1 - \alpha.$$

If Σ^0 is unknown, using the approach above we need to estimate lower and upper bounds for $\|\cdot\|_{\Sigma^0}$.

References

1. Aitkin, M., Rubin, D.: Estimation and hypothesis testing in finite mixture models. J. R. Stat. Soc. Ser. B **47**, 67–75 (1985)
2. Breiman, L.: Bagging predictors. Mach. Learn. **24**, 123–140 (1996)
3. Bühlmann, P., Meinshausen, N.: Magging: maximin aggregation for inhomogeneous large-scale data. IEEE Proc. (2014, preprint). arxiv:1409.2638
4. DeSarbo, W., Cron, W.: A maximum likelihood methodology for clusterwise linear regression. J. Classif. **5**, 249–282 (1988)
5. Fan, J., Zhang, W.: Statistical estimation in varying coefficient models. Ann. Stat. **27**, 1491–1518 (1999)
6. Figueiredo, M., Jain, A.: Unsupervised learning of finite mixture models. IEEE Trans. Pattern Anal. Mach. Intell. **24**, 381–396 (2002)
7. Hastie, T., Tibshirani, R.: Varying-coefficient models. J. R. Stat. Soc. Ser. B **55**, 757–796 (1993)
8. McLachlan, G., Peel, D.: Finite Mixture Models. Wiley, New York (2004)
9. Meinshausen, N., Bühlmann, P.: Maximin effects in inhomogeneous large-scale data. Ann. Stat. **43**(4), 1801–1830 (2015)
10. Pinheiro, J., Bates, D.: Mixed-Effects Models in S and S-PLUS. Springer, New York (2000)
11. Van de Geer, S., Bühlmann, P., Ritov, Y., Dezeure, R.: On asymptotically optimal confidence regions and tests for high-dimensional models. Ann. Stat. **42**(3), 1166–1202 (2014)
12. Zhang, C.H., Zhang, S.S.: Confidence intervals for low dimensional parameters in high dimensional linear models. J. R. Stat. Soc. Ser. B (Stat Methodol.) **76**(1), 217–242 (2014)

χ^2-Confidence Sets in High-Dimensional Regression

Sara van de Geer and Benjamin Stucky

Abstract We study a high-dimensional regression model. Aim is to construct a confidence set for a given group of regression coefficients, treating all other regression coefficients as nuisance parameters. We apply a one-step procedure with the square-root Lasso as initial estimator and a multivariate square-root Lasso for constructing a surrogate Fisher information matrix. The multivariate square-root Lasso is based on nuclear norm loss with ℓ_1-penalty. We show that this procedure leads to an asymptotically χ^2-distributed pivot, with a remainder term depending only on the ℓ_1-error of the initial estimator. We show that under ℓ_1-sparsity conditions on the regression coefficients β^0 the square-root Lasso produces to a consistent estimator of the noise variance and we establish sharp oracle inequalities which show that the remainder term is small under further sparsity conditions on β^0 and compatibility conditions on the design.

1 Introduction

Let X be a given $n \times p$ input matrix and Y be a random n-vector of responses. We consider the high-dimensional situation where the number of variables p exceeds the number of observations n. The expectation of Y (assumed to exist) is denoted by $f^0 := \mathbb{E}Y$. We assume that X has rank n ($n < p$) and let β^0 be any solution of the equation $X\beta^0 = f^0$. Our aim is to construct a confidence interval for a pre-specified group of coefficients $\beta_J^0 := \{\beta_j^0 : j \in J\}$ where $J \subset \{1, \ldots, p\}$ is a subset of the indices. In other words, the $|J|$-dimensional vector β_J^0 is the parameter of interest and all the other coefficients $\beta_{-J}^0 := \{\beta_j^0 : j \notin J\}$ are nuisance parameters.

For one-dimensional parameters of interest ($|J| = 1$) the approach in this paper is closely related to earlier work. The method is introduced in [20]. Further references are [8, 18]. Related approaches can be found in [3–5].

For confidence sets for groups of variables ($|J| > 1$) one usually would like to take the dependence between estimators of single parameters into account. An

S. van de Geer (✉) • B. Stucky
Seminar for Statistics, ETH Zürich, Rämistrasse 101, 8092 Zürich, Switzerland
e-mail: geer@stat.math.ethz.ch; stucky@stat.math.ethz.ch

A. Frigessi et al. (eds.), *Statistical Analysis for High-Dimensional Data*, Abel Symposia 11, DOI 10.1007/978-3-319-27099-9_13

important paper that carefully does this for confidence sets in ℓ_2 is [12]. Our approach is related but differs in an important way. As in [12] we propose a de-sparsified estimator which is (potentially) asymptotically linear. However, [12] focus at a remainder term which is small also for large groups. Our goal is rather to present a construction which has a small remainder term after studentizing and which does not rely on strong conditions on the design X. In particular we do not assume any sparsity conditions on the design.

The construction involves the square-root Lasso $\hat{\beta}$ which is introduced by [2]. See Sect. 2 for the definition of the estimator $\hat{\beta}$. We present a a multivariate extension of the square-root Lasso which takes the nuclear norm of the multivariate residuals as loss function. Then we define in Sect. 3.1 a de-sparsified estimator $\hat{b}_J$ of β_J^0 which has the form of a one-step estimator with $\hat{\beta}_J$ as initial estimator and with multivariate square-root Lasso invoked to obtain a surrogate Fisher information matrix. We show that when $Y \sim \mathcal{N}_n(f^0, \sigma_0^2 I)$ (with both f^0 and σ_0^2 unknown), a studentized version of $\hat{b}_J - \beta_J^0$ has asymptotically a $|J|$-dimensional standard normal distribution.

More precisely we will show in Theorem 1 that for a given $|J| \times |J|$ matrix $M = M_\lambda$ depending only on X and on a tuning parameter λ, one has $M_\lambda(\hat{b}_J - \beta_J^0)/\sigma_0 = \mathcal{N}_{|J|}(0, I) +$ rem where the remainder term "rem" can be bounded by $\|\text{rem}\|_\infty \leq \sqrt{n}\lambda \|\hat{\beta}_{-J} - \beta_{-J}^0\|_1/\sigma_0$. The choice of the tuning parameter λ is "free" (and not depending on σ_0), it can for example be taken of order $\sqrt{\log p/n}$. The unknown parameter σ_0^2 can be estimated by the normalized residual sum of squares $\hat{\sigma}^2 := \|Y - X\hat{\beta}\|_2^2/n$ of the square-root Lasso $\hat{\beta}$. We show in Lemma 3 that under sparsity conditions on β^0 one has $\hat{\sigma}^2/\sigma_0^2 = 1 + o_{\mathbb{P}}(1)$ and then in Theorem 2 an oracle inequality for the square-root Lasso under further sparsity conditions on β^0 and compatibility conditions on the design. The oracle result allows one to "verify" when $\sqrt{n}\lambda\|\hat{\beta}_{-J} - \beta_{-J}^0\|_1/\sigma_0 = o_{\mathbb{P}}(1)$ so that the remainder term rem is negligible. An illustration assuming weak sparsity conditions is given in Sect. 5. As a consequence

$$\|M_\lambda(\hat{b}_J - \beta_J^0)\|_2^2/\hat{\sigma}^2 = \chi_{|J|}^2(1 + o_{\mathbb{P}}(1)),$$

where $\chi_{|J|}^2$ is a random variable having a χ^2-distribution with $|J|$ degrees of freedom. For $|J|$ fixed one can thus construct asymptotic confidence sets for β_J^0 (we will also consider the case $|J| \to \infty$ in Sect. 8). We however do not control the size of these sets. Larger values for λ makes the confidence sets smaller but will also give a larger remainder term.

In Sect. 6 we extend the theory to structured sparsity norms other than ℓ_1, for example the norm used for the (square-root) group Lasso, where the demand for ℓ_2-confidence sets for groups comes up quite naturally. Section 8 contains a discussion. The proofs are in Sect. 9.

1.1 Notation

The mean vector of Y is denoted by f^0 and the noise is $\epsilon := Y - f^0$. For a vector $v \in \mathbb{R}^n$ we write (with a slight abuse of notation) $\|v\|_n^2 := v^T v/n$. We let $\sigma_0^2 := \mathbb{E}\|\epsilon\|_n^2$ (assumed to exist).

For a vector $\beta \in \mathbb{R}^p$ we set $S_\beta := \{j : \beta_j \neq 0\}$. For a subset $J \subset \{1, \ldots, p\}$ and a vector $\beta \in \mathbb{R}^p$ we use the same notation β_J for the $|J|$-dimensional vector $\{\beta_j : j \in J\}$ and the p-dimensional vector $\{\beta_{j,J} := \beta_j \mathrm{l}\{j \in J\} : j = 1, \ldots, p\}$. The last version allows us to write $\beta = \beta_J + \beta_{-J}$ with $\beta_{-J} = \beta_{J^c}$, J^c being the complement of the set J. The jth column of X is denoted by X_j ($j = 1, \ldots, p$). We let $X_J := \{X_j : j \in J\}$ and $X_{-J} := \{X_j : j \notin J\}$.

For a matrix A we let $\|A\|_{\text{nuclear}} := \text{trace}((A^T A)^{1/2})$ be its nuclear norm. The ℓ_1-norm of the matrix A is defined as $\|A\|_1 := \sum_k \sum_j |a_{k,j}|$. Its ℓ_∞-norm is $\|A\|_\infty := \max_k \max_j |a_{k,j}|$.

2 The Square-Root Lasso and Its Multivariate Version

2.1 The Square-Root Lasso

The square-root Lasso [2] $\hat{\beta}$ is

$$\hat{\beta} := \arg\min_{\beta \in \mathbb{R}^p} \left\{ \|Y - X\beta\|_n + \lambda_0 \|\beta\|_1 \right\}. \tag{1}$$

The parameter $\lambda_0 > 0$ is a tuning parameter. Thus $\hat{\beta}$ depends on λ_0 but we do not express this in our notation.

The square-root Lasso can be seen as a method that estimates β^0 and the noise variance σ_0^2 simultaneously. Defining the residuals $\hat{\epsilon} := Y - X\hat{\beta}$ and letting $\hat{\sigma}^2 := \|\hat{\epsilon}\|_n^2$ one clearly has

$$(\hat{\beta}, \hat{\sigma}^2) = \arg \min_{\beta \in \mathbb{R}^p,\ \sigma^2 > 0} \left\{ \frac{\|Y - X\beta\|_n^2}{\sigma} + \sigma + 2\lambda_0 \|\beta\|_1 \right\} \tag{2}$$

provided the minimum is attained at a positive value of σ^2.

We note in passing that the square-root Lasso is *not* a quasi-likelihood estimator as the function $\exp[-z^2/\sigma - \sigma]$, $z \in \mathbb{R}$, is not a density with respect to a dominating measure not depending on $\sigma^2 > 0$. The square-root Lasso is moreover not to be confused with the scaled Lasso. The latter *is* a quasi-likelihood estimator. It is studied in e.g. [14].

We show in Sect. 4.1 (Lemmas 2 and 3) that for the case where $\epsilon \sim \mathcal{N}_n(0, \sigma_0^2 I)$ for example one has $\hat{\sigma} \to \sigma_0$ under ℓ_1-sparsity conditions on β^0. In Sect. 4.2

we establish oracle results for $\hat{\beta}$ under further sparsity conditions on β^0 and compatibility conditions on X (see Definition 2 for the latter). These results hold for a "universal" choice of λ_0 provided an ℓ_1-sparsity condition on β^0 is met.

In the proof of our main result in Theorem 1, the so-called *Karush-Kuhn-Tucker conditions*, or KKT-conditions, play a major role. Let us briefly discuss these here. The KKT-conditions for the square-root Lasso say that

$$\frac{X^T(Y - X\hat{\beta})/n}{\hat{\sigma}} = \lambda_0 \hat{z} \tag{3}$$

where $\hat{z}$ is a p-dimensional vector with $\|\hat{z}\|_\infty \leq 1$ and with $\hat{z}_j = \text{sign}(\hat{\beta}_j)$ if $\hat{\beta}_j \neq 0$. This follows from sub-differential calculus which defines the sub-differential of the absolute value function $x \mapsto |x|$ as

$$\{\text{sign}(x)\}\{x \neq 0\} + [-1, 1]\{x = 0\}.$$

Indeed, for a fixed $\sigma > 0$ the sub-differential with respect to β of the expression in curly brackets given in (2) is equal to

$$-\frac{2X^T(Y - X\beta)/n}{\sigma} + 2\lambda_0 z(\beta)$$

with, for $j = 1, \ldots, p$, $z_j(\beta)$ the sub-differential of $\beta_j \mapsto |\beta_j|$. Setting this to zero at $(\hat{\beta}, \hat{\sigma})$ gives the above KKT-conditions (3).

2.2 *The Multivariate Square-Root Lasso*

In our construction of confidence sets we will consider the regression of X_J on X_{-J} invoking a multivariate version of the square-root Lasso. To explain the latter, we use here a standard notation with X being the input and Y being the response. We will then replace X by X_{-J} and Y by X_J in Sect. 3.1.

The matrix X is as before an $n \times p$ input matrix and the response Y is now an $n \times q$ matrix for some $q \geq 1$. We define the multivariate square-root Lasso

$$\hat{B} := \arg\min_B \left\{ \|Y - XB\|_{\text{nuclear}} / \sqrt{n} + \lambda_0 \|B\|_1 \right\} \tag{4}$$

with $\lambda_0 > 0$ again a tuning parameter. The minimization is over all $p \times q$ matrices B. We consider $\hat{\Sigma} := (Y - X\hat{B})^T (Y - X\hat{B})/n$ as estimator of the noise co-variance matrix.

The KKT-conditions for the multivariate square-root Lasso will be a major ingredient of the proof of the main result in Theorem 1. We present these KKT-conditions in the following lemma in Eq. (5).

Lemma 1 *We have*

$$(\hat{B}, \hat{\Sigma}) = \arg \min_{B,\ \Sigma>0} \left\{ \text{trace}\left((Y - XB)^T (Y - XB) \Sigma^{-1/2} \right) / n \right.$$
$$\left. + \text{trace}(\Sigma^{1/2}) + 2\lambda_0 \|B\|_1 \right\}$$

where the minimization is over all symmetric positive definite matrix Σ (this being denoted by $\Sigma > 0$) and where it is assumed that the minimum is indeed attained at some $\Sigma > 0$. The multivariate Lasso satisfies the KKT-conditions

$$X^T (Y - X\hat{B}) \hat{\Sigma}^{-1/2} / n = \lambda_0 \hat{Z}, \tag{5}$$

where $\hat{Z}$ is a $p \times q$ matrix with $\|\hat{Z}\|_\infty \leq 1$ and with $\hat{Z}_{k,j} = \text{sign}(\hat{B}_{k,j})$ if $\hat{B}_{k,j} \neq 0$ ($k = 1, \ldots, p, j = 1, \ldots, q$).

3 Confidence Sets for β_J^0

3.1 The Construction

Let $J \subset \{1, \ldots, p\}$. We are interested in building a confidence set for $\beta_J^0 := \{\beta_j^0 : j \in J\}$. To this end, we compute the multivariate ($|J|$-dimensional) square root Lasso

$$\hat{\Gamma}_J := \arg \min_{\Gamma_J} \left\{ \|X_J - X_{-J}\Gamma_J\|_{\text{nuclear}} / \sqrt{n} + \lambda \|\Gamma_J\|_1 \right\} \tag{6}$$

where $\lambda > 0$ is a tuning parameter. The minimization is over all $(p - |J|) \times |J|$ matrices Γ_J. We let

$$\tilde{T}_J := (X_J - X_{-J}\hat{\Gamma}_J)^T X_J / n \tag{7}$$

and

$$\hat{T}_J := (X_J - X_{-J}\hat{\Gamma}_J)^T (X_J - X_{-J}\hat{\Gamma}_J) / n, \tag{8}$$

We assume throughout that the "hat" matrix $\hat{T}_J$ is non-singular. The "tilde" matrix $\tilde{T}_J$ only needs to be non-singular in order that the de-sparsified estimator $\hat{b}_J$ given below in Definition 1 is well-defined. However, for the normalized version we need not assume non-singularity of $\tilde{T}_J$.

The KKT-conditions (5) appear in the form

$$X_{-J}^T(X_J - X_{-J}\hat{\Gamma}_J)\hat{T}_J^{-1/2}/n = \lambda \hat{Z}_J, \tag{9}$$

where $\hat{Z}_J$ is a $(p - |J|) \times |J|$ matrix with $(\hat{Z}_J)_{k,j} = \text{sign}(\hat{\Gamma}_J)_{k,j}$ if $(\hat{\Gamma}_J)_{k,j} \neq 0$ and $\|\hat{Z}_J\|_\infty \leq 1$.

We define the normalization matrix

$$M := M_\lambda := \sqrt{n}\hat{T}_J^{-1/2}\tilde{T}_J. \tag{10}$$

Definition 1 The *de-sparsified* estimator of β_J^0 is

$$\hat{b}_J := \hat{\beta}_J + \tilde{T}_J^{-1}(X_J - X_{-J}\hat{\Gamma}_J)^T(Y - X\hat{\beta})/n,$$

with $\hat{\beta}$ the square-root Lasso given in (1), $\hat{\Gamma}_J$ the multivariate square-root Lasso given in (6) and the matrix $\tilde{T}_J$ given in (7). The normalized de-sparsified estimator is $M\hat{b}_J$ with M the normalization matrix given in (10).

3.2 The Main Result

Our main result is rather simple. It shows that using the multivariate square-root Lasso for de-sparsifying, and then normalizing, results in a well-scaled "asymptotic pivot" (up to the estimation of σ_0 which we will do in the next section). Theorem 1 actually does not require $\hat{\beta}$ to be the square-root Lasso but for definiteness we have made this specific choice throughout the paper (except for Sect. 6).

Theorem 1 *Consider the model $Y \sim \mathcal{N}_n(f^0, \sigma_0^2)$ where $f^0 = X\beta^0$. Let $\hat{b}_J$ be the de-sparsified estimator given in Definition 1 and let $M\hat{b}_J$ be its normalized version. Then*

$$M(\hat{b}_J - \beta_J^0)/\sigma_0 = \mathcal{N}_{|J|}(0, I) + \text{rem}$$

where $\|\text{rem}\|_\infty \leq \sqrt{n}\lambda\|\hat{\beta}_{-J} - \beta_{-J}^0\|_1/\sigma_0$.

To make Theorem 1 work we need to bound $\|\hat{\beta} - \beta^0\|_1/\hat{\sigma}$ where $\hat{\sigma}$ is an estimator of σ_0. This is done in Theorem 2 with $\hat{\sigma}$ the estimator $\|\hat{\epsilon}\|_n$ from the square-root Lasso. A special case is presented in Lemma 5 which imposes weak sparsity conditions for β^0. Bounds for $\sigma_0/\hat{\sigma}$ are also given.

Theorem 1 is about the case where the noise ϵ is i.i.d. normally distributed. This can be generalized as from the proof we see that the "main" term is linear in ϵ. For independent errors with common variance σ_0^2 say, one needs to assume the Lindeberg condition for establishing asymptotic normality.

4 Theory for the Square Root Lasso

Let $f^0 := \mathbb{E}Y$, β^0 be a solution of $X\beta^0 = f^0$ and define $\epsilon := Y - f^0$. Recall the square-root Lasso $\hat{\beta}$ given in (1). It depends on the tuning parameter $\lambda_0 > 0$. In this section we develop theoretical bounds, which are closely related to results in [15] (who by the way use the term scaled Lasso instead of square-root Lasso in that paper). There are two differences. Firstly, our lower bound for the residual sum of squares of the square-root Lasso requires, for the case where no conditions are imposed on the compatibility constants, a smaller value for the tuning parameter (see Lemma 3). These compatibility constants, given in Definition 2, are required only later for the oracle results. Secondly, we establish an oracle inequality that is sharp (see Theorem 2 in Sect. 4.2 where we present more details).

Write $\hat{\epsilon} := Y - X\hat{\beta}$ and $\hat{\sigma}^2 := \|\hat{\epsilon}\|_n^2$. We consider bounds in terms of $\|\epsilon\|_n^2$, the "empirical" variance of the unobservable noise. This is a random quantity but under obvious conditions it convergences to its expectation σ_0^2. Another random quantity that appears in our bounds is $\epsilon/\|\epsilon\|_n$, which is a random point on the n-dimensional unit sphere. We write

$$\hat{R} := \frac{\|X^T\epsilon\|_\infty}{n\|\epsilon\|_n}.$$

When all X_j are normalized such that $\|X_j\|_n = 1$, the quantity $\hat{R}$ is the maximal "empirical" correlation between noise and input variables. Under distributional assumptions $\hat{R}$ can be bounded with large probability by some constant R. For completeness we work out the case of i.i.d. normally distributed errors.

Lemma 2 *Let $\epsilon \sim \mathcal{N}_n(0, \sigma_0^2 I)$. Suppose the normalized case where $\|X_j\|_n = 1$ for all $j = 1, \ldots, p$. Let α_0, $\underline{\alpha}$ and $\bar{\alpha}$ be given positive error levels such that $\alpha_0 + \underline{\alpha} + \bar{\alpha} < 1$ and $\log(1/\underline{\alpha}) < n/4$. Define*

$$\underline{\sigma}^2 := \sigma_0^2\left(1 - 2\sqrt{\frac{\log(1/\underline{\alpha})}{n}}\right),$$

$$\bar{\sigma}^2 := \sigma_0^2\left(1 + 2\sqrt{\frac{\log(1/\bar{\alpha})}{n}} + \frac{2\log(1/\bar{\alpha})}{n}\right)$$

and

$$R := \sqrt{\frac{\log(2p/\alpha_0)}{n - 2\sqrt{n\log(1/\underline{\alpha})}}}.$$

We have

$$\mathbb{P}(\|\epsilon\|_n \le \underline{\sigma}) \le \underline{\alpha},\ \mathbb{P}(\|\epsilon\|_n \ge \bar{\sigma}) \le \bar{\alpha}$$

and

$$\mathbb{P}(\hat{R} \geq R \cup \|\epsilon\|_n \leq \underline{\sigma}) \leq \alpha_0 + \underline{\alpha}.$$

4.1 Preliminary Lower and Upper Bounds for $\hat{\sigma}^2$

We now show that the estimator of the variance $\hat{\sigma}^2 = \|\hat{\epsilon}\|_n^2$, obtained by applying the square-root Lasso, converges to the noise variance σ_0^2. The result holds without conditions on compatibility constants (given in Definition 2). We do however need the ℓ_1-sparsity condition (11) on β_0. This condition will be discussed below in an asymptotic setup.

Lemma 3 *Suppose that for some $0 < \eta < 1$, some $R > 0$ and some $\underline{\sigma} > 0$, we have*

$$\lambda_0(1-\eta) \geq R$$

and

$$\lambda_0 \|\beta^0\|_1 / \underline{\sigma} \leq 2\Big(\sqrt{1 + (\eta/2)^2} - 1 \Big). \tag{11}$$

Then on the set where $\hat{R} \leq R$ and $\|\epsilon\|_n \geq \underline{\sigma}$ we have $\Big| \|\hat{\epsilon}\|_n / \|\epsilon\|_n - 1 \Big| \leq \eta$.

We remark here that the result of Lemma 3 is also useful when using a square-root Lasso for constructing an asymptotic confidence interval for a single parameter, say β_j^0. Assuming random design it can be applied to show that without imposing compatibility conditions the residual variance of the square root Lasso for the regression of X_j on all other variables X_{-j} does not degenerate.

Asymptotics Suppose $\epsilon_1, \ldots, \epsilon_n$ are i.i.d. with finite variance σ_0^2. Then clearly $\|\epsilon\|_n / \sigma_0 \to 1$ in probability. The normalization in (11) by $\underline{\sigma}$—which can be taken more or less equal to σ_0—makes sense if we think of the standardized model

$$\tilde{Y} = X\tilde{\beta}^0 + \tilde{\epsilon},$$

with $\tilde{Y} = Y/\sigma_0$, $\tilde{\beta}^0 = \beta^0/\sigma_0$ and $\tilde{\epsilon} = \epsilon/\sigma_0$. The condition (11) is a condition on the normalized $\tilde{\beta}^0$. The rate of growth assumed there is quite common. First of all, it is clear that if $\|\beta^0\|_1$ is very large then the estimator is not very good because of the penalty on large values of $\|\cdot\|_1$. The condition (11) is moreover closely related to standard assumptions in compressed sensing. To explain this we first note that

$$\|\beta^0\|_1/\sigma_0 \leq \sqrt{s_0}\|\beta^0\|_2/\sigma_0$$

when s_0 is the number of non-zero entries of β^0 (observe that s_0 is a scale free property of β^0). The term $\|\beta^0\|_2/\sigma_0$ can be seen as a signal-to-noise ratio. Let us assume this signal-to-noise ratio stays bounded. If λ_0 corresponds to the standard choice $\lambda_0 \asymp \sqrt{\log p/n}$ the assumption (11) holds with $\eta = o(1)$ as soon as we assume the standard assumption $s_0 = o(n/\log p)$.

4.2 An Oracle Inequality for the Square-Root Lasso

Our next result is an oracle inequality for the square-root Lasso. It is as the corresponding result for the Lasso as established in [6]. The oracle inequality of Theorem 2 is sharp in the sense that there is a constant 1 in front of the approximation error $\|X(\beta - \beta^0)\|_n^2$ in (12). This sharpness is obtained along the lines of arguments from [9], who prove sharp oracle inequalities for the Lasso and for matrix problems. We further have extended the situation in order to establish an oracle inequality for the ℓ_1-estimation error $\|\hat{\beta} - \beta^0\|_1$ where we use arguments from [17] for the Lasso. For the square-root Lasso, the paper [15] also has oracle inequalities, but these are not sharp.

Compatibility constants are introduced in [16]. They play a role in the identifiability of β^0.

Definition 2 Let $L > 0$ and $S \subset \{1, \dots, p\}$. The compatibility constant is

$$\hat{\phi}^2(L, S) = \min\left\{ |S| \|X\beta\|_n^2 : \ \|\beta_S\|_1 = 1, \ \|\beta_{-S}\|_1 \le L \right\}.$$

We recall the notation $S_\beta = \{j : \ \beta_j \neq 0\}$ appearing in (12).

Theorem 2 *Let λ_0 satisfy for some $R > 0$*

$$\lambda_0(1 - \eta) > R$$

and assume the ℓ_1-sparsity (11) for some $0 < \eta < 1$ and $\underline{\sigma} > 0$, i.e.

$$\lambda_0 \|\beta^0\|_1/\underline{\sigma} \le 2\left(\sqrt{1 + (\eta/2)^2} - 1 \right).$$

Let $0 \le \delta < 1$ be arbitrary and define

$$\underline{\lambda} := \lambda_0(1 - \eta) - R,$$
$$\bar{\lambda} := \lambda_0(1 + \eta) + R + \delta\underline{\lambda}$$

and

$$L := \frac{\bar{\lambda}}{(1-\delta)\underline{\lambda}}.$$

Then on the set where $\hat{R} \le R$ *and* $\|\epsilon\|_n \ge \underline{\sigma}$, *we have*

$$2\delta\underline{\lambda}\|\hat{\beta} - \beta^0\|_1\|\epsilon\|_n + \|X(\hat{\beta} - \beta^0)\|_n^2$$

$$\le \min_S \left\{ \min_{\beta \in \mathbb{R}^p,\ S_\beta = S} \left[2\delta\underline{\lambda}\|\beta - \beta^0\|_1\|\epsilon\|_n + \|X(\beta - \beta^0)\|_n^2 \right] + \bar{\lambda}^2 \frac{|S|\|\epsilon\|_n^2}{\hat{\phi}^2(L,S)} \right\}. \quad (12)$$

The result of Theorem 2 leads to a trade-off between the approximation error $\|X(\beta - \beta^0)\|_n^2$, the ℓ_1-error $\|\beta - \beta^0\|_1$ and the sparseness[1] $|S_\beta|$ (or rather the *effective sparseness* $|S_\beta|/\hat{\phi}^2(L, S_\beta)$).

5 A Bound for the ℓ_1-Estimation Error Under (Weak) Sparsity

In this section we assume

$$\sum_{j=1}^{r} |\beta_j^0|^r \le \rho_r^r, \quad (13)$$

where $0 < r < 1$ and where $\rho_r > 0$ is a constant that is "not too large". This is sometimes called *weak sparsity* as opposed to *strong sparsity* which requires "not too many" non-zero coefficients $s_0 := \#\{\beta_j^0 \ne 0\}$. We start with bounding the right hand side of the oracle inequality (12) in Theorem 2.

We let $S_0 := S_{\beta^0}$ be the active set $S_0 := \{j : \beta_j^0 \ne 0\}$ of β_0 and let $\hat{\Lambda}_{\max}^2(S_0)$ be the largest eigenvalue of $X_{S_0}^T X_{S_0}/n$. The cardinality of S_0 is denoted by $s_0 = |S_0|$. We assume in this section the normalization $\|X_j\|_n = 1$ so that that $\hat{\Lambda}_{\max}(S_0) \ge 1$ and $\hat{\phi}(L, S) \le 1$ for any L and S.

Lemma 4 *Suppose* β^0 *satisfies the weak sparsity condition (13) for some* $0 < r < 1$ *and* $\rho_r > 0$. *For any positive* δ, $\underline{\lambda}$, $\bar{\lambda}$ *and* L

$$\min_S \left\{ \min_{\beta \in \mathbb{R}^p,\ S_\beta = S} \left[2\delta\underline{\lambda}\|\beta - \beta^0\|_1\|\epsilon\|_n + \|X(\beta - \beta^0)\|_n^2 \right] + \bar{\lambda}^2 \frac{|S|\|\epsilon\|_n^2}{\hat{\phi}^2(L,S)} \right\}$$

[1]Or non-sparseness actually.

$$\leq 2\bar{\lambda}^{2-r}\left(\delta\underline{\lambda}/\bar{\lambda} + \frac{\hat{\Lambda}_{\max}^r(S_0)}{\hat{\phi}^2(L,\hat{S}_*)}\right)\left(\frac{\rho_r}{\|\epsilon\|_n}\right)^r \|\epsilon\|_n^2,$$

where $\hat{S}_* := \{j: \ |\beta_j^0| > \bar{\lambda}\|\epsilon\|_n/\hat{\Lambda}_{\max}(S_0)\}$.

As a consequence, we obtain bounds for the prediction error and ℓ_1-error of the square-root Lasso under (weak) sparsity. We only present the bound for the ℓ_1-error as this is what we need in Theorem 1 for the construction of asymptotic confidence sets.

To avoid being taken away by all the constants, we make some arbitrary choices in Lemma 5: we set $\eta \leq 1/3$ in the ℓ_1-sparsity condition (11) and we set $\lambda_0(1-\eta) = 2R$. We choose $\delta = 1/7$.

We include the confidence statements that are given in Lemma 2 to complete the picture.

Lemma 5 *Suppose* $\epsilon \sim \mathcal{N}_n(0, \sigma_0^2 I)$. *Let* α_0 *and* $\underline{\alpha}$ *be given positive error levels such that* $\alpha_0 + \underline{\alpha} < 1$ *and* $\log(1/\underline{\alpha}) < n/4$. *Define*

$$\underline{\sigma}^2 := \sigma_0^2\left(1 - 2\sqrt{\frac{\log(1/\underline{\alpha})}{n}}\right), \ R := \sqrt{\frac{\log(2p/\alpha_0)}{n - 2\sqrt{n\log(1/\underline{\alpha})}}}.$$

Assume the ℓ_1*-sparsity condition*

$$R\|\beta^0\|_1/\underline{\sigma} \leq (1-\eta)\left(\sqrt{1+(\eta/2)^2} - 1\right), \ \textit{where } 0 < \eta \leq 1/3$$

and the ℓ_r*-sparsity condition (13) for some* $0 < r < 1$ *and* $\rho_r > 0$. *Set*

$$S_* := \{j: \ |\beta_j^0| > 3R\underline{\sigma}/\hat{\Lambda}_{\max}(S_0)\}.$$

Then for $\lambda_0(1-\eta) = 2R$, *with probability at least* $1-\alpha_0-\underline{\alpha}$ *we have the* ℓ_r*-sparsity based bound*

$$(1-\eta)\frac{\|\hat{\beta}-\beta^0\|_1}{\hat{\sigma}} \leq \frac{\|\hat{\beta}-\beta^0\|_1}{\|\epsilon\|_n} \leq (6R)^{1-r}\left(1 + \frac{6^2\hat{\Lambda}_{\max}^r(S_0)}{\hat{\phi}^2(6,S_*)}\right)\left(\frac{\rho_r}{\underline{\sigma}}\right)^r,$$

the ℓ_0*-sparsity based bound*

$$(1-\eta)\frac{\|\hat{\beta}-\beta^0\|_1}{\hat{\sigma}} \leq \frac{\|\hat{\beta}-\beta^0\|_1}{\|\epsilon\|_n} \leq 3R\left(\frac{6^2 s_0}{\hat{\phi}^2(6,S_0)}\right)$$

and moreover the following lower bound for the estimator $\hat{\sigma}$ of the noise level:

$$(1-\eta)\sigma_0/\hat{\sigma} \le \left(1 - 2\sqrt{\frac{\log(1/\underline{\alpha})}{n}}\right)^{-1/2}.$$

Asymptotics Application of Theorem 1 with σ_0 estimated by $\hat{\sigma}$ requires that $\sqrt{n}\lambda\|\hat{\beta} - \beta^0\|_1/\hat{\sigma}$ tends to zero in probability. Taking $\lambda \asymp \sqrt{\log p/n}$ and for example $\alpha_0 = \alpha = 1/p$, we see that this is the case under the conditions of Lemma 5 as soon as for some $0 < r < 1$ the following ℓ_r-sparsity based bound holds:

$$\left(\frac{\hat{\Lambda}^r_{\max}(S_0)}{\hat{\phi}^2(6, S_*)}\right)\left(\frac{\rho_r}{\sigma_0}\right)^r = \frac{o(n/\log p)^{\frac{1-r}{2}}}{(\log p)^{\frac{1}{2}}}.$$

Alternatively, one may require the ℓ_0-sparsity based bound

$$\left(\frac{1}{\hat{\phi}^2(6, S_0)}\right)s_0 = \frac{o(n/\log p)^{\frac{1}{2}}}{(\log p)^{\frac{1}{2}}}.$$

6 Structured Sparsity

We will now show that the results hold for norm-penalized estimators with norms other than ℓ_1. Let Ω be some norm on $\mathbb{R}^{p-|J|}$ and define for a $(p-|J|) \times |J|$ matrix $A := (a_1, \ldots, a_{|J|})$

$$\|A\|_{1,\Omega} := \sum_{j=1}^{|J|} \Omega(a_j).$$

For a vector $z \in \mathbb{R}^{p-|J|}$ we define the dual norm

$$\Omega_*(z) = \sup_{\Omega(a)\le 1} |z^T a|,$$

and for a $(p-|J|) \times |J|$ matrix $Z = (z_1, \ldots, z_{|J|})$ we let

$$\|Z\|_{\infty,\Omega_*} = \max_{1\le j\le |J|} \Omega_*(z_j).$$

Thus, when Ω is the ℓ_1-norm we have $\|A\|_{1,\Omega} = \|A\|_1$ and $\|Z\|_{\infty,\Omega_*} = \|Z\|_\infty$. We let the multivariate square-root Ω-sparse estimator be

$$\hat{\Gamma}_J := \arg\min_{\Gamma_J}\left\{ \|X_J - X_{-J}\Gamma_J\|_{\text{nuclear}}/\sqrt{n} + \lambda\|\Gamma\|_{1,\Omega}\right\}.$$

This estimator equals (6) when Ω is the ℓ_1-norm.

We let, as in (7), (8) and (10) but now with the new $\hat{\Gamma}_J$, the quantities $\tilde{T}_J$, $\hat{T}_J$ and M be defined as

$$\tilde{T}_J := (X_J - X_{-J}\hat{\Gamma}_J)^T X_J/n,$$
$$\hat{T}_J := (X_J - X_{-J}\hat{\Gamma}_J)^T (X_J - X_{-J}\hat{\Gamma}_J)/n$$

and

$$M := M_\lambda := \sqrt{n}\hat{T}_J^{-1/2}\tilde{T}_J.$$

The Ω-de-sparsified estimator of β_J^0 is as in Definition 1

$$\hat{b}_J := \hat{\beta}_J + \tilde{T}_J^{-1}(X_J - X_{-J}\hat{\Gamma}_J)^T (Y - X\hat{\beta})/n,$$

but now with $\hat{\beta}$ not necessarily the square root Lasso but a suitably chosen initial estimator and with $\hat{\Gamma}_J$ the multivariate square-root Ω-sparse estimator. The normalized de-sparsified estimator is $M\hat{b}_J$ with normalization matrix M given above. We can then easily derive the following extension of Theorem 1.

Theorem 3 *Consider the model $Y \sim \mathcal{N}_n(f^0, \sigma_0^2)$ where $f^0 = X\beta^0$. Let $\hat{b}_J$ be the Ω-de-sparsified estimator depending on some initial estimator $\hat{\beta}$. Let $M\hat{b}_J$ be its normalized version. Then*

$$M(\hat{b}_J - \beta_J^0)/\sigma_0 = \mathcal{N}_{|J|}(0, I) + \text{rem}$$

where $\|\text{rem}\|_\infty \le \sqrt{n}\lambda\Omega(\hat{\beta}_{-J} \quad \beta_{-J}^0)/\sigma_0$.

We see from Theorem 3 that confidence sets follow from fast rates of convergence of the Ω-estimation error. The latter is studied in [1, 13, 17] for the case where the initial estimator is the least squares estimator with penalty based on a sparsity inducing norm $\bar{\Omega}$ (say). Group sparsity [19] is an example which we shall now briefly discuss.

Example 1 Let $G_1, \ldots, G_T$ be given mutually disjoint subsets of $\{1, \ldots, p\}$ and take as sparsity-inducing norm

$$\bar{\Omega}(\beta) := \sum_{t=1}^{T} \sqrt{|G_t|}\|X\beta_{G_t}\|_2, \ \beta \in \mathbb{R}^p.$$

The group Lasso is the minimizer of least squares loss with penalty proportional to $\bar{\Omega}$. Oracle inequalities for the $\bar{\Omega}$-error of the group Lasso have been derived in [11] for example. For the square-root version we refer to [7]. With group sparsity, it lies at hand to consider confidence sets for one of the groups G_t i.e., to take $J = G_{t_0}$ for a given t_0. Choosing

$$\Omega(a) = \sum_{t \neq t_0} \sqrt{|G_t|}\|Xa_{G_t}\|_2, \ a \in \mathbb{R}^{p-|G_{t_0}|}$$

will ensure that $\Omega(\hat{\beta}_{-G_{t_0}} - \beta_{-G_{t_0}}) \leq \bar{\Omega}(\hat{\beta} - \beta^0)$ which gives one a handle to control the remainder term in Theorem 3. This choice of Ω for constructing the confidence set makes sense if one believes that the group structure describing the relation between the response Y and the input X is also present in the relation between $X_{G_{t_0}}$ and $X_{-G_{t_0}}$.

7 Simulations

Here we denote by $\widetilde{Y} = \widetilde{X}B_0 + \epsilon$ an arbitrary linear multivariate regression. In a similar fashion to the square-root Algorithm in Bunea et al. [7] we propose the following algorithm for the multivariate square-root Lasso:

Algorithm 1 msrL

Require: Take a constant K big enough, and choose an arbitrary starting matrix $B(0) \in \mathbb{R}^{p \times q}$.
1: $Y \leftarrow \widetilde{Y}/K$
2: $X \leftarrow \widetilde{X}/K$
3: **for** $t = 0, 1, 2, ...t_{stop}$ **do**
4: $\quad B(t+1) := \overline{\Phi}\left(B(t) + X^T \cdot (Y - XB(t));\ \lambda \|Y - XB(t)\|_{nuclear}\right)$
5: **return** $B(t_{stop} + 1)$

Here we denote

$$\overline{\Phi}(a; \eta) := \begin{cases} 0, & \text{if } a = 0 \\ \frac{a}{\|a\|_2}(\|a\|_2 - \eta)_+, & \text{if } a > 0 \end{cases}.$$

The value t_{stop} can be chosen in such a way that one gets the desired accuracy for the algorithm. This algorithm is based on a Fixpoint equation from the KKT conditions. The square root Lasso is calculated via the algorithm in Bunea et al. [7].

We consider the usual linear regression model:

$$Y = X\beta + \epsilon.$$

In our simulations we take a design matrix X, where the rows are fixed i.i.d. realizations from $\mathcal{N}(0, \Sigma)$. We have n observations, and p explanatory variables. The covariance matrix Σ has the following toeplitz structure $\Sigma_{i,j} = 0.9^{|i-j|}$. The errors are i.i.d. Gaussian distributed, with variance $\sigma^2 = 1$. A set of points J is also chosen. J denotes the set of indices of the parameter vector β that we want to find asymptotic group confidence intervals for. Define as $q = |J|$ the number of indices of interest. For each different setting of p and n we do $r = 1000$ simulations. In each repetition we calculate the teststatistic χ^2. A significance level of 0.05 is chosen. The lambda of the square root LASSO λ_{srL} in the simulations is the theoretical lambda λ_{srLt} scaled by 3. For the lambda of the multivariate square root LASSO λ_{msrL} we do not have theoretical results yet. That is why we use cross-validation where we minimize the error expressed in nuclear norm, to define λ_{msrL}. It is important to note, that the choice of λ_{msrL} is very crucial, especially for cases where n is small. One could tune λ_{msrL} in such a fashion that even cases like $n = 100$ work much better, see Fig. 2. But the point here is to see what happens to the chi-squared test statistic with a fixed rule for the choice of λ_{msrL}. This basic set up is used throughout all the simulations below.

7.1 Asymptotic Distribution

First let us look at the question how the histogram of the teststatistic looks like for different n. Here we use $p = 500$ and $q = 6$ with $J = (1, 3, 4, 8, 10, 33)$, where the entries in β_J are chosen randomly from a Uniform distribution on $[1, 4]$. We also specify β_{-J} to be the zero vector. So the set J that we are interested in, is in fact the same set as the active set of β. Furthermore $p - q$ gives the amount of sparsity. Here we look at a sequence of $n = 100, 200, 300, 400, 500, 600, 800$. As above, for each setting we calculate 1000 simulations. For each setting we plot the histogram for the teststatistic and compare it with the theoretical chi-squared distribution on $q = 6$ degrees of freedom. Figures 1 and 2 show the results.

The histograms show that with increasing n, we get a fast convergence to the true asymptotic chi-squared distribution. It is in fact true that we could multiply the teststatistic with a constant $C_n \leq 1$ in order to get the histogram match the chi-squared distribution. This reflects the theory. Already with $n = 400$ we get a very good approximation of the chi-squared distribution. But we see that the tuning of λ_{msrL} is crucial for small n, see Fig. 2.

Next we try the same procedure but we are interested in what happens if we let J and the active set S_0 not be the same set. Here we take $J = (1, 3, 4, 8, 10, 33)$ and β_0 is taken from the uniform distribution on $[1, 4]$ on the set $S_0 = (2, 3, 5, 8, 11, 12, 14, 31)$. So only the indices $J \cap S_0 = \{3, 8\}$ coincide. Figure 3 shows the results.

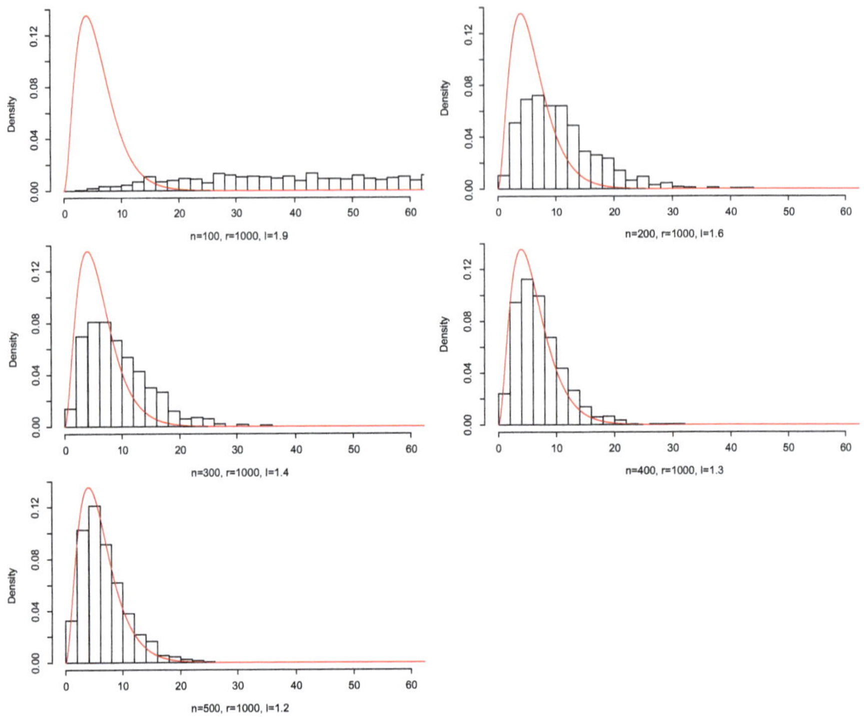

Fig. 1 Histogram of the Teststatistic, where the underlying active set is the index set for the parameter of interest. Here $l = \lambda$ denotes the cross-validation lambda

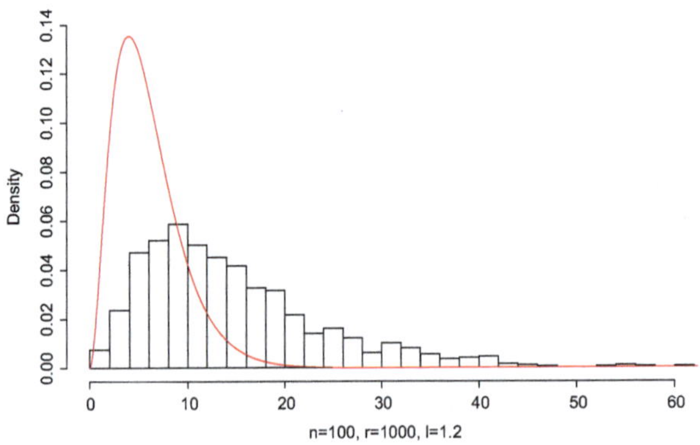

Fig. 2 Histogram of Teststatistic with a tuned $\lambda_{msrL} = l = 1.2$ for $n = 100$

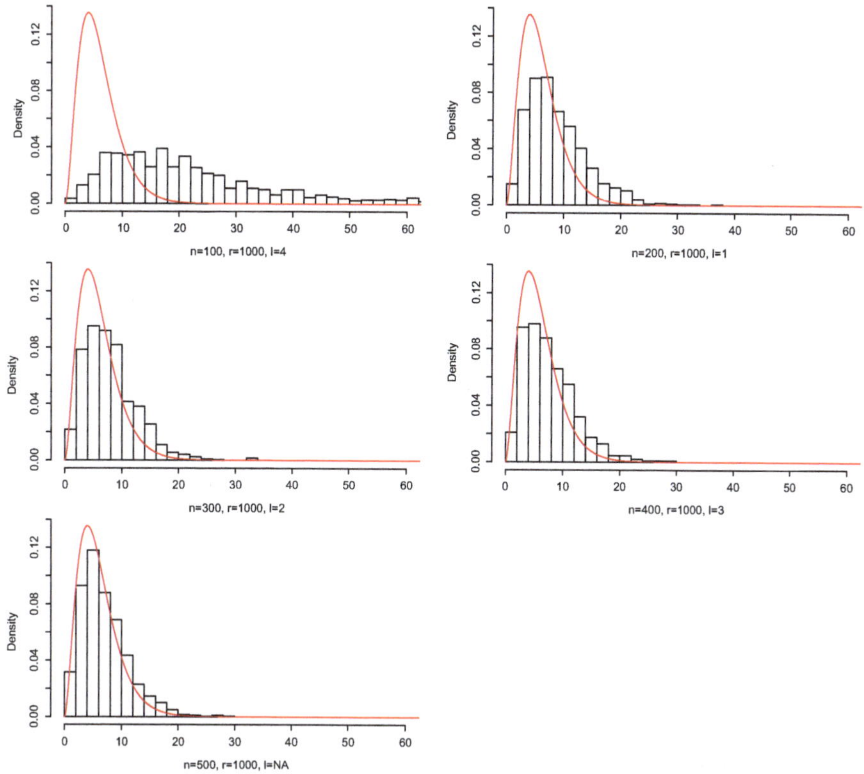

Fig. 3 Histogram of the Teststatistic, where the index set of the parameter of interest is different from the active set. Here $l = \lambda$ denotes the cross-validation lambda

Compared to the case where J and S_0 are the same set, it seems that this setting can handle small n better than in the case where all the elements of J are the nonzero indices of β_0. So the previous case seems to be the harder case. Therefore we stick with $J = S_0 = (1, 3, 4, 8, 10, 33)$ for all the other simulations in Sects. 7.2 and 7.3.

7.2 *Confidence Level for an Increasing* $\boldsymbol{\lambda_{msrL}}$

Up until now we have not looked at the behaviour for different λ. We only used the cross-validation λ. So here we look at $n = 400, p = 500$ and we take $\lambda_{msrL} = (0.01, 0.11, 0.21, \ldots, 2.91)$ a fixed sequence. Figure 4 shows the results.

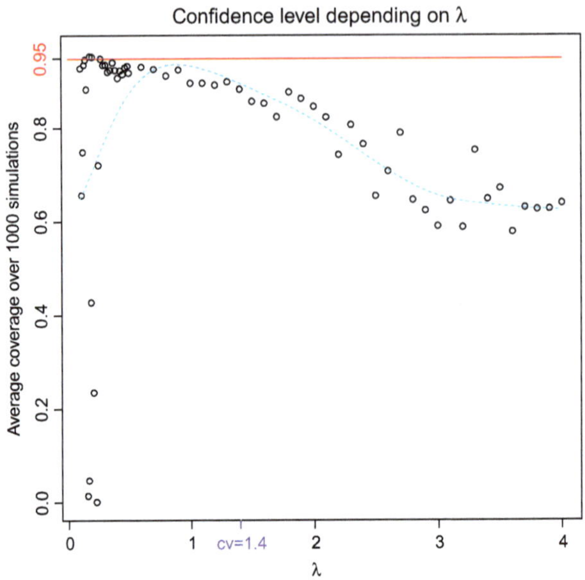

Fig. 4 Average confidence level with fixed $n = 400$ and $p = 500$, increased λ

If we take λ too low the behaviour breaks down. On the other hand, if λ is too big, we will not achieve a good average confidence level. The cross-validation λ seems to be still a bit to high. So the cross-validation λ could be better.

7.3 *Levelplot for n and p*

Not let us look at an overview of plot of different settings. We will use the levelplot to present the results Here we use the cross-validation λ. We let n and p increase and look again at the average coverage of the confidence interval (average over the 1000 simulations for each gridpoint). The border between high and low dimensional cases is marked by the white line in Fig. 5. Increasing p does not worsen the procedure too much, which is very good. And, as expected, increasing the number of observations n increases "the accuracy" of the average confidence interval.

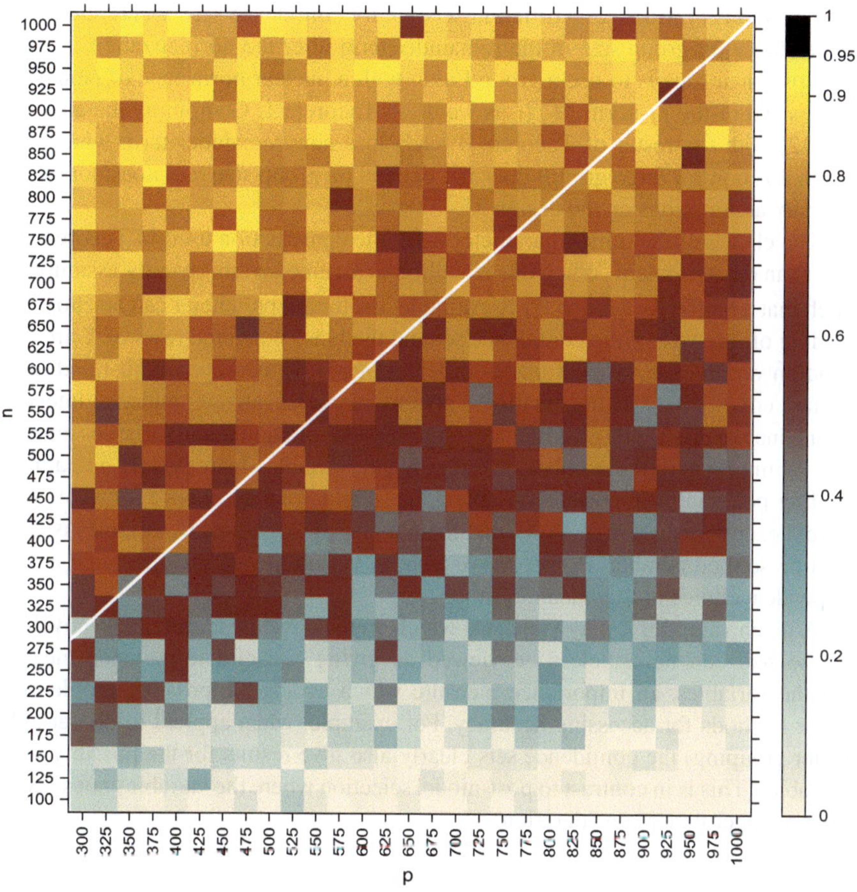

Fig. 5 Levelplot of average confidence level for a grid n, p

8 Discussion

We have presented a method for constructing confidence sets for groups of variables which does not impose sparsity conditions on the input matrix X. The idea is to use a loss function based on the nuclear norm of the matrix of residuals. We called this the multivariate square-root Lasso as it is an extension of the square-root Lasso in the multivariate case.

It is easy to see that when the groups are large, one needs the ℓ_2-norm of the remainder term $\|\text{rem}\|^2$ in Theorem 1 to be of small order $\sqrt{|J|}$ in probability, using the representation $\chi^2_{|J|} = |J| + O_{\mathbb{P}}(\sqrt{J})$. This leads to the requirement that $\sqrt{n}\lambda\|\hat{\beta}_{-J} - \beta_j^0\|_1/\sigma_0 = o_{\mathbb{P}}(1/|J|^{1/4})$, i.e., that it decreases faster for large groups.

The paper [12] introduces a different scheme for confidence sets, where there is no dependence on group size in the remainder term after the normalization for large groups. Their idea is to use a group Lasso with a nuclear norm type of penalty on Γ_J instead of the ℓ_1-norm $\|\Gamma_J\|_1$ as we do in Theorem 1. Combining the approach of [12] with the result of Theorem 3 leads to a new remainder term which after normalization for large groups does not depend on group size *and* does not rely on sparsity assumptions on the design X.

The choice of the tuning parameter λ for the construction used in Theorem 1 is as yet an open problem. When one is willing to assume certain sparsity assumptions such that a bound for $\|\hat{\beta} - \beta^0\|_1$ is available, the tuning parameter can be chosen by trading off the size of the confidence set and the bias. When the rows of X are i.i.d. random variables, a choice for λ of order $\sqrt{\log p/n}$ is theoretically justified under certain conditions. Finally, smaller λ give more conservative confidence intervals. Thus, increasing λ will give one a "solution path" of significant variables entering and exiting, where the number of "significant" variables increases. If one aims at finding potentially important variables, one might want to choose a cut-off level here, i.e. choose λ in such a way that the number of "significant" variables is equal to a prescribed number. However, we have as yet no theory showing such a data-dependent choice of λ is meaningful.

A given value for λ may yield sets which do not have the approximate coverage. These sets can nevertheless be viewed as giving a useful importance measure for the variables, an importance measure which avoids the possible problems of other methods for accessing accuracy. For example, when applied to all variables (after grouping) the confidence sets clearly also give results for the possibly weak variables. This is in contrast to post-model selection where the variables not selected are no longer under consideration.

9 Proofs

9.1 Proof for the Result for the Multivariate Square-Root Lasso in Sect. 2.2

Proof of Lemma 1 Let us write, for each $p \times q$ matrix B, the residuals as $\Sigma(B) := (Y - XB)^T(Y - XB)/n$. Let $\Sigma_{\min}(B)$ be the minimizer of

$$\text{trace}(\Sigma(B)\Sigma^{-1/2}) + \text{trace}(\Sigma^{1/2}) \tag{14}$$

over Σ. Then $\Sigma_{\min}(B)$ equals $\Sigma(B)$. To see this we invoke the reparametrization $\Omega := \Sigma^{-1/2}$ so that $\Sigma^{1/2} = \Omega^{-1}$. We now minimize

$$\text{trace}(\Sigma(B)\Omega) + \text{trace}(\Omega^{-1})$$

over $\Omega > 0$. The matrix derivative with respect to Ω of trace$(\Sigma(B)\Omega)$ is $\Sigma(B)$. The matrix derivative of trace(Ω^{-1}) with respect to Ω is equal to $-\Omega^{-2}$. Hence the minimizer $\Omega_{\min}(B)$ satisfies the equation

$$\Sigma(B) - \Omega_{\min}^{-2}(B) = 0,$$

giving

$$\Omega_{\min}(B) = \Sigma^{-1/2}(B).$$

so that

$$\Sigma_{\min}(B) = \Omega_{\min}^{-2}(B) = \Sigma(B).$$

Inserting this solution back in (14) gives 2trace$(\Sigma^{1/2}(B))$ which is equal to $2\|Y - XB\|_{\text{nuclear}}/\sqrt{n}$. This proves the first part of the lemma.

Let now for each $\Sigma > 0$, $B(\Sigma)$ be the minimizer of

$$\text{trace}(\Sigma(B)\Sigma^{-1/2}) + 2\lambda_0\|B\|_1.$$

By sub-differential calculus we have

$$X^T(Y - XB)\Sigma^{-1/2}/n = \lambda_0 Z(\Sigma)$$

where $\|Z(\Sigma)\|_\infty \leq 1$ and $Z_{k,j}(\Sigma)) = \text{sign}(B_{k,j}(\Sigma))$ if $B_{k,j}(\Sigma) \neq 0$ ($k = 1, \ldots, p$, $j = 1, \ldots q$). The KKT-conditions (5) follow from $\hat{B} = B(\hat{\Sigma})$. □

9.2 Proof of the Main Result in Sect. 3.2

Proof of Theorem 1 We have

$$\begin{aligned} M(\hat{b}_J - \hat{\beta}_J) &= \hat{T}_J^{-1/2}(X_J - X_{-J}\hat{\Gamma}_J)^T\epsilon/\sqrt{n} - \hat{T}_J^{-1/2}(X_J - X_{-J}\hat{\Gamma}_J)^T X(\hat{\beta} - \beta^0)/\sqrt{n} \\ &= \hat{T}_J^{-1/2}(X_J - X_{-J}\hat{\Gamma}_J)^T\epsilon/\sqrt{n} - \hat{T}_J^{-1/2}(X_J - X_{-J}\hat{\Gamma}_J)^T X_J(\hat{\beta}_J - \beta_J^0)/\sqrt{n} \\ &\quad -\hat{T}_J^{-1/2}(X_J - X_{-J}\hat{\Gamma}_J)^T X_{-J}(\hat{\beta}_{-J} - \beta_{-J}^0)/\sqrt{n} \\ &= \hat{T}_J^{-1/2}(X_J - X_{-J}\hat{\Gamma}_J)^T\epsilon/\sqrt{n} - M(\hat{\beta}_J - \beta_J^0) - \sqrt{n}\lambda\hat{Z}_J^T(\hat{\beta}_{-J} - \beta_{-J}^0) \end{aligned}$$

where we invoked the KKT-conditions (9). We thus arrive at

$$M(\hat{b}_J - \beta_J^0) = \hat{T}_J^{-1/2}(X_J - X_{-J}\hat{\Gamma}_J)^T\epsilon/\sqrt{n} + \sigma_0\text{rem}, \tag{15}$$

where

$$\text{rem} = -\sqrt{n}\lambda \hat{Z}_J^T(\hat{\beta}_{-J} - \beta_{-J}^0)/\sigma_0.$$

The co-variance matrix of the first term $\hat{T}_J^{-1/2}(X_J - X_{-J}\hat{\Gamma}_J)^T\epsilon/\sqrt{n}$ in (15) is equal to

$$\sigma_0^2\hat{T}_J^{-1/2}(X_J - X_{-J}\hat{\Gamma}_J)^T(X_J - X_{-J}\hat{\Gamma}_J)\hat{T}_J^{-1/2}/n = \sigma_0^2 I$$

where I is the identity matrix with dimensions $|J|\times|J|$. It follows that this term is $|J|$-dimensional standard normal scaled with σ_0. The remainder term can be bounded using the dual norm inequality for each entry:

$$|\text{rem}_j| \leq \sqrt{n}\lambda \max_{k\notin J} |(\hat{Z}_J)_{kj}|\|\hat{\beta}_{-J} - \beta_{-J}^0\|_1/\sigma_0 \leq \sqrt{n}\lambda\|\hat{\beta}_{-J} - \beta_{-J}^0\|_1/\sigma_0$$

since by the KKT-conditions (9), we have $\|\hat{Z}_J\|_\infty \leq 1$. □

9.3 Proofs of the Theoretical Result for the Square-Root Lasso in Sect. 4

Proof of Lemma 2 Without loss of generality we can assume $\sigma_0^2 = 1$. From [10] we know that for all $t > 0$

$$\mathbb{P}\left(\|\epsilon\|_n^2 \leq 1 - 2\sqrt{t/n}\right) \leq \exp[-t]$$

and

$$\mathbb{P}\left(\|\epsilon\|_n^2 \geq 1 + 2\sqrt{t/n} + 2t/n\right) \leq \exp[-t].$$

Apply this with $t = \log(1/\underline{\alpha})$ and $t = \log(1/\bar{\alpha})$ respectively. Moreover $X_j^T\epsilon/n \sim \mathcal{N}(0, 1/n)$ for all j. Hence for all $t > 0$

$$\mathbb{P}\left(|X_j^T\epsilon|/n \geq \sqrt{2t/n}\right) \leq 2\exp[-t], \ \forall\, j.$$

It follows that

$$\mathbb{P}\left(\|X^T\epsilon\|_\infty/n \geq \sqrt{2(t + \log(2p))/n}\right) \leq \exp[-t].$$

□

Proof of Lemma 3 Suppose $\hat{R} \leq R$ and $\|\epsilon\|_n \geq \underline{\sigma}$. First we note that the inequality (11) gives

$$\lambda_0\|\beta^0\|_1/\|\epsilon\|_n \leq 2\Big(\sqrt{1+(\eta/2)^2}-1\Big).$$

For the upper bound for $\|\hat{\epsilon}\|_n$ we use that

$$\|\hat{\epsilon}\|_n + \lambda_0\|\hat{\beta}\|_1 \leq \|\epsilon\|_n + \lambda_0\|\beta^0\|_1$$

by the definition of the estimator. Hence

$$\|\hat{\epsilon}\|_n \leq \|\epsilon\|_n + \lambda_0\|\beta^0\|_1 \leq \Big[1+2\Big(\sqrt{1+(\eta/2)^2}-1\Big)\Big]\|\epsilon\|_n \leq (1+\eta)\|\epsilon\|_n.$$

For the lower bound for $\|\hat{\epsilon}\|_n$ we use the convexity of both the loss function and the penalty. Define

$$\alpha := \frac{\eta\|\epsilon\|_n}{\eta\|\epsilon\|_n + \|X(\hat{\beta}-\beta^0)\|_n}.$$

Note that $0 < \alpha \leq 1$. Let $\hat{\beta}_\alpha$ be the convex combination $\hat{\beta}_\alpha := \alpha\hat{\beta} + (1-\alpha)\beta^0$. Then

$$\|X(\hat{\beta}_\alpha-\beta^0)\|_n = \alpha\|X(\hat{\beta}-\beta^0)\|_n = \frac{\eta\|\epsilon\|_n\|X(\hat{\beta}-\beta^0)\|_n}{\eta\|\epsilon\|_n + \|X(\hat{\beta}-\beta^0)\|_n} \leq \eta\|\epsilon\|_n.$$

Define $\hat{\epsilon}_\alpha := Y - X\hat{\beta}_\alpha$. Then, by convexity of $\|\cdot\|_n$ and $\|\cdot\|_1$,

$$\begin{aligned}\|\hat{\epsilon}_\alpha\|_n + \lambda_0\|\hat{\beta}_\alpha\|_1 &\leq \alpha\|\hat{\epsilon}\|_n + \alpha\lambda_0\|\hat{\beta}\|_1 + (1-\alpha)\|\epsilon\|_n + (1-\alpha)\lambda_0\|\beta^0\|_1\\ &\leq \|\epsilon\|_n + \lambda_0\|\beta^0\|_1\end{aligned}$$

where in the last step we again used that $\hat{\beta}$ minimizes $\|Y-X\beta\|_n + \lambda_0\|\beta\|_1$. Taking squares on both sides gives

$$\|\hat{\epsilon}_\alpha\|_n^2 + 2\lambda_0\|\hat{\beta}_\alpha\|_1\|\hat{\epsilon}_\alpha\|_n + \lambda_0^2\|\hat{\beta}_\alpha\|_1^2 \leq \|\epsilon\|_n^2 + 2\lambda_0\|\beta^0\|_1\|\epsilon\|_n + \lambda_0^2\|\beta^0\|_1^2. \quad (16)$$

But

$$\begin{aligned}\|\hat{\epsilon}_\alpha\|_n^2 &= \|\epsilon\|_n^2 - 2\epsilon^T X(\hat{\beta}_\alpha-\beta^0)/n + \|X(\hat{\beta}_\alpha-\beta^0)\|_n^2\\ &\geq \|\epsilon\|_n^2 - 2R\|\hat{\beta}_\alpha-\beta^0\|_1\|\epsilon\|_n + \|X(\hat{\beta}_\alpha-\beta^0)\|_n^2\\ &\geq \|\epsilon\|_n^2 - 2R\|\hat{\beta}_\alpha\|_1\|\epsilon\|_n - 2R\|\beta^0\|_1\|\epsilon\|_n + \|X(\hat{\beta}_\alpha-\beta^0)\|_n^2.\end{aligned}$$

Moreover, by the triangle inequality

$$\|\hat{\epsilon}_\alpha\|_n \geq \|\epsilon\|_n - \|X(\hat{\beta}_\alpha - \beta^0)\|_n \geq (1-\eta)\|\epsilon\|_n.$$

Inserting these two inequalities into (16) gives

$$\|\epsilon\|_n^2 - 2R\|\hat{\beta}_\alpha\|_1\|\epsilon\|_1 - 2R\|\beta^0\|_1\|\epsilon\|_n + \|X(\hat{\beta}_\alpha - \beta^0)\|_n^2 + 2\lambda_0(1-\eta)\|\hat{\beta}_\alpha\|_1\|\epsilon\|_n$$
$$+\lambda_0^2\|\hat{\beta}_\alpha\|_1^2 \leq \|\epsilon\|_n^2 + 2\lambda_0\|\beta^0\|_1\|\epsilon\|_n + \lambda_0^2\|\beta^0\|_1^2$$

which implies by the assumption $\lambda_0(1-\eta) \geq R$

$$\|X(\hat{\beta}_\alpha - \beta^0)\|_n^2 \leq 2(\lambda_0 + R)\|\beta^0\|_1\|\epsilon\|_1 + \lambda_0^2\|\beta^0\|_1^2.$$
$$\leq 4\lambda_0\|\beta^0\|_1\|\epsilon\|_1 + \lambda_0^2\|\beta^0\|_1^2$$

where in the last inequality we used $R \leq (1-\eta)\lambda_0 \leq \lambda_0$. But continuing we see that we can write the last expression as

$$4\lambda_0\|\beta^0\|_1\|\epsilon\|_1 + \lambda_0^2\|\beta^0\|_1^2 = \left((\lambda_0\|\beta_0\|_1/\|\epsilon_n\|_n + 2)^2 - 4\right)\|\epsilon\|_n^2.$$

Again invoke the ℓ_1-sparsity condition

$$\lambda_0\|\beta^0\|_1/\|\epsilon\|_n \leq 2\left(\sqrt{1+(\eta/2)^2} - 1\right)$$

to get

$$\left((\lambda_0\|\beta_0\|_1/\|\epsilon_n\|_n + 2)^2 - 4\right)\|\epsilon\|_n^2 \leq \frac{\eta^2}{4}\|\epsilon\|_n^2.$$

We thus established that

$$\|X(\hat{\beta}_\alpha - \beta^0)\|_n \leq \frac{\eta\|\epsilon\|_n}{2}.$$

Rewrite this to

$$\frac{\eta\|\epsilon\|_n\|X(\hat{\beta} - \beta^0)\|_n}{\eta\|\epsilon\|_n + \|X(\hat{\beta} - \beta^0)\|_n} \leq \frac{\eta\|\epsilon\|_n}{2},$$

and rewrite this in turn to

$$\eta\|\epsilon\|_n\|X(\hat{\beta} - \beta^0)\|_n \leq \frac{\eta^2\|\epsilon\|_n^2}{2} + \frac{\eta\|\epsilon\|_n\|X(\hat{\beta} - \beta^0)\|_n}{2}$$

or

$$\|X(\hat{\beta} - \beta^0)\|_n \leq \eta \|\epsilon\|_n.$$

But then, by repeating the argument, also

$$\|\hat{\epsilon}\|_n \geq \|\epsilon\|_n - \|X(\hat{\beta} - \beta^0)\|_n \geq (1-\eta)\|\epsilon\|_n.$$

□

Proof of Theorem 2 Throughout the proof we suppose $\hat{R} \leq R$ and $\|\epsilon\|_n \geq \underline{\sigma}$. Define the Gram matrix $\hat{\Sigma} := X^T X/n$. Let $\beta \in \mathbb{R}^p$ and $S := S_\beta = \{j : \beta_j \neq 0\}$. If

$$(\hat{\beta} - \beta)^T \hat{\Sigma} (\hat{\beta} - \beta^0) \leq -\delta \underline{\lambda} \|\hat{\beta} - \beta\|_1 \|\epsilon\|_n$$

we find

$$\begin{aligned} &2\delta\underline{\lambda}\|\hat{\beta} - \beta\|_1 \|\epsilon\|_n + \|X(\hat{\beta} - \beta^0)\|_n^2 \\ &= 2\delta\underline{\lambda}\|\hat{\beta} - \beta\|_1 \|\epsilon\|_n + \|X(\beta - \beta^0)\|_n^2 - \|X(\beta - \hat{\beta})\|_n^2 + 2(\hat{\beta} - \beta)^T \hat{\Sigma} (\hat{\beta} - \beta^0) \\ &\leq \|X(\beta - \beta^0)\|_n^2. \end{aligned}$$

So then we are done.

Suppose now that

$$(\hat{\beta} - \beta)^T \hat{\Sigma} (\hat{\beta} - \beta^0) \geq -\delta \underline{\lambda} \|\hat{\beta} - \beta\|_1 \|\epsilon\|_n.$$

By the KKT-conditions (3)

$$(\hat{\beta} - \beta)^T \hat{\Sigma} (\hat{\beta} - \beta^0) + \lambda_0 \|\hat{\beta}\|_1 \|\hat{\epsilon}\|_n \leq \epsilon^T X(\hat{\beta} - \beta)/n + \lambda_0 \|\beta\|_1 \|\hat{\epsilon}\|_n.$$

By the dual norm inequality and since $\hat{R} \leq R$

$$|\epsilon^T X(\hat{\beta} - \beta)|/n \leq R \|\hat{\beta} - \beta\|_1 \|\epsilon\|_n.$$

Thus

$$(\hat{\beta} - \beta)^T \hat{\Sigma} (\hat{\beta} - \beta^0) + \lambda_0 \|\hat{\beta}\|_1 \|\hat{\epsilon}\|_n \leq R \|\hat{\beta} - \beta\|_1 \|\epsilon\|_n + \lambda_0 \|\beta\|_1 \|\hat{\epsilon}\|_n.$$

This implies by the triangle inequality

$$(\hat{\beta} - \beta)^T \hat{\Sigma} (\hat{\beta} - \beta^0) + (\lambda_0 \|\hat{\epsilon}\|_n - R\|\epsilon\|_n) \|\hat{\beta}_{-S}\|_1 \leq (\lambda_0 \|\hat{\epsilon}\|_n + R\|\epsilon\|_n) \|\hat{\beta}_S - \beta\|_1.$$

We invoke the result of Lemma 3 which says that $(1-\eta)\|\epsilon\|_n \leq \|\hat{\epsilon}\|_n \leq (1+\eta)\|\epsilon\|_n$. This gives

$$(\hat{\beta}-\beta)^T\hat{\Sigma}(\hat{\beta}-\beta^0) + \underline{\lambda}\|\hat{\beta}_{-S}\|_1\|\epsilon\|_n \leq (\lambda_0(1+\eta)+R)\|\hat{\beta}_S-\beta\|_1\|\epsilon\|_n. \tag{17}$$

Since $(\hat{\beta}-\beta)^T\hat{\Sigma}(\hat{\beta}-\beta^0) \geq -\delta\underline{\lambda}\|\epsilon\|_n\|\hat{\beta}-\beta\|_1$ this gives

$$(1-\delta)\underline{\lambda}\|\hat{\beta}_{-S}\|_1\|\epsilon\|_n \leq (\lambda_0(1+\eta)+R+\delta\underline{\lambda})\|\hat{\beta}_S-\beta\|_1\|\epsilon\|_n = \bar{\lambda}\|\hat{\beta}_S-\beta\|_1\|\epsilon\|_n.$$

or

$$\|\hat{\beta}_{-S}\|_1 \leq L\|\hat{\beta}_S-\beta\|_1.$$

But then

$$\|\hat{\beta}_S-\beta\|_1 \leq \sqrt{|S|}\|X(\hat{\beta}-\beta)\|_n/\hat{\phi}(L,S). \tag{18}$$

Continue with inequality (17) and apply the inequality $ab \leq (a^2+b^2)/2$ which holds for all real valued a and b:

$$\begin{aligned}(\hat{\beta}-\beta)\hat{\Sigma}(\hat{\beta}-\beta^0) &+ \underline{\lambda}\|\hat{\beta}_{-S}\|_1\|\epsilon\|_n + \delta\underline{\lambda}\|\hat{\beta}_S-\beta\|_1\|\epsilon\|_n \\ &\leq \bar{\lambda}\|\epsilon\|_n\sqrt{|S|}\|X(\hat{\beta}-\beta)\|_n/\hat{\phi}(L,S) \\ &\leq \frac{1}{2}\bar{\lambda}^2\frac{|S|\|\epsilon\|_n^2}{\hat{\phi}^2(L,S)} + \frac{1}{2}\|X(\hat{\beta}-\beta)\|_n^2.\end{aligned}$$

Since

$$2(\hat{\beta}-\beta)^T\hat{\Sigma}(\hat{\beta}-\beta^0) = \|X(\hat{\beta}-\beta^0)\|_n^2 - \|X(\beta-\beta^0)\|_n^2 + \|X(\hat{\beta}-\beta)\|_n^2,$$

we obtain

$$\begin{aligned}\|X(\hat{\beta}-\beta^0)\|_n^2 &+ 2\underline{\lambda}\|\hat{\beta}_{-S}\|_1\|\epsilon\|_n + 2\delta\underline{\lambda}\|\hat{\beta}_S-\beta\|_1\|\epsilon\|_n \\ &\leq \|X(\beta-\beta^0)\|_n^2 + \bar{\lambda}^2|S|\|\epsilon\|_n^2/\hat{\phi}^2(L,S).\end{aligned}$$

□

9.4 Proofs of the Illustration Assuming (Weak) Sparsity in Sect. 5

Proof of Lemma 4 Define $\lambda_* := \bar{\lambda}\|\epsilon\|_n/\hat{\Lambda}_{\max}(S_0)$ and for $j = 1,\ldots,p$,

$$\beta_j^* = \beta_j^0 1\{|\beta_j^0| > \lambda_*\}.$$

Then

$$\begin{aligned}\|X(\beta^* - \beta^0)\|_n^2 &\le \hat{\Lambda}_{\max}^2(S_0)\|\beta^* - \beta^0\|_2^2 \le \hat{\Lambda}_{\max}^2(S_0)\lambda_*^{2-r}\rho_r^r \\ &= \bar{\lambda}^{2-r}\hat{\Lambda}_{\max}^r(S_0)\rho_r^r\|\epsilon\|_n^{2-r} \le \bar{\lambda}^{2-r}\hat{\Lambda}_{\max}^r(S_0)\rho_r^r\|\epsilon\|_n^{2-r}/\hat{\phi}^2(L, S_*)\end{aligned}$$

where in the last inequality we used $\hat{\phi}(L, S_*) \le 1$. Moreover, noting that $S_{\beta^*} = \hat{S}_* = \{j : |\beta_j^0| > \lambda^*\}$ we get

$$|S_{\beta^*}| \le \lambda_*^{-r}\rho_r^r = \bar{\lambda}^{-r}\|\epsilon\|_n^{-r}\hat{\Lambda}_{\max}^r(S_0).$$

Thus

$$\bar{\lambda}^2|S_{\beta^*}|\|\epsilon\|_n^2/\hat{\phi}^2(L, S_{\beta^*}) \le \bar{\lambda}^{2-r}\hat{\Lambda}_{\max}^r(S_0)\rho_r^r\|\epsilon\|_n^{2-r}/\hat{\phi}^2(L, \hat{S}_*).$$

Moreover

$$\|\beta^* - \beta_0\|_1 \le \lambda_*^{1-r}\rho_r^r = \bar{\lambda}^{1-r}\|\epsilon\|_n^{1-r}\hat{\Lambda}_{\max}^r(S_0)/\hat{\phi}^2(L, \hat{S}_*),$$

since $\hat{\phi}^2(L, \hat{S}_*)/\hat{\Lambda}_{\max}(S_0) \le 1$. □

Proof of Lemma 5 The ℓ_1-sparsity condition (11) holds with $\eta \le 1/3$. Theorem 2 with $\lambda_0(1-\eta) = 2R$ gives $\underline{\lambda} = \lambda_0(1-\eta) - R = R$ and $3R \le \bar{\lambda} = \lambda_0(1+\eta) + R + \delta\underline{\lambda} \le (5+\delta)R$. We take $\delta = 1/7$. Then $L = \bar{\lambda}/((1-\delta)\underline{\lambda}) \le (5+\delta)/(1-\delta) = 6$. Set $\hat{S}_* := \{j : |\beta_j^0| > \bar{\lambda}\|\epsilon\|_n/\hat{\Lambda}_{\max}(S_0)\}$. On the set where $\|\epsilon\|_n \ge \underline{\sigma}$ we have $\hat{S}_* \subset S_*$ since $\bar{\lambda} \ge 3R$. We also have $\bar{\lambda}/(\delta\underline{\lambda}) \le 6^2$. Hence, using the arguments of Lemma 4 and the result of Theorem 2, we get on the set $\hat{R} \le R$ and $\|\epsilon\|_n \ge \underline{\sigma}$,

$$\frac{\|\hat{\beta} - \beta^0\|_1}{\|\epsilon\|_n} \le \bar{\lambda}^{1-r}\left(1 + \frac{6^2\hat{\Lambda}_{\max}^r(S_0)}{\hat{\phi}^2(6, S_*)}\right)\left(\frac{\rho_r}{\|\epsilon\|_n}\right)^r.$$

Again, we can bound here $1/\|\epsilon\|_n$ by $1/\underline{\sigma}$. We can moreover bound $\bar{\lambda}$ by $6R$. Next we see that on the set where $\hat{R} \le R$ and $\|\epsilon\|_n \ge \underline{\sigma}$, by Lemma 3,

$$\hat{\sigma} \ge (1-\eta)\|\epsilon\|_n \ge (1-\eta)\underline{\sigma}.$$

The ℓ_0-bound follows in the same way, inserting $\beta = \beta^0$ in Theorem 1. Invoke Lemma 2 to show that the set $\{\hat{R} \le R \cap \|\epsilon\|_n \ge \underline{\sigma}\}$ has probability at least $1 - \alpha_0 - \underline{\alpha}$. □

9.5 Proof of the Extension to Structured Sparsity in Sect. 6

Proof of Theorem 3 This follows from exactly the same arguments as used in the proof of Theorem 1 as the KKT-conditions (9) with general norm Ω imply that

$$\|X_{-J}^T(X_J - X_{-J}\hat{\Gamma}_J)\hat{T}_J^{-1/2}/n\|_{\infty,\Omega_*} \le \lambda. \qquad \square$$

References

1. Bach, F.: Structured sparsity-inducing norms through submodular functions. In: Advances in Neural Information Processing Systems (NIPS), vol. 23, pp. 118–126 (2010)
2. Belloni, A., Chernozhukov, V., Wang, L.: Square-root Lasso: pivotal recovery of sparse signals via conic programming. Biometrika **98**(4), 791–806 (2011)
3. Belloni, A., Chernozhukov, V., Kato, K.: Uniform postselection inference for LAD regression models (2013). arXiv:1306.0282
4. Belloni, A., Chernozhukov, V., Wei, Y.: Honest confidence regions for logistic regression with a large number of controls (2013). arXiv:1306.3969
5. Belloni, A., Chernozhukov, V., Hansen, C.: Inference on treatment effects after selection among high-dimensional controls. Rev. Econ. Stud. **81**(2), 608–650 (2014)
6. Bickel, P., Ritov, Y., Tsybakov, A.: Simultaneous analysis of Lasso and Dantzig selector. Ann. Stat. **37**, 1705–1732 (2009)
7. Bunea, F., Lederer, J., She, Y.: The group square-root Lasso: theoretical properties and fast algorithms (2013). arXiv:1302.0261
8. Javanmard, A., Montanari, A.: Hypothesis testing in high-dimensional regression under the Gaussian random design model: asymptotic theory (2013). arXiv:1301.4240v1
9. Koltchinskii, V., Lounici, K., Tsybakov, A.B.: Nuclear-norm penalization and optimal rates for noisy low-rank matrix completion. Ann. Stat. **39**(5), 2302–2329 (2011)
10. Laurent, B., Massart, P.: Adaptive estimation of a quadratic functional by model selection. Ann. Stat. **28**(5), 1302–1338 (2000)
11. Lounici, K., Pontil, M., van de Geer, S., Tsybakov, A.B.: Oracle inequalities and optimal inference under group sparsity. Ann. Stat. **39**, 2164–2204 (2011)
12. Mitra, R., Zhang, C.-H.: The benefit of group sparsity in group inference with de-biased scaled group Lasso (2014). arXiv:1412.4170
13. Obozinski, G., Bach, F.: Convex relaxation for combinatorial penalties (2012). arXiv:1205.1240
14. Sun, T., Zhang, C.-H.: Scaled sparse linear regression. Biometrika **99**, 879–898 (2012)
15. Sun, T., Zhang, C.-H.: Sparse matrix inversion with scaled lasso. J. Mach. Learn. Res. **14**(1), 3385–3418 (2013)
16. van de Geer, S.A.: The deterministic Lasso. In: JSM Proceedings, p. 140. American Statistical Association, Alexandria, VA (2007)
17. van de Geer, S.: Weakly decomposable regularization penalties and structured sparsity. Scand. J. Stat. **41**(1), 72–86 (2014)
18. van de Geer, S., Bühlmann, P., Ritov, Y., Dezeure, R.: On asymptotically optimal confidence regions and tests for high-dimensional models. Ann. Stat. **42**, 1166–1202 (2014)
19. Yuan, M., Lin, Y.: Model selection and estimation in regression with grouped variables. J. R. Stat. Soc. Ser. B **68**, 49 (2006)
20. Zhang, C.-H., Zhang, S.S.: Confidence intervals for low dimensional parameters in high dimensional linear models. J. R. Stat. Soc. Ser. B Stat. Methodol. **76**(1), 217–242 (2014)

MIX
Papier aus verantwortungsvollen Quellen
Paper from responsible sources
FSC® C105338

If you have any concerns about our products,
you can contact us on
ProductSafety@springernature.com

In case Publisher is established outside the EU,
the EU authorized representative is:
Springer Nature Customer Service Center GmbH
Europaplatz 3, 69115 Heidelberg, Germany

Printed by Libri Plureos GmbH
in Hamburg, Germany